MEDICINE
AND ITS
TECHNOLOGY

Contributions in Medical History
Series Editor: John Burnham

Women & Men Midwives
Medicine, Morality, and Misogyny in Early America
Jane B. Donegan

American Midwives 1860 to the Present
Judy Barrett Litoff

Speech and Speech Disorders in Western Thought
Before 1600
Ynez Violé O'Neill

Sex, Diet, and Debility in Jacksonian America:
Sylvester Graham and Health Reform
Stephen Nissenbaum

Shock, Physiological Surgery, and George
Washington Crile: Medical Innovation in the
Progressive Era
Peter C. English

Professionalizing Modern Medicine: Paris Surgeons
and Medical Science and Institutions in the
18th Century
Toby Gelfand

MEDICINE
AND ITS
TECHNOLOGY

An Introduction to the History of Medical Instrumentation

AUDREY B. DAVIS

CONTRIBUTIONS IN MEDICAL HISTORY, NUMBER 7

Greenwood Press
Westport, Connecticut • London, England

Library of Congress Cataloging in Publication Data

Davis, Audrey B
  Medicine and its technology.

  (Contributions in medical history ; no. 7
ISSN 0147-1058)
  Includes bibliographical references and index.
  1. Medical instruments and apparatus—History.
2. Medical innovations—History. I. Title.
II. Series. [DNLM: 1. Equipment and supplies—
History. 2. Technology, Medical—History. W1 Co778NH
no. 7/ W 26 D2605m]
R856.A5D38   610'.28   80-25202
ISBN 0-313-22807-8 (lib. bdg.)

Library of Congress Catalog Card Number: 80-25202
ISBN: 0-313-22807-8
ISSN: 0147-1058

First published in 1981

Greenwood Press
A division of Congressional Information Service, Inc.
88 Post Road West, Westport, Connecticut 06881

Printed in the United States of America

10 9 8 7 6 5 4 3 2 1

To Miles, Laura, and Allan,
and to my museum colleagues, Uta and Silvio,
who inspired this book

CONTENTS

Illustrations   ix
Preface   xiii

Part I. Historiography

  1. Introduction   3
  2. Literature Sources of
    Medical Instruments   15
  3. Collections of Medical Instruments   37

Part II. Significant Instrumentation

  4. Medical Thermometry   61

  5. The Stethoscope   87
  6. Concepts of the Pulse and Instruments 117

**Part III. Exploring the Impact of
Medical Technology**

  7. Diagnosis and Instruments   141
  8. Medical Standards and Instruments   185
  9. The Social Implications of Standards 211
  10. Conclusion   233

Notes   245
Index   275

ILLUSTRATIONS

FIGURES

1.1	Massachusetts General Hospital operating room after 1900	8
1.2	Massachusetts General Hospital delivery room after 1900	9
1.3	Sewell heart pump used in 1950	12
2.1	Order of tracheal tubes	19
2.2	Manufacturing tracheal tubes in the twentieth century	19
2.3	Assembling plastic tracheal tubes in the twentieth century	19
2.4	Dental cabinet circa 1910-1920	24
2.5	Cabinet for instruments of the nose and throat specialist circa 1910-1920	25
2.6	Dr. Black working at his lathe in his laboratory circa 1890	26
2.7	Assortment of handles for various surgical and diagnostic instruments	28
2.8	Illustration of splints applied in 1893 to various body sites	34
3.1	Revolutionary War surgical set	38
3.2	Kolff-Brigham kidney machine circa 1949	38
3.3	Crude drugs on exhibit circa 1880	41
3.4	Nineteenth-century (1860) dental chair	45
3.5	Seventeenth-century Italian majolica drug jar	46
3.6	Jerome Kidder's tip battery patented in 1871	49
3.7	Trepanning set	50
3.8	1933 incubator for premature infants	50
3.9	Another photograph of the 1933 incubator	50
3.10	Facial prosthetics in case	51
3.11	Plethysmograph	52
3.12	Bronchoscope and accessories circa 1925	52
3.13	Dissecting instruments	54
4.1	Axial thermometer and case	67
4.2	1865 thermometer	70
4.3	Four types of clinical thermometers in 1889 advertisement	71
4.4	Clinical thermometer owned in 1883	72
4.5	Dr. Clifford Albutt's short clinical thermometer (self-registering)	72
4.6	One-minute thermometer	74
4.7	Taylor Instrument Company medical thermometer and case circa 1900	76
4.8	Clinical thermometer in centigrade degrees	76
4.9	Apex rectal thermometer	77
4.10	1882 Immisch thermometer	78
4.11	Thermometer circa 1800	83
4.12	Taylor Monroe thermometer	84
4.13	Two Tycos thermometers	84
4.14	1889 John Barry's clinical thermometer	85
5.1	Cardiometer from 1893	94
5.2	Bowles patent chest piece	95
5.3	Modern binaural stethoscope	96
5.4	Nineteenth-century wood monaural stethoscope	98
5.5	Same monaural stethoscope disassembled	98

5.6   Monaural stethoscope with ivory ear pieces and wooden insert for bell   99
5.7   Wood stethoscope with ivory tip and hollowed-out bell   100
5.8   Silver two-piece monaural stethoscope   100
5.9   Wood monaural stethoscope   100
5.10   Wood monaural stethoscope with ivory earpiece   100
5.11   Conversation tube and hearing aid   101
5.12   Conversation tube and hearing aid circa 1893   101
5.13   1829 Illustration   103
5.14   Illustration of binaural stethoscope with parts labeled   104
5.15   Illustration of Cammann-type stethoscope circa 1889   105
5.16   1889 Illustrations   106
5.17   Multiple electrical stethoscope used to instruct a small group   111
5.18   The See-Hear, a combined fluoroscope and stethoscope   112
5.19   Assortment of 1889 monaural stethoscopes   113
5.20   Diagnostic equipment for mediate auscultation   114
5.21   Binaural Stethoscope   115
6.1   Pulse scale from Robert Fludd   121
6.2   1710 Illustration   124
6.3   Illustration of Marey sphygmograph applied to the wrist circa 1893   126
6.4   Illustration of Dugeon's sphygmograph circa 1893   127
6.5   1889 illustration of Dudgeon sphygmograph   127
6.6   Pond's sphygmograph   128
6.7   Keeler polygraph circa 1950   132
6.8   Marey and Pond sphygmographs illustrated in 1889   133
6.9   Display of Frank Wilson's electrocardiographic equipment   134
6.10   Original electrocardiograph of Frank Wilson   134
6.11   Galvanometer of Frank Wilson's electrocardiographic machine   135
6.12   Original American string galvanometer   135
6.13   Carbon arc lamp   136
6.14   Beck-Lee electrocardiograph   136
6.15   Victor electrocardiograph in the 1930s   137
7.1   Urinalysis equipment circa 1893   150
7.2   Fehling's urine test set   151
7.3   Ureometer circa 1893   151
7.4   Nineteenth-century Nitze cystoscope   155
7.5   Caliper compass   165
7.6   Measuring the length of the right ear   166
7.7   Measuring the length of the left foot   167
7.8   Measuring the length of the left little finger   168
7.9   Late nineteenth-century dynamometer   169
7.10   Large caliper rule   170
7.11   Measuring the furniture collection   171
7.12   Galton's whistles   172
7.13   Dynamometer   172
7.14   Salter dynamometer   173
7.15   Dynamometer circa 1893   173
7.16   Dynamometer suspended from two supports   174
7.17   Mid-nineteenth century dynamometer   175
7.18   Dynamometer made by Charrière   175
7.19   Spearman aesthesiometer   177
8.1   1918 Faught pocket sphygmomanometer   194
8.2   Dr. Oliver's portable mercurial compressed air manometer circa 1910   195
8.3   Barnes dry spirometer circa 1893   196
8.4   Standard wet spirometer circa 1893   196
8.5   Late nineteenth-century cyrtometer   197
8.6   Portable recording apparatus   198
8.7   Scales for grading the sizes of urethral instruments circa 1893   202
8.8   Dr. Roger's Tycos sphgmomanometer dials patented in 1915 and 1917   205
8.9   1896 Riva Rocci sphygmomanometer   207
8.10   Replica of Von Basch's sphygmomanometer, 1880   208
9.1   Snellen's 1862 eye test   218
9.2   Green's astigmatic dial circa 1893   219
9.3   Pray's letters for testing vision circa 1893   220

9.4   Self-recording perimeter   222
9.5   Javal-Schiötz ophthalmometer circa
       1893   222
9.6   Thomson's interchangeable disc circa
       1893   223
9.7   Charts advertised in 1897   227

10.1 . Medical students in 1892 dissecting a
       cadaver   234
10.2 Nineteenth-century obstetrical kit   234
10.3 Dr. Charles Kell's office   242
10.4 Dr. Green Vardiman Black's office   243
10.5 Dr. Edward Angle's office   243

PREFACE

When a study grows out of the everyday concerns of a historian, there is an enormous satisfaction in seeing it evolve into a publication. I planned to write at least one book on the development of the technology of medicine soon after joining the staff of the National Museum of American History (until recently the National Museum of History and Technology) in 1967 as Assistant Curator of Medical Sciences. In this museum in which Medical Sciences is only one of twenty-one collecting areas, the resources for storing, exhibiting, and augmenting the collection are always limited. However, research in the literature and objects of the collection are limited only by the curator's energy. The history of medical technology not only appealed to my sense of curiosity, but also it seemed a lacuna in the history of medicine and American history that someone in my enviable position should and must undertake to fill.

As a nonmedically educated historian I have brought a perspective that transcends any medical specialist's interests and have relied on the goodwill and helpfulness of medical practitioners and medical historians with a background in medicine who are interested in the history of medical technology. I am especially grateful to Drs. George Burch, Chester Burns, John Crellin and William Rosenthal.

In an area with relatively few historical publications and currently involved students, I have been acutely aware of the lack of collegial stimulation. Therefore, I am grateful to curators of other areas who happily shared with me their excitement and frustration with the keeping of National collections. At one time or another everyone on the museum staff has contributed to my evolution as a curator, but I can single out several who unselfishly responded to my repeated requests, namely Uta C. Merzbach, who

has a perfect record of offering correct and sound advice; Silvio Bedini, who as an object historian has no peer and whose enthusiasm for his discoveries is contagious; Jon B. Eklund with whom I co-authored several papers; Virginia Beets, who as Museum Registrar taught me with grace and style the never ending vigilance required of museum curators; and Ben Lawless whose unmatched exhibit creativity makes all the drudgery of keeping objects so worthwhile.

Stanley Reiser in our too infrequent conversations has offered insight. My contacts with the staff and students of The Johns Hopkins Institute of the History of Medicine have been a constant source of stimulation, and I am thankful to them for letting me wander onto their institutional turf. Genevieve Miller as a pioneer in the curating of medical objects has always given me good counsel.

For financial support I thank the Smithsonian Research Foundation, the Commonwealth Foundation, the Burroughs-Wellcome Foundation, the Houston Endowment, and the Bausch and Lomb and Becton and Dickinson companies who contributed to aspects of the study that allowed me to do some of the spadework necessary before writing this book.

The institutions with libraries and object treasures that I have used repeatedly include the National Library of Medicine, the Medical-Chirurgical Library in Baltimore, The Johns Hopkins Medical Library, the Wellcome Museum of the History of Medicine at the Science Museum, and the Smithsonian Institution Library. To their staffs who assisted and even welcomed my inquiries over the past decade I am deeply indebted and mention Dorothy Hanks, Pat Munoz, and Doris Thibodeau as the most helpful. Linda Deer of the Wellcome Museum was especially cordial and helpful. Edwin Clark, who permitted me to camp with the Wellcome Museum Collection to photograph and study its objects afforded me a particularly rich period of discovery. Since I studied the Wellcome Collection and prepared this text the medical objects have been transferred to the London Science Museum. The reader is advised to check with the Wellcome and Science Museum for the up-to-date location and condition of the vast Wellcome Collections. Much has been accomplished in cataloguing and changing the exhibition of these objects since I wrote this text. Frank Pietropaoli, Ellen Wells, and Lucien Rossignol of the Smithsonian Institution Library have been constant sources of expertise. Mr. Rossignol relentlessly pursued references on my behalf and is responsible for considerably shortening the time I had to spend seeking out sources.

For editorial and seemingly endless amounts of duties in preparing the manuscript for publication I thank John Burnham and of the Greenwood Press James Sabin, Margaret Brezicki, Mildred Vasan, and Judith Dodson.

Finally I am most appreciative of the Smithsonian Institution for giving me the freedom to pursue my research with the necessary support in travel allowances, staff to process and care for the objects (Everett Jackson, Mariko Murray, and Michael Harris), photographic services (Al Harrell and Rolfe Baggert), and fellows to further the intellectual process (Nan Knight, Jonathan Lebenau, Barbara Melosh, Emily Savage-Smith, William Simon, and Michael Sokal). The academic climate of the museum has especially benefited from the competent steward-ship of Barney Finn, Department Chairman, Robert Multhauf and Daniel Boorstin, past Directors of the Museum, and Roger Kennedy, Director.

Medical museums have developed sporadically over the past century in the United States. Cities with first-rate medical centers, such as Baltimore, Boston, Charleston, Cleveland, and Philadelphia, have estab-lished museums and are continuing to support them, albeit in a small way. Collecting the medical mate-rials scattered about medical schools, hospitals, attics, basements, pawnshops, and junkyards is the lot of the medical museum curator. Perhaps it is time to make a public statement with parts of all these col-lections in a National Medical Museum. Bringing together the medical momentoes from all parts of the country and exhibiting a great variety of objects for all visitors to view and study could most effectively teach Americans about their medical heritage.

PART I

HISTORIOGRAPHY

1

INTRODUCTION

SCOPE OF THE TEXT:

Medical practice in the Western world underwent fundamental changes in the nineteenth and twentieth centuries. In altering practice to maintain good health, relieve disease, and prolong life, physicians used instruments, devices, and aids to prevent, uncover, delineate, and cure diseases. This book is an introduction to the history of those technological devices and the methods and ideas from which they sprang and to which they led. Such technological innovations were a part of the scientific, economic, and sociological dimensions of medicine, and the history of medical technology, while easily delineated as a narrow theme in itself, thus involved the whole broad history of medicine. Medical technology is a term that has been adopted by a group of twentieth-century professionals, medical technologists, who are specially trained to assist physicians through various laboratory and other instrumentally controlled tests. In this volume, however, the term is employed specifically to signify the physician's use of instruments, devices, and appliances in the diagnosis and treatment of disease.

A technology of medicine arose in the nineteenth century with the direct application of devices and instruments to a part of the body for the purpose of diagnosis and treatment. Therefore, this aspect of the history of medicine involves another special field of study, the history of technology. Technology is understood to be an intermediary between science and mechanics, translating the discussions of science into the uses of mechanics. Of the classical professions, medicine was the first to employ technology extensively.

Many aspects of medical practice constitute applied science.[1] Even the most mechanical elements of medicine, however, are rarely, if ever, described as technology by its practitioners. Physicians are reluctant to see themselves as technicians or applied scientists, although they have come to place immense value on their scientific training and its techniques. The tension between the physician's self-image and his methodology continues to permeate medicine. By the twentieth century, medicine no longer could be practiced without special facilities and apparatus that was not entirely under the control of the physician. The wise physician combined a flexible approach, using a variety of instruments and appliances, whether labeled as technological or not, and that same wise physician worked with an awareness of the patient's ability to understand the procedure and influence the outcome by his or her own efforts.

The roots of technology in medicine may be divided into those developments that dealt with the type of medicine practiced with instruments and those that related directly to the shape, form, and construction of the instrument. Medical technology requires analysis both as a technical development and as a factor in the evolution of medical practice, drawing upon two main types of literature, medical and historical. The articles, lectures, textbooks, and other information contributed by many of the pioneers in the development of medical technology—the primary sources—are listed in the Index Catalogue of the Surgeon-General's Office of the U.S. Army, beginning with the first volume in 1872 and continuing into the twentieth century. This literature, supplemented with other aspects of Victorian medicine, society, science, and technology[2], provides a basis for the study of the development of medical technology.

Secondary accounts, frequently written by medical practitioners, often discuss the major discoveries, such as the stethoscope and other instruments, and their immediate impact on medical procedures. This basic information makes a further synthesis feasible. However, an assessment of various instruments in still broader medical and other contexts remained for the historian who is not caught up in the daily routine of designing and applying instruments and who may reflect on the wide range of implements introduced in the nineteenth century. My purpose in this book is to point out the kind of history that has been written and to indicate what might be done in the future. Therefore, I draw further on medical and auxiliary literature, including technical and scientific descriptions, patent specifications, and historical reviews, attempting to illustrate how it is possible to place the development of instruments applied to medicine in a historical sequence that combines a narrative of their discoveries and technological refinements with an analysis of their applications and effects.

A recent and successful book, the only one of its kind, which assesses the rise of medical technology is Stanley J. Reiser's *Medicine and the Reign of Technology*[3] In a text with an excellent bibliography, Reiser traces the history of the early diagnostic instruments and laboratory tests as they were understood by medical professionals and concludes that these instruments and tests placed a barrier between the physician and the patient that has continued to widen. He is alarmed about the consequences for present-day medical practice, which he believes suffers from an overabundance of technologically oriented procedures delivered with a minimum of the physician's personal concern and attention. Remoteness between the physician and patient is the most objectionable effect of medical technology; it is, however, only one of the consequences of using instruments to identify and alleviate disease. Fast and efficient diagnoses, effective and alternative treatments, and, in some instances, preventive measures are other results of medical technology that need to be analyzed and understood.

Aside from Reiser's book and the specific treatments of individual instruments, the history of technology is a neglected subject. It is my objective, using the special resources and literature available, to show that the neglect is undeserved.

Much of the literature related to technology in medicine and its assessment is scattered among sources that are overlooked or not readily available, and a special effort is often required to locate and retrieve them. One purpose of this introductory work is to cite a variety of sources to consult in a study of the technology of medicine. I have also tried to footnote major references which will lead the reader to the literature that I have not drawn upon, particularly references in languages other than English, French, and German, since most of my references emphasize Anglo-American medical literature.

The bulk of the literature on the technology used in Western medicine up to the early twentieth century was, in fact, developed by or used in England, France, Germany, or the United States, thus most medical instruments and the issues that they raised are discussed in the medical and other literature of these countries. References are also given for specific objects which may be found in museums in Europe and the United States so that researchers will be encouraged to analyze these objects and their collections as a whole, recognizing the importance of making evaluations and distinctions about the quality, intrinsic worth, and relationship of each item to specific physical diagnosis and medical treatment.

I have depended for illustrative material largely on British and American writings and museum instrument collections. This sampling of material is designed essentially to call attention to the nature of some of the issues that are involved in the history of medical technology. The literature includes texts and articles published to explain the rationale and effects of medical instruments and devices, editorials, notes, book reviews, addresses, letters to the editors of journals, patents, and comments in the general nonmedical literature on various aspects of medical technology. I have sampled all of this material to show how it might be used, but I have by no means exhausted the potential for an analysis of these matters. The major texts, articles, and instruments are discussed in the first two chapters on sources but these chapters cannot be considered complete. The notes to all the other chapters provide additional literature to direct the reader to other sources I have utilized.

This essay is intended as an initial history of medical practice, society, and the culture in which it is utilized. I have tried to present my discussion so that it will be meaningful and accessible to the scholar, the lay reader, the nonspecialist, the physician, and the technologist. Thus, I risk offending all these readers either by not providing enough detail or by including too much. The notes are intended to serve the needs of all readers who wish to explore the subject further. The basic questions and issues remain constant regardless of the area of the Western world under survey. Subsequent historians may study not only the recent decades, after the definitions of the problems were established in ways that I shall suggest, but also local cultural variations that would be inappropriate for detailed discussions in an introductory work such as this one.

Most of the relevant technological and social developments, in fact, appeared in some stage during the nineteenth century; I therefore emphasize Victorian-era medicine. I have not followed events in a strictly chronological sequence because I wish to discuss a few conceptual issues in depth. In raising questions, I have not brought the discussion up into the twentieth century, but occasionally examples from the twentieth-century literature will appear merely to illustrate the point under examination. The nineteenth century, in fact, suffices very well to introduce the whole subject.

ORGANIZATION OF THE TEXT:

To elucidate some of the themes threading through the history of the technology of medicine, I have selected the earliest instruments to be widely adopted —thermometers, stethoscopes, and cardiac and pulse-related devices—and discussed them in separate chapters. The medical milieu in which these instruments were adopted and to which they contributed involves the history of the technology of diagnostic medicine. Other more specialized and less well-known instruments, together with a few therapeutic devices, are discussed less intensively to illustrate some of the issues raised by the use of instruments in medicine.

Instruments such as endoscopes and sensory, neurological, and blood-testing equipment are not discussed in the depth that a full survey of the history of medical technology would suggest. The recent appearance of Reiser's book, in which many of these instruments are included, permits a more selective discussion of the specific instruments included in my text. I instead preferred to concentrate on issues raised by the use of instruments, as well as changes imposed upon medical practitioners who have responded in a myriad of ways to the challenges introduced along with medical instruments. A number of myths and unanalyzed truths pervade the history of medical technology because historians have not explored adequately the invention and application of medical instruments. Yet it is important to determine the broader issues and institutions directly related to medical instruments so as to delineate their lineage and indicate the physical changes made in a significant implement, in distinction from the social and intellectual background factors.

Taken as a whole, medical instruments are significant for the concepts they raised and controverted. These broader issues include the standardization of the physiologic functions measured by instruments, the selection of specific criteria to distinguish health and disease, the changing concepts of disease, and the stage in an illness at which the patient sought the advice of the physician and he recognized the disease. Some technology provided a means to record and define disease patterns such as abnormal blood pressure, unusual kidney function, and irregular heart action, and other technology indicated other functional changes of lesser importance or not apparent as an acute episode of disease. In two chapters, one on standardization and the other on the impact of instrumentation on the study and understanding of physiology and pathology, I explore important components of the interaction between instruments and medicine up to the end of the nineteenth century.

One important result of medical technology was a greater reliance on medically derived criteria to select individuals for jobs and for buying life insurance. Some of the factors that brought the physician into an active consultantship with various economic and social institutions are discussed in a third chapter devoted to the social implications of medical standards.

To provide a background for the study of the technology of medicine and to orient the reader to the wide range of items employed in the practice of medicine, I have discussed in the second chapter the status of collections of medical instruments. The rationale for bringing specific collections together into a museum setting has varied. A few collectors have preserved objects that are unique today. Many items have not survived or are imperfect and can be studied only by comparison with existent devices or through descriptions in the literature.

IMPACT OF INSTRUMENTATION ON PRACTICE:

All professions are practiced according to special knowledge (theories and laws) and techniques, which are best known to those qualified through education and apprenticeship. Of all professions, medicine most extensively has emphasized the assistance and intervention of agents or forces besides the physician's personal contacts to redirect the unhealthy body to function normally. Ancient healers turned to the application of heat, cold, water, sunlight, and other easily accessible agents to facilitate the healing process within the body and to encourage natural forces to work their powers to rid the body of disease. Wet cloths, mud baths, sun baths, drying concoctions, special diets, and drugs are among the earliest ways that physicians used physical agents to curtail disease. Their use inaugurated a type of medicine that developed over several thousand years into diagnosis and treatment relying heavily on technological devices and appliances. Beginning with the use of natural forces, which were focused directly on the source of an illness, medicine evolved its methodology into one dependent on instruments to discover the source of illness, and then, to cure it.

INSTRUMENTATION AND SURGERY:

Operations on the body presented the earliest opportunities for a medical practitioner, who was a surgeon, to apply a special instrument in the treatment of disease. Instruments were used to extract foreign bodies penetrating the skin, eyes, ears, and nose, to remove the dead fetus from the womb and to remove a diseased appendage, ulcer, or tumor. Through most of the history of medicine, treating internal diseases by surgical procedures was often unsuccessful or only temporarily effective. Removal of cataracts and other operations requiring superficial incisions were more effective. The surgeon developed the tools and skills to cut into the body quickly and safely, but the pain, blood, pus, and disfigurement associated with surgery undermined acceptance of this form of treatment by physicians and patients for millenia. By the fifteenth century, English surgeons were separated from physicians, received less formal education, and were generally regarded as inferior medical practitioners. Physicians confined their intervention during illness to the prescription of chemical and botanical drugs, or when no other alternative procedures existed, to surgical procedures, which the surgeon, not the physician, carried out.

In 1785 the Italian surgeon Giovanni Alessandro Brambilla had proposed to "ransom . . . surgery from the condition of being the maid of medicine and raise it to a sister level,"[4] a goal which surgery achieved and surpassed in a little more than a century after his death. Instrumentation and technology played an important role in equalizing these two branches of medicine. Two discoveries—effective anesthesia and bacterial control through antisepsis—enabled the nineteenth-century surgeon to equal and eventually surpass the physician in the successful treatment of disease. The surgeon thereupon learned

to apply a greater variety of instruments at a more leisurely pace when the patient was made insensitive to pain. His optimism about the success of the operation and the life of the patient encouraged the surgeon to experiment with innovative procedures until, by the twentieth century, it was assumed by professionals and patients in Western society that surgery offered the best methods of curing many diseases.

INSTRUMENTATION AND DIAGNOSIS:

Physicians began to form closer bonds with surgeons, since medical treatment so often included and depended on surgery. In Britain and on the Continent, technology induced closer association between the two major medical professions, which had been unequal rivals for centuries. The surgeon matched the brilliance of the diagnostician, and both depended on manipulation of their instruments for their prowess measured in scientific terms. In the United States and in some rural parts of Europe, the roles of surgeon and physician were never effectively separated. It was during the period that surgery was rising to the pinnacle of medical treatment that diagnostic and therapeutic instruments were introduced and applied to the diagnosis and nonsurgical treatment of diseases. While surgical instruments served as an extension of the surgeon's hands, diagnostic instruments provided additional functions as extensions of the eyes, ears, and nose, as well as the hands and mind, of the physician. Diagnostic instruments opened medicine up to a greater variety of practitioners by enhancing their basic skills, supplementing their observational abilities, and structuring the diagnostic interview with the patient. Therapeutic devices and machines, such as electric, exercise, and body manipulation tools greatly extended the choice of treatment procedures.

Medical instruments for diagnosis included mechanical aids, which were designated as devices, machines, tools, appliances, hardware, and occasionally toys and gadgets. From the sixteenth century, the word *toy*[5] has been used to categorize things of little or no practical value, and for those physicians who could not reconcile an instrument like a stethoscope with more efficient or effective diagnosis, this instrument and others remained in the category of a toy. Some diagnostic instruments were difficult to apply, but others could be learned by an interested person seeking the source of disease, especially when refinements in instruments became feasible after the invention of incandescent lamps and the introduction of a range of new materials, including hard and soft rubber, plastic, compacted wood, veneers, and aluminum and other metallic alloys.

Medical instruments used by the surgeon and diagnostician have evolved out of the tools and hardware existing in various crafts, industries, and sciences. Modifications proposed by the physician and surgeon have been essential, but technological facility and social attitudes also determined the shape, style, quality, and the extent of use of the final apparatus employed by the medical professional.

INSTRUMENTATION AND NONSURGICAL THERAPY:

Medicine in the technological era acquired many of the characteristics that marked other institutions at the same time. So, by adopting procedures based on information obtained with instruments and devices, medicine developed an approach to illness that transformed it into a special form of technology. From being only minimally a part of medical practice, and confined primarily to surgery until the nineteenth century, technology became an integral part of general medicine. Not only did the methods of disease, discovery, and treatment become mechanized, but also the possibilities for treatment were broadened to include devices originally made for other purposes. For instance, new exercise apparatus such as the bicycle led the physician to prescribe cycling to alleviate nervous disorders, which were previously treated by horseback riding and drugs.[6] Exercise and other forms of physical stimulation, including electric shocking, were delivered with apparatus from laboratory science on which the physician began to depend more and more for the rationale and interpretation of disease.

The instruments of diagnosis that were recommended and taught to most physicians by the end of the nineteenth century included the stethoscope, thermometer, pulse writer, microscope, blood pressure recorder (sphygmomanometer), and devices to carry out chemical tests to analyze bodily fluids. Other instruments that were applied both for diagnosis and therapy, however, were used by the medical professional in different periods. Pressure chambers, color blindness tests, anthropometrical equipment, electrical machines, and other devices and instruments taken as a whole were more numerous than earlier in the century and reflect aspects of the mechanization of medicine that the basic diagnostic instruments do not reveal. It is in studying the development and impact of the whole panoply of these varied instruments that the historian may come to grips with some of the problems that the nineteenth-century practitioner faced and learned to solve.

Qualities in the practice of medicine changed also. The application of instruments imparted information such as "the feel" of inserting a needle, and "the give" of it as it entered a spinal cavity or a vein, and the resistance encountered when an urethral stricture was explored with a catheter.[7] One of the frustrations of the historian is that, except in a few instances, it is impossible to reconstruct what instruments felt like to the operator or the patient. However, at least I have tried to inform the reader of the range of instruments manufactured and to give an accurate impression of the actual instruments the physician and surgeon employed in specific instances during the nascent period of medical instrumentation.

The collective effect of instrumentation merits consideration and offers the historian opportunities for interpreting the interactions between physicians, surgeons, and their patients in other than scientific and technological terms; the social, economic, and cultural ramifications were experienced by nearly everyone and placed medical practice in focus as an integral part of everyday life. For instance, when instruments and devices were developed for testing and classifying color blindness and other visual impairments, groups of workers like the railroad employees were expected to pass specific vision tests in order to qualify for, obtain, and retain their jobs. The custom of administering the tests, of ensuring their accuracy, and of placing the visually handicapped employee in an appropriate position arose and carried over into other situations as the physical and mental standards for other jobs became amenable to specific physical diagnostic tests, which were administered by instruments. The impact of the diagnostic and therapeutic instrument on the laboring community cannot be overestimated.

For three different purposes then, diagnosis, surgical therapy, and nonsurgical therapy, instruments in the nineteenth century shaped the approach of the physician to disease and his relationship to the patient. Accurate diagnosis with the aid of the stethoscope, microscope, chemical analysis, and other instruments enabled the physican to select a specific type of treatment and to recognize those diseases for which no effective therapy existed by the late nineteenth century. The physician's application of mechanical agents and instruments to define, prevent, curtail, and eliminate diseases had, therefore, become essential to the most acceptable form of medical practice.

Technology changed the very location of physicians' activities. Medical instruments and special equipment to perform a myriad of surgical procedures found a natural focus in the physician's office and hospital (see figures 1.1 and 1.2). Of course, along with technology other factors contributing to the rise of hospital and medical office practice included changing modes of transportation, social acceptance of disease and how it is to be cured, unavailability of family members to care for the sick, and the regulations stipulated by health insurance companies, all of which in turn reflected available technology.[8]

This process was most extreme in the United States. In 1873, only 200 hospitals could be counted. By 1910, over 4,000 existed and by 1920 more than 6,000, a figure that has remained relatively constant since then.[9] Some doctors' offices supplemented the hospital and came to rival it in the types of special equipment supported by physicians, who had joined with their colleagues to share the cost of expensive apparatus by the mid-twentieth century.[10]

INSTRUMENTATION AND THE GERM THEORY:

In addition to the uses to which medical technology was put, the very construction of instruments and devices used to diagnose and cure disease and maintain health was influenced by basic biological discoveries. The most significant was the germ theory of disease. The bacterial cause of disease not only played a major role in the diagnosis, treatment, and prevention of disease, but also determined the materials and construction of instruments used by the physician and surgeon.

The germ theory led to a radical change in the shape and construction of instruments. In the fourth quarter of the nineteenth century when medical instruments became essential, the bacterial origin of disease revolutionized the construction and application of them. Instruments were no longer only extensions of the physician's senses, they became the link that, if not handled carefully, transferred bacteria from doctor to patient, patient to doctor, and patient to patient.

Before it was realized that they should be sterilized, instruments passed through a stage in which they

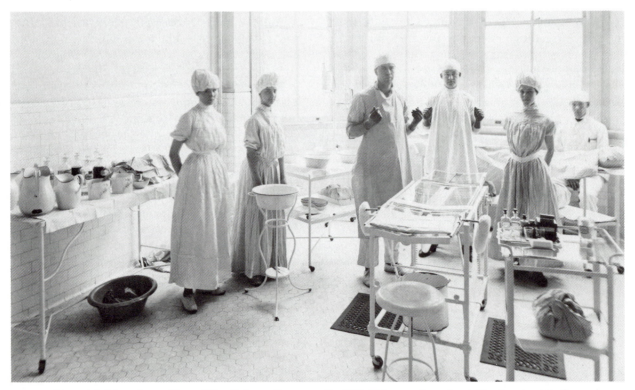

Figure 1.1. Massachusetts General Hospital operating room after 1900. This scene shows the staff and equipment of an up-to-date operating room. Note the white enameled pitchers, basins, stools, and glass table characteristic of a sterile environment in this period. From the *Archives of the Masschusetts General Hospital.* S.I. Photo No. 77-5515.

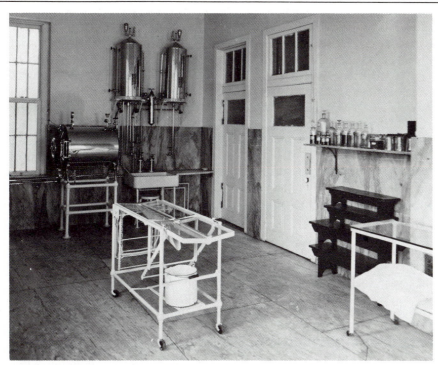

Figure 1.2. Massachusetts General Hospital delivery room after 1900. Note the brass steam sterilizer, distilled water containers, and delivery table. From the *Archives of the Massachusetts General Hospital. S.I. Photo No. 77-5512.*

became the agents of bacterial dispersion. Mucus-laden thermometers, contaminated spatulas for inspecting the throat, sweat-stained stethoscopes, rusty, chipped, and blood-stained scalpels, amputating saws, picks, probes, tonsillotomes, and mouth gags were among the offending devices. Gradually physicians and surgeons learned or were forced to clean up or dispose of their instruments after each use. As the germ theory was put into practice, the styles and shapes of instruments were changed to make them easier to clean, as well as capable of withstanding the rigors of sterilization. Within the last decade, frequently used items have been made cheaply enough so that they could be disposed of after one application, the ultimate method of controlling the spread of infection by medical instruments.

In the process of becoming sterile, instruments changed vastly in appearance. Medical instruments, like medical literature, displayed the signs of the scientific changes in medicine. When disease descriptions became more scientific, they were expressed in language divested of color and increasingly burdened with technical terms strung together in a bald style. In a parallel way in the same period handsome instruments with handles of pearl, ivory, carved ebony,

mahogany, and engraved metals, contained in cases lined with velvet were replaced with plain, unadorned medical utensils, stored in plain boxes. As a medical writer noted in 1883, "Formerly . . . instrument cases were generally of wood, covered with leather, and lined with velvet. But this bright picture has its shadows; the handsome velvet retains dirt too easily, and the luxurious interior of the box is absolutely opposed to a radical cleaning, and to an antisepsis in harmony with the doctrine of modern surgery. The simple box of wood has now come into vogue. . . ."[11] By the end of the nineteenth century, medical instruments had lost their elaborate decoration and their lavish beauty to become plain, unadorned, utilitarian, and sanitary.

Instrument design changes were reflected in basic and widely applied instruments. Wooden tongue depressors that had to be burned after use or were fixed with removable and easily sterilized glass bodies replaced metallic spatulas that needed to be boiled after each use.[12] Thermometers were sterilized in alcohol and marked so that their surfaces remained smooth. They were carried in cases stripped of their customary plushy or velvet linings, leaving no hiding places for bacteria. Metallic and flexible stethoscopes were carried in separate cases and no longer mingled with other instruments or transported in the physician's tall hat. Exceptions occurred for other than scientific reasons. The stethoscope developed a symbolic nature which led even a physician fully aware of the germ theory to carry it suspended from his or her neck. Rigid but detachable surgical tools were also among the necessary design changes instituted for maintaining bacteria-free instruments. The change to newer materials—chip-proof steel, aluminum and metallic alloys, hardened rubber, and plastics—that could withstand heat and constant care required to keep instruments clean served as continual reminders that instruments were a regular part of medical practice.

Practice was merely changed, rather than eased, however. With perception rare for his profession, S. Weir Mitchell of Philadelphia by 1891 equated the physician to a mechanic in the quantity of tools he used. These instruments were not laborsaving, he pointed out. Instruments demanded time and care from the physician if they were to be used effectively. Those physicians prone to take shortcuts in using an instrument were apt to be misled in their diagnoses. The physician, he continued, had to guard against being complacent when employing an instrument, and perhaps, drawing conclusions without considering all symptoms. Even the simplest procedures demanded careful application; for instance, taking the temperature in one place or at one time was not sufficient to understand the change in body temperature during the course of a disease.[13]

The practice of sterilizing medical equipment, tools, surgical instruments, dressings, hospital garments, and linen stimulated a new industry important to the medical profession. Companies arose to meet the demand for all types and sizes of steam and hot water sterilizers and to provide chemical and antibacterial solutions for cleaning medical equipment and hospital rooms. Sensing the economic goals to be achieved, a number of manufacturers of medical apparatus installed sterilization departments in their factories.

Pressurized sterilizers were made in Germany and France in response to the bacteriological discoveries of Lister, Pasteur, and Koch. In the United States, the American Sterilizer Company of Erie, Pennsylvania, founded in 1894, was largely supported by government contracts during World War I to produce portable bulk disinfectors and field sterilizers for the armed services. By 1950, the company had become the largest American distributor of medical sterilizers, employing 670 people.[14]

One of the most dramatic applications of technological change in response to the germ theory of disease was made in dentistry. The dentist employed a great variety of small tools to scrape, shape, prepare, and fill teeth. Many elegant sets of dental instruments with highly decorative handles, stored in handsome mahogany and oak cabinets, testify to the dentist's mechanical skill with and pride in these implements. The dentist is usually considered to have been among the last of the medical professionals to sterilize equipment systematically in order to eliminate and minimize the spread of disease bacteria, although it should have been relatively simple to keep dental instruments in sterile solutions in an office. However, the dentist was not taught to understand the need for sterilized instruments until the Americans, Willoughby Dayton Miller and Frank Billings, and others, proved conclusively that mouth bacteria could cause serious diseases. Some of these diseases spread to other parts of the body and led to chronic ailments with devastating effects. Keeping the mouth germ-free is difficult, which placed a burden on the dentist, especially when extracting a tooth, drilling deep cavities, and treating gum diseases. In 1894 William Hunter of England praised American dentists for their extraordinary skills and berated them for their poor habits of cleanliness and lack of appreciation for preventive dentistry.[15] Hunter claimed that

The dentists of America are the best in the world, but they are, nevertheless, away behind the mark. We appreciate their ingenuity, their skill, their drills and dams, their composite fillings and artificial teeth, [but] they do not sterilize themselves or teach their patients how to prevent caries. They are wonderful patchers-up of things half-gone; but they do not show us how to prevent the going. There is hardly a dentist [there are a few] who works in an aseptic way or uses aseptic instruments.[16]

Dentists used their instruments in some of the most sensitive parts of the body, which demanded a feel for delicate instruments. As Roswell O. Stebbins observed in 1893,

Sharp, well-tempered instruments, of proper shape, in the hands of a careful operator, will cause less pain in excavating the cavity of a tooth, than the best local anesthetic or obtundent applied to the tooth, if dull, ill-shaped instruments are used with force enough to crush down the tooth structure, which is generally the case, as the majority of dentists are not mechanics, or do not care to soil their hands and take the time to make, or obtain, the proper instrument to be used. The dental engine, so often looked upon as an invention of torture, has gained this unenviable reputation by the improper use to which it has been put.[17]

These deficiencies were apparent to patients and created a dread of the dentist, which is beginning to be overcome by the use of modern dental instruments that produce little pain. Stebbins concluded that, "When the regulation of the speed of the wheel is under absolute control of the operator, the excavating of a cavity by the use of a sharp drill or burr, of proper size, causes so little pain or discomfort that the most sensitive patient does not object to its use."[18]

INSTRUMENTATION AND CULTURE:

The acceptance and application of technology by a medical community depended, in part, on the prevailing conditions in the society. The social and cultural factors that impinge on the technology of medicine and grow from it are manifold. One way to understand some of the changes introduced with and stemming from instruments is to compare a culture that used medical instruments with one that rejected them.

Consider briefly the differences between Oriental and Western medicine. Western medicine was most clearly severed from Eastern medicine by the use of the instruments in the nineteenth century. A few instruments (acupuncture implements) have been and continue to be used by Eastern practitioners, but the intent of acupuncture is quite different from the reasons for which Western physicians and surgeons employ instruments. Chinese "surgery is based upon the theory that there are intimate connections between the external surface of the body and the structures within, and that treatment applied externally not only affects the immediate tissues but their deep connections as well. Charts of the body surface have been made, mapping out three hundred and sixty-seven distinct areas, with their minute inner connections elaborately detailed."[19] These are the acupuncture sites into which the acupuncture needle is placed.

Chinese surgery was not challenged in the nineteenth century as it had been in the industrializing West, "owing to the almost entire absence of complicated machinery in mine, factory and transit, where there are comparatively few of the severer accidents characteristic of the densely populated regions of the Occident."[20] Chinese physicians possessed little mechanical skill and could not ligate a bleeding vessel. The Chinese laborers who came to the United States to work on railroads and who suffered acci-

dents were treated by American physicians and surgeons.[21]

Western physicians have attributed their success in diagnosis and treatment to their increasing adoption of scientific methods, which in practice meant the use of medical technology to apply scientific principles for exploring and assisting bodily functions. Scientific principles and the equipment to execute them changed the focus of the physician from the patient as an individual to that of his body cells, tissues, organs, and systems. This shift in interpretation took many forms but one illustration indicates how medicine and engineering were blended in the West to bring about changes in the attitude toward the body and in the teaching of medicine. H. A. Huntington suggested in 1899 that a gas engine or electric motor with synthetic pipes be installed on the dissecting table so that students could "perform surgical operations on the cadaver under more nearly natural conditions."[22] He explained that "instead of injecting the arteries as at present, attach a rubber tube to a pump whose force and strokes shall be such to send a red antiseptic fluid into the arteries of the cadaver, imitating as nearly as possible the conditions of life. Students can then perform all sorts of surgical operations under far more interesting and instructive conditions than on the dead cadaver."[23] The dead body was not the only subject of laboratory experimentation. For the study of living organs, all sorts of artificial steps were taken to outline, describe, and test the organs' functional abilities (see figure 1.3).

The dramatic difference between Western and Eastern methods of diagnosis is illustrated by Richard Selzer who tells of "Grand Rounds" in which he participated as an observer a few years ago, which was conducted by Yeshi Dhonden, personal physician to the Dalai Lama. Dhonden and his Western colleague both diagnosed a patient's heart disease, using their respective observational and instrument-supported methods.[24]

INSTRUMENTATION AND PRECISION:

It would be difficult to overestimate the importance of instruments of precision in the practice of medicine. In many instances, technology intensified the quest for describing in numerical terms the limits between health and disease. Measurement of physiologic and anatomic characteristics, especially body temperature, volume of air inhaled and exhaled, the pressure of the blood in the arteries, the rate of the beat of the pulse, sensitivity to pressure and pain on the skin, sensitivity to colors, sounds, and tastes, and

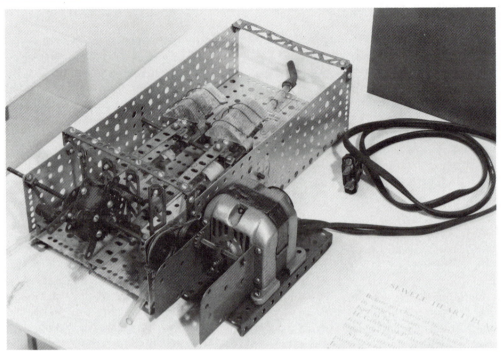

Figure 1.3. Sewell heart pump used in 1950. One of the experimental heart pumps made by William H. Sewell while a medical student at Yale. Constructed from an erector set, the device controlled delivery of air pressure and suction to the pumping mechanism where alternate contraction and expansion of a rubber tube forced the blood to circulate. *NMAH No. M 8015, S.I. Photo No. 74-10389.*

the tension in the eyeball were among aspects of the human body described with the aid of numbers. The physician compared the standards established for each of these instrumentally measurable physical characteristics with those of a patient being examined. The instrument revealed the varying amounts of disorder and "abnormal" functions tolerated by the body. Some of these were previously unnoted or may have seemed irrelevant. Occasionally, the behavior of the individual did not bear out the conclusions drawn from diagnostic measurements made in the course of a physical examination. Individuals could appear to function normally while suffering from serious disease. Standards, like any other aspect of diagnosis, did not in themselves suggest or guarantee modes of treatment.

Precision was sought by physicians with the methods and instruments employed to measure body structures and fluids. The scientific ambiance articulated by William Whewell's analysis of the inductive sciences, which was exemplified by scientists of the caliber of James Clerk Maxwell, enticed physicians aspiring to become scientific to adopt methods of precision and to quantify their diagnoses. Numerical constants (degrees of temperature, beats of the pulse

per minute, millimeters of pressure in the blood vessels, vital capacity of gases in the lungs, blood cell counts, visual acuity, and color sensitivity) are among the forms of precision measurements nineteenth-century physicians employed in performing diagnosis with instruments.

Standards were being established in the sciences and in the machine shops where instruments were produced. In Europe, organizations like the Société Genèvoise d'Instruments de Physique, founded in 1862, improved and produced extremely accurate instruments for scientific measurements, which were adopted by the most precision-conscious industries such as the watchmaking industry. The "American system" of manufacturing, which grew out of the demands for precision by the gun manufacturers, developed into a method of mass production of interchangeable mechanical parts. Precision was the key to the interchangeability of parts; it was essential to achieve close tolerances in shaping and sizing each piece. From a tolerance equal to the thickness of a sixpence to one-thousandth of an inch in 1880, and one ten-thousandth of an inch by 1890, the sizes of instruments became more critical.[25] While the manufacture of automobiles consumed the largest number of precision machines and tools, all other industries, including the production of medical instruments, also required the use of precision tools.

CONCLUSION:

Few medical instrument manufacturers have remained in business since the nineteenth century, and those who have did not retain a full collection of all their instruments or their promotional literature. The instruments produced in the nineteenth and early twentieth centuries survived mainly as objects of value to collectors or as documents of the type of medicine delivered by them. Many of these instruments are preserved in national, local, and private medical museums. In the next two chapters, the historiography of medical technology and museums, as well as the literature pertaining to medical instruments as museum objects, is discussed in order to provide a basis for understanding the role of the museum and other institutions in preserving original objects as primary documents for the historian of medical technology.

2

LITERATURE SOURCES OF MEDICAL INSTRUMENTS

SECONDARY LITERATURE:

There is a long and honorable literature that describes medical technology, but it is scattered. Since it is less abundant and presents fewer points for discussion, I will first review the standard secondary literature, then discuss major examples of the primary literature, followed by a discussion of some of the issues brought out by the literature related to medical trade catalogues, which describe medical instruments most explicitly. The special secondary literature produced to record instrument collections includes instrument catalogues and exhibition catalogues, which are discussed in the final section.

S. Weir Mitchell, in his classic lecture given in 1891 on precision in medical instruments, provides some important references for the student of medical technology for the period up to the mid-nineteenth century. He described the sources he consulted to write the history of instruments used to measure the pulse, respiration, and body temperature. He explained that the literature he used was ". . . not in the books of medical history. It is here and there in memoirs, journals, lay-biographies, rare old folios and forgotten essays."[1] His excellent essay became a model for other historians who published monographs on other instruments.

Surgical instruments employed in ancient India by the Hindus are described from Hindu medical sources by Girindrenath Mukhopadhyoya in his Griffith Prize Essay for 1909 and in a successive volume on surgical instruments. Many of these instruments are similar to the instruments used by the ancient Greeks, which were discussed by John Stewart Milne in his volume *Surgical Instruments in Greek and Roman Times* published in 1907. Milne's and Mukhopadyhoya's volumes[2] make use of archeological discoveries from the nineteenth century that were preserved in the museums of Athens, Naples, and other European cities, although no Indian instruments were among these collections of ancient specimens.

A thorough historical review of all surgical instruments up to the seventeenth century is presented in Ernst Julius Guerlt's three-volume *Geschichte der Chirurgie und ihrer Ausuebung.*[3] Guerlt's texts provide line drawings of the instruments discussed and list the public museums and institutions where examples of these instruments could be located. His commentary was based on an exhaustive search of the literature of surgeons, supplemented by secondary accounts, primarily written by nineteenth-century German authors. Guerlt's volumes are essential for anyone with an interest in the history of ancient, medieval, and early Renaissance surgery.

By the mid-twentieth century, scholars were expecting more comprehensive historical accounts of medical instruments. In 1951, for instance, Henry Sigerist demanded a more intensive, analytical, and social history of instruments and of the technology of medicine. He wrote: "The history of medicine is to a large extent the history of its tools; this is particularly true in the case of surgery and the surgical specialties . . . It goes without saying that the history of the surgical instrument is closely related to and must be studied in relation to the general history of technology."[4] Since that time, little has been written to bear out his statement, and no publication known to him had met his expectations for relating medical tools to technology in its broadest context. Sigerist was aroused by the missed opportunities apparent in C. J. S. Thompson's *The History and Evolution of Surgical Instruments*[5] and V. Moeller-Christensen's *The History of the Forceps.*[6] These remain useful repertories (Sigerist's apt word meaning lists) but do not discuss the questions the tools may suggest; no less do the books seek answers to the tools' modes of use and existence other than they were fashioned and applied.

I know of no studies that fulfill Sigerist's desiderata, although Ruth and Edward Brecher's *The Rays: A History of Radiology in the U.S. and Canada*[7] comes closer to the ideal text Sigerist had hoped would appear in print. The Brechers discuss and document the apparatus related to the medical applications of X-radiation and include the supporting theories, practices, episodes, and institutions that shaped the applications of radiation in twentieth-century medical practice. Another example of a discussion of medicine and its technology in antiquity that would have appealed to Sigerist is Guido Majno's book *The Healing Hand: Man and Wound in the Ancient World*. Without claiming to have written a history of the technology of medicine, Majno has published a well-illustrated history of wounds and their treatment in ancient cultures.[8] In an effort to be clear and complete, he has brought to bear all the relevant evidence on wounds represented in carvings, paintings, and artifacts, as well as the literature, which makes his book a type of "museological reader." The wounds inflicted by blows from assorted objects, insect bites, microbes, chemicals, and other agents are illustrated in drawings and photographs of the evidence on which their history is traced, including ancient trephined skulls, carious teeth reputed to be several million years old, ancient drugs, and graphics made in stone, marble, clay, or applied to coins and various containers and vessels. The probes, stitches, cauteries, and ointments used to clean and fix these wounds are depicted and explained so that the technology of ancient wound healing has been made an integral part of this well-written historical essay.[9]

Makers of tools were, as will be developed, fundamentally involved in medical instrumentation, especially surgical implements. Yet, little literature on the subject exists, which is the more remarkable in that historians of technology have not turned their attention to the subject. For instance, in Eugene Ferguson's *Bibliography of Sources for the Study of the History of Technology*,[10] medicine, surgery, and their subdivisions are not even indexed and only two minor references even mention medicine. Even classic medical bibliographies such as the one by Garrison and Morton, compiled in the twentieth century and reprinted in multiple editions,[11] do not include more than a few entries for medical or surgical instruments. Garrison and Morton's book has only three references listed under the category Surgical Instruments, with a few additional ones scattered among the listings for the bodily systems. One surprising oversight is the text with the most thoroughly documented discussion of an instrument: Sir Kedarnath Das' *Obstetric Forceps, its History and Evolution* of 1929.[12] It is the first English language treatise on the history of the obstetrical forceps, containing over 2,000 references and 878 illustrations. The author's diligence is so marked that it might have been expected that others would have been inspired to publish studies of other important groups of medical instruments.

Fundamental to the historical study of instruments is a rationale for tackling and coming to terms with medically related objects. Straightforward studies of the development of a specialty and its tools, such as Leonard Murphy's chronologically organized assessment *The History of Urology*[13] and George Burch and N. P. Pasquale's *A History of Electrocardiography*,[14] are available in monographic and serial form. These publications range from the ridiculous, containing misinformation wrapped in an unappealing style with little focus other than that of a chronicle, to competent summaries intended for the practitioner who wants to know "a little something" or more about the history of his specialty. Authors of medical texts occasionally include a chapter or two on the history of their subject and its technical devices. One good example is a book by Arthur Master, Charles I. Garfield, and Max B. Walters,[15] which explains the development of instruments used to measure blood pressure. The best of these studies are essential and it is hoped that more of them will appear, especially related to twentieth-century instrumentation.

PRIMARY LITERATURE:

The primary literature on medical technology presents several viewpoints regarding descriptions of medical and surgical instruments and the techniques to which they led that should be discussed in the published literature. A basic guide to the important surgical treatises up to the mid-nineteenth century from the standpoint of the manufacturer and the application of instruments is the two-volume work of Gustav Gaujot, *Arsenal de la Chirurgie Contemporaine*.[16] Gaujot, whose texts are largely primary sources, discusses all the important European instrument makers and manufacturers of surgical, orthopedic, prosthetic, obstetrical, and diagnostic equipment. The construction, application, and effectiveness of each instrument is included. Almost all of the early texts mentioned below were noted by Gaujot. Clear instructions about the construction, functions, and applications of medical instruments have repeatedly been called for since Albucasis made this appeal in the tenth-century treatise *On Surgery and Instruments*, which was translated into Latin at Toledo by Gerard of Cremona in the second half of the twelfth century.[17] Albucasis, in the earliest remaining treatise to provide drawings of surgical instruments, acknowledged that operative surgery was poorly taught and practiced in his time. Therefore, he "decided to revive the art by expounding, elucidating and epitomizing it in his treatise; and to present the forms of cauterizing irons and other operative instruments since this is an adjunct to explanation and a vital necessity."[18] Hippocrates, Celsus, and Paulus Aeginata, among others, discussed specific instruments, but no illustrations are contained in the manuscripts of their writings or in those manuscripts through which their writings are known to us, except for figures depicting the techniques of bone setting, which appear in a Greek manuscript of Appolonius also transcribed in the tenth century.[19] Celsus in the first century B.C. briefly had described thirty-five surgical instruments. Albucasis drew on descriptions provided by Greek physicians and recommended some instruments of his own. In chapter forty-six, "On the shapes of the instruments used for incising and perforating," a number of standard surgical instruments, such as probes, knives, and hooks, are illustrated.[20]

Among the earliest surgical procedures Albucasis discussed were those involving cauterization with hot iron rods to which were appended variously shaped points, and other procedures including bloodletting, bandaging sprains, setting dislocations and broken bones, and perforating the skin. Stylized illustrations of the instruments under discussion are inserted between the lines of the text. Without indicating perspective or scale, these illustrations show the parts and shapes of instruments. Often the whole of a shaft or a point is colored or inked in like a silhouette, and therefore, the details of the implement are distorted. At the time these Islamic illustrations appeared, Moorish art was heavily involved with geometric ornamentation,[21] thus, these drawings bear witness to the period and culture in which they originated.

Given the model of Albucasis, surgical treatises in the fifteenth through eighteenth centuries also were published with the intention of correcting past errors, including new instruments, and supplying fuller information on their design and use. Natural-sized illustrations, in woodcuts and copper plate engravings or intaglios, appeared initially during the Renaissance.

Eugene Ferguson has emphasized the novelty of providing drawings to scale in other technological treatises published in these centuries. He claims that "the ambiguity of object size and location in space shown in earlier drawings were swept away by the Renaissance invention of perspective."[22] Among surgical treatises that attest to this statement are Hans von Gersdorff's *Feldtbuch der Wundtartzney*,[23] which depicted surgical tools in three-dimensional engravings. Of special note is a retractor (der Loucher), which was shown being applied to the body for keeping a narrow wound open during surgery, an application that was not obvious from the construction of the instrument.[24] A sixteenth-century French surgical text by Jacques Guilleneau, which was translated into English and Dutch, emphasized its author's views that the range of surgeon's tools should not be extensive. God had given humans two appendages to perform many actions and it seemed appropriate that only a few instruments could provide the flexibility needed to carry out all medical procedures. Guilleneau presented illustrations of instruments with their dimensions and their parts in proportional drawings to provide the instrument maker or smith with the information he needed to construct them.[25] The most beautifully illustrated sixteenth-century surgical texts were published by Andreas Vesalius and Vidus Vidius.[26]

Some outstanding illustrated surgical texts appeared in the post-Renaissance period, and therefore, escaped Guerlt's attention. For instance, there is the book by the German, Johannes Scultetus, which was posthumously published by his nephew in 1655. Scultetus' *Armamentarium Chirurgicum*, which contains forty-three copper plate engravings of instruments, presents detailed versions of surgical methods and procedures, including the extraction of a dead fetus with a "crooks,"[27] an implement undepicted since its description by Soranus and Paulus Aeginata, although it was illustrated in cruder form in Albucasis' volume.[28] Scultetus' text is enriched with the details of instrument construction and application, as well as with enlarged views of instrument components.[29] The more common operations performed at the time, including treatment for dislocations, operations on the eyes, teeth, and other organs, amputations, and trephining were among the procedures depicted. The book displays the advantage gained in using copperplate engravings to express detail, and to a lesser extent, perspective to inform the reader about the technological details of surgical instruments. The last illustration in the *Armamentarium* represents the figure of a man to which many of the surgeon's instruments were applied, indicating how they were to be used to treat various diseases and wounds likely to inflict an individual. The figure represents a replication of an earlier illustration of a human figure that displayed the major types of wounds produced by weapons. Some of the wounding instruments were not unlike the knives, scalpels, and other tools used by the surgeon. A similarly illustrated figure was used to show the various sites on the body selected for bloodletting.[30]

In 1723 the Parisian surgeon, Réné Jacques Croissant de Garengeot published an improved text on surgical instruments, which was issued in later editions. Garengeot aspired to fill the gap left in the literature after the publication of Scultetus' book. Garengeot noted that the mechanical advances of the past thirty or forty years, which were being applied to other crafts and trades, had not yet been utilized in the construction of surgical instruments. The quality of surgical treatment was deteriorating with the result that some operations were not performed successfully and others not undertaken at all. In Garengeot's text the engravings corresponded exactly to his description of the instruments. The terms applied to instruments were those employed by respected instrument makers of his acquaintance such as G. Vigneron Jr. of Paris.[31]

Laurence Heister of Germany shared the laurels for excellence with Garengeot in the publication of eighteenth-century surgical texts. Heister was extolled for providing exceptional and explicit instructions on the design and uses of instruments. His text published in 1719 was issued in German, and later, in Latin and English. The text illustrated the actual sizes of instruments, a feature Heister carried to a fine art among authors of surgical texts.[32]

Often, the same woodcuts and intaglio engravings were used in more than one publication. The first anthology of the engravings of surgical instruments that had appeared in other publications during the previous half century was published in 1610. Peter Uffenbach of Frankfurt selected engravings from the publications of the surgeons Ambroise Paré, Fabritius Hildanus, and others to produce the *Thesaurus Chirurgiae*.[33] By the early nineteenth century, a number of illustrated surgical texts were composed of graphics taken from previously published books and journals. These compilations depicted important operations, instruments, bandages, and other apparatus used by the most esteemed practitioners in European countries. The historian Julius Guerlt provided line drawings based on the graphics of most of the important Renaissance surgeons including Della Croce, Ryff, Paré, Fabrizio d'Aquapendente, and Fabritius Hildanus to mention a few of them. An American reviewer noted the thoroughness of the surgical text produced by the German compiler, L. F. V. Froriep, who included colored engravings and original drawings taken from the surgical literature in a number of languages.[34]

A distinguished American folio-sized treatise on surgical operations was composed by Joseph Pancoast, professor of anatomy and surgery at Jefferson Medical College in Philadelphia. It was published in 1844, one year prior to the introduction of anesthesia. The procedures portrayed reflect some of the operating room drama of the pre-anesthetic era and introduce Pancoast's original surgical techniques and types of instruments.[35] Originality and novelty in instruments were the hallmarks of many surgical books, which, on the other hand, sometimes neglected to provide some of the fundamentals of surgical techniques.

By the third quarter of the nineteenth century, a United States naval surgeon succeeded in assuaging the curiosity of some of those searching for specific details about simple and common surgical practices that had been taken for granted by the authors of surgical texts. Philip S. Wade published a text on *Mechanical Therapuetics* in 1867, which received praise from a commentator in the *Medical Record* of 1868. The reviewer explained why the book was so helpful to the neophyte surgeon.

We have never seen any work of its kind that can compete with it in real utility and extensive adaptability. But it is particularly in regard to the detailing of minor matters connected with dressings, trivial operations and the like, that the excellence of the work consists. These are in fact most important subjects to the tyro, for the reason that they are not treated of either in the lecture-room or in the most advanced textbooks. How often has a young graduate to get his first idea of the best manner to make a poultice, and to do many other simple things, from some hint judiciously and perhaps courteously dropped by the nurse, and all this for the reason of the very simplicity of the maneuvres. Many a young practitioner has been more puzzled over the proper dressing of a stump than the operation which created it; and many a fledgling would rather attempt Caesarian section than the passage of a female catheter. Our author seems to have understood the extent of this ignorance in all of the various departments of elementary surgery, and has made a very elaborate and successful effort to dispel it.[36]

Medical instruments introduced primarily in the nineteenth century were not always described in sufficient detail, although some noteworthy review articles appeared explaining the derivation and application of diagnostic and therapeutic instruments. An extensive article of this type was written in 1898 by W. P. Northrup, who described the practical tracheal tubes invented by Joseph O'Dwyer.[37] (See figures 2.1, 2.2, and 2.3.) In other areas, manufacturers, teachers, and practitioners were accused of being responsible for the lack of adequate descriptions of instruments. Medical teachers, such as A. L. Ranney, recognized the inadequacies of many texts in explaining the design and function of mechanical devices. Ranney taught a course in the Post-graduate Medical School of New York in 1884 and was obliged to supplement the available texts on nervous diseases in his lectures. He quoted the words of a young practitioner, which inspired his lectures on instruments:

I feel, doctor, that textbooks upon nervous affections abound in pictures of instruments employed in diagnosis, such as batteries, thermoelectric apparatus, galvanometers, dynamometers, dynamographs, etc., but they are scanty in the descriptions of the uses of these instruments and their value in diagnosis. I presume that it is impossible to correctly interpret the various phenomena of nervous affections without these costly appliances, so I am often forced to guess at the disease and let it go at that.[38]

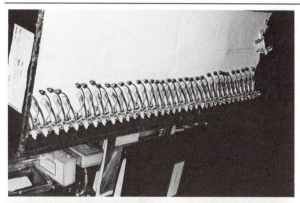

Figure 2.1. Order of tracheal tubes, from George P. Pilling Co. of Philadelphia ready for shipment to the hospital. Manufactured in the 1970s as they have been over the past half century. *Photo by author at the factory.*

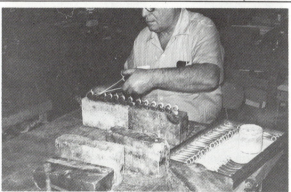

Figure 2.2. Manufacturing tracheal tubes in the twentieth century. *Photo by author at George P. Pilling Co. of Philadelphia.*

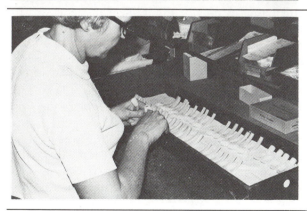

Figure 2.3. Assembling plastic tracheal tubes in the twentieth century. *Photo by author at George P. Pilling Co. of Philadelphia.*

Physicians began to study at least elementary physics by the second half of the nineteenth century. Physics texts offering scientific and engineering information in a form that relied minimally on mathematics were most successful in teaching medical students the basic principles of the subject. Arnott's *Elements of Physics, General and Medical* and John C. Draper's *A Text Book on Medical Physics for the Use of Students and Practitioners of Medicine* were the American texts noted for their "clear and untechnical explanation of physical phenomena."[39] Physicians were attracted to these authors because these texts demonstrated the functions of the microscope, electric battery, and pressure gauge and elucidated theories related to light and sound, all of which were essential to an understanding of diagnosis and treatment in medicine administered by devices, instruments, and appliances.

Inadequate descriptions and insufficient explanations of medical instruments were still found in the medical literature of the 1970s. In the volume *Chest Tubes and Chest Bottles* by Arndt Von Hippel appears this criticism:

Nowhere in the present literature can be found an explanation for the rational use of intrapleural drainage tubes under various circumstances. Underwater sealed drainage is essentially simple, both in theory and practice; however, I know of no other procedures which can be misunderstood by so many people—the blame, of course, lies in the fact that thoracic surgeons do not take the time to explain the simple working of the apparatus so that it is understood.[40]

TRADE CATALOGUES:

Instrument manufacturers had realized, since the nineteenth century, that they could gain the confidence of their prospective customers by appearing to fill the lacunae in the medical technology literature. In 1889 the manufacturer George Tiemann of New York summed up the deficiencies in the literature pertaining to instruments, which he recognized and promised to help eliminate. He claimed that "in surgical works many of the instruments for performing operations are not illustrated. In illustrated catalogues, on the other hand, a description of the *modus operandi* is wanting. A good drawing of an instrument imparts an accurate conception of its form and construction. A description of the application added to this gives a clearer idea of its suitableness to the end proposed."[41] To make the bridge between the instrument and its application, Tiemann produced an 846-page trade catalogue. In his enlarged instrument

catalogue designed to sell medical and surgical instruments, Tiemann proposed to describe "the use of the instruments and appliances by accompanying the illustrations with pertinent quotations from the writings of inventors and authors, as published in medical periodicals, recent works on surgery, and from other sources. . . . By consulting the following pages and comparing the observations and experiments of the various authors, practitioners of surgery may form their own opinions, and be assisted in the choice of the most approved instruments and apparatus for the accomplishment of their purposes."[42] Tiemann remains a supplier of instruments to the present.

Another major American supplier of medical instruments echoed Tiemann's sentiments a decade later and attempted to publish an improved text. Charles Truax of Chicago, Illinois, summed up the deficiencies in the medical literature by explaining that "the practitioner who desires information relative to any particular instrument or appliance and searches in the standard textbook for descriptions and recommendations is soon lost in a maze of unsatisfactory and confusing suggestions. Accurate descriptions are few, differentiations of patterns are almost unknown, and definite reasons for preferring one model rather than another are often absolutely wanting."[43] The descriptions and illustrations provided by Truax were exemplary.

Manufacturers have long boasted of the instructive nature of their trade catalogues and other advertising literature. Among the most lavishly illustrated catalogues to be published in the nineteenth century were those supplied by George Tiemann and E. B. Meyrowitz of New York, M. F. Charrière of Paris, Arnold and Sons of London, Codman and Shurtleff of Boston, and George Pilling of Philadelphia.[44] These manufacturers were also the most careful in making instruments to exacting specifications and in attempting to provide the refinements requested by surgeons and physicians, as well as those that appeared necessary to the maker, after difficulties were reported by those who used them. The most outstanding of all these firms was the one founded in 1820 by M. F. Charrière, which continued to manufacture instruments until 1930. Charrière, who made the most beautiful and precise medical and surgical instruments, traveled to England in 1836 to study British techniques of manufacturing hand tools to lay the basis for producing the best surgical implements. He brought back a method of tempering steel that was used in making scissors, which soon was adopted by all the producers of his region around Nogent in France.[45] Upon mastering the manufacturing techniques associated with surgical instruments, Charrière studied the manual dexterity of surgeons to produce instruments which could be used with greater ease and convenience. Popular demand led Charrière to produce a preliminary catalogue of his instruments in 1843, while he continued to work on a more definitive version, which appeared in 1867 under the guidance of two of his students, Robert and Adolph Collin.

Among the innovations he introduced were the application of glazing, silver plating, and platinage of steel, lead, and tin to surgical instruments, and the development of instruments that spared the surgeon some effort, such as a forceps that could be left in the closed position so that it would not have to be held continuously. By substituting German silver for silver, he reduced the cost of instruments. Charrière's advertisement for instruments and devices of use to the recuperating or self-medicating patient as well as the physician were among the earliest commercially available items of this type. Such items included ivory-tipped nursing bottles, bloodletting instruments, hearing aids, syringes, pumps, sounds, pessaries, bandages, and orthopedic apparatus. He outlined the evolution of each piece, discussed the material used in its construction, listed the available sizes and types, and indicated their costs.

Charrière's catalogues served Europeans and Americans throughout the nineteenth and twentieth centuries, not only as a source of premium quality manufactured implements, but equally as texts to supplement instruction in medical technology.[46] For instance, as early as 1840, an unidentified English surgeon published a description of those surgical instruments which most impressed him during his travels in France and Germany. The instruments illustrated in the English text were those manufactured by Charrière. The traveling surgeon revealed that:

Some of them [instruments] were curious from their novelty in the ingenuity displayed in their construction, while the greater number recommended themselves chiefly as being the instruments used by those surgeons from France and Germany who had acquired eminence in the treatment of special classes of surgical diseases. As most of them are comparatively unknown in this country, the author has published the present Manual in the belief that a work exhibiting their form and explaining their use may be serviceable to the junior members of his profession. Such a work will enable them to understand more easily the publications of the continental surgeons, whether in the original or when

quoted by English authors; and may, at the same time, be useful in throwing out hints for the improvement or alteration of instruments suited to the circumstances of individual cases.[47]

The text was arranged with descriptions corresponding to a number assigned to each instrument which, in turn, was illustrated in a plate placed at the back of the volume. Each piece, including its parts, was briefly described with a few details about its construction and use.

Manufacturers soon supplied more instruments and different models of an instrument with a single function than the average practitioner required. Manufacturers whose marketing techniques were enhanced by the increasingly detailed trade catalogues thus began to control the design of instruments to an extent not possible previously.

In the twentieth century, manufacturers, aware of the limitations of their physician and surgeon clients' mechanical skills, attempted to simplify instruments by limiting the number of their parts and to advertise instruments on this basis. E. B. Meyrowitz of New York, in reference to an implement for eye surgery called a tendon tucker, in his Bulletin for 1931 wrote that "there is hardly any mechanism on the instrument which would confuse the surgeon."[48]

Trade catalogues are an obvious but neglected source of primary information on medical instruments manufactured since the nineteenth century, but with few exceptions they have not been systematically collected by medical libraries or instrument collectors. Medical trade catalogues are usually classified as ephemeral and not saved by libraries or, if stored, are not catalogued. An annotated bibliography of extant medical instrument trade catalogues, beginning with the earliest ones from the eighteenth and nineteenth centuries, extending to those published around 1930, and prefaced with an introductory chapter, would provide a valuable, and as yet, unavailable medical instrument research source. The bibliography of trade catalogues should contain the titles, dates, number of pages, and range of instruments advertised. Special features potentially useful to the historical researcher and the location of the catalogues should be included. Presently, a listing of catalogues for about 2,000 manufacturers and distributors has been assembled and is on file in the National Museum of American History. These data have been gathered from medical libraries and museums in the United States, Great Britain, and Canada and from a few continental libraries. The best controlled medical trade catalogue collections are owned by the New York Academy of Medicine and the Yale Beineke Rare Book and Manuscript Library. Other large collections exist in the Wellcome Museum of the History of Medicine at the Science Museum, the Royal College of Surgeons Library of England, the Armed Forces Institute of Pathology Museum, the Bausch and Lomb Company Collection in the Rush Rhees Library in Rochester, New York, and the Smithsonian Institution. The Smithsonian Institution acquired the extensive collection of X-ray equipment trade catalogues owned by the American College of Radiology.

Catalogues designed to sell a product for use by the physician, medical assistant, nurse, or patient range in size from a single sheet flyer to over a thousand pages in one volume bound between hard covers. By the end of the nineteenth century, most large instrument manufacturers published new catalogues each year. Special products, new designs in basic equipment, and improvements in instruments were advertised. Small publications issued throughout the year, such as the *Monthly Bulletin* published by the New York-based E. B. Meyrowitz Company, which specialized in optical instruments, kept customers informed of the latest models and up-to-date equipment.

Almost all trade catalogues contain illustrations, diagrams, and from the end of the nineteenth century, photographs which show the structure and sometimes the function of an object. The technical terms for implements and their parts are often found only in catalogues[49] designed to sell equipment to physicians. The more successful manufacturers exhibited a pride in the knowledge and craftsmanship of their products, which they displayed in the design and organization of their trade catalogues. Occasionally, the history of a device was traced along with its role in medical practice. Trade exhibitions inspired some manufacturers to publish special catalogues depicting their best instruments. Trade catalogues are especially useful to compare with exhibition and museum catalogues as well as with descriptions of instruments in the medical literature to discover those instruments that were adopted by medical practitioners. The commercially successful items were repeatedly advertised and discussed in the medical literature and frequently endorsed by respected medical practitioners.

Trade catalogues adopted more of the characteristics of the medical literature as manufacturers provided a greater variety of instruments and a more extensive medical technology. Among the topics touched on in trade catalogues were aspects of the interpersonal relationships created by the use of medical technology among different medical specialists. The medical equipment manufacturer understood the professional pride and jealousies existing among physicians, surgeons, pharmacists, and dentists and sometimes offered to bridge the information gap separating specialists. For example, King sold anesthesia apparatus to dentists, who were skillful at operating the dispensing units. The company offered to teach physicians, who often were unfamiliar with these anesthesia devices, how to operate a dental anesthesia machine, so that physicians might not find themselves embarrassed in front of their dental colleagues.[50]

The growth of a few medical specialties may be traced in the trade catalogue literature of the producers who supplied medical instruments to these specialists. A series of trade catalogues issued over a number of years provides documentation for the technological changes encouraged by medical specialists and to which they adapted. The best example is the specialty of physical medicine, which grew in importance as a variety of equipment became available. Physical medicine flourished after a spectacular range of devices were introduced for applying heat, electricity, water, X rays, and various motions and vibrations to the body in the period beginning at the end of the nineteenth century. Aspects of physical medicine had been practiced since antiquity, but a resurgence in medical technology resulted in the design and production of a variety of devices and instruments, which changed the nature of physical medicine and led to the separation of physical medicine from general medicine and the creation of a specialized medical profession.[51]

In the early twentieth century, electric equipment and X-ray manufacturers like Reinhold Wappler of New York responded to the increasing scientific awareness of physical medicine specialists who attributed their increasing success in treatment to medical equipment. Scientific and technological astuteness on the part of the physician forced manufacturers to provide better instruments and to explain their functions in scientifically derived and approved terms. By the twentieth century, physicians would no longer tolerate shoddy equipment such as glass measuring tubes marked by eye and unchecked for their accuracy of calibration.[52] Catalogues became specific and technical and occasionally included explanations of the techniques employed to make better medical equipment.

Trade catalogues changed their character to reflect the state of the industry and were subdivided as one or more subgroups of instruments, devices, or aids became sufficiently complex and numerous to require many pages of description and illustration in a separate publication. For instance, James Swift and Son of London in 1909-1910 produced the twenty-third edition of their microscope catalogue by separating the petrological microscopes from biological and medical models. When medical specialists began to use primarily one type of instrument, as in urology, gynecology, or ophthalmology, trade catalogues were designed to include all the models and types of available instruments of the medical specialty. The larger and more complete catalogues were organized into sections corresponding to the medical practitioner's specialization. Institutions such as hospitals and nursing homes demanded yet other types of items from the medical instrument manufacturer. (See figures 2.4 and 2.5.) Larger quantities of items, such as surgical dressings, surgical instruments, thermometers, bed pans, and linen were required regularly by the hospital. Rugged items were designed that could stand up to constant use and impersonal care to cope with the wear and tear of constant use within the hospital.[53]

Trade catalogues fill a void in the medical literature related to medical technology. The nature of medicine and surgery has led some medical professionals to keep detailed aspects of diagnosis and treatment from the public and even their potential patients, thus greatly limiting the printed primary sources available to the nonspecialist reader. It is apparent from reading editorials in medical journals published over the last century that the issue of educating the lay person about the technical details of medical procedures has been controversial and has taken a toll, in that medical technology has not been discussed as fully or as openly as it might have been. George Shrady, the editor of *The Medical Record*, an influential nineteenth-century American medical journal, argued against the publication of technical medical and surgical facts in lay publications. In 1887 he criticized the New York daily paper, *The Tribune*, for reporting medical news including the details of surgical operations. Medical practitioners, the editor claimed, understand that "the less the public knows about details of surgical operations, the better. Only the first year medical student revels in knife, saw and blood."[54] Shrady defended his position on the grounds that reverence for the body before, during, and after surgery should be maintained. Surgical

procedures were becoming successful and surgeons were beginning to have reason to be proud of their accomplishments by this time. Dignified reporting included technical description and assessment without emphasizing the gory details, which the medical practitioner writer was best equipped to do. Medical reports in the daily papers seemed to violate the bounds of decorum tolerated by surgeons and even some patients. A few years later, a popular account of surgical operations that were reported to have been performed as part of an entertainment program before an audience at the People's Theatre in Omaha, Nebraska strained the imagination and tolerance of the medical writer who commented on the article and the event. Could the public have witnessed surgical operations and enjoyed them as a spectacle, he pondered?[55]

While the physician and surgeon were expected by their colleagues to guard against publicity that could be construed as a form of advertising, medical trade catalogue producers freely used the names and inventions of physicians in their publications. Editorials repeatedly cautioned physicians about the unethical and nonprofessional aspects of any form of advertising.[56] One commentator noted "the severe attack of publicity" a medical practitioner (unnamed of course) had suffered, and it was hoped that the physician had not triggered off the attack by presenting the news to the press himself.[57] At the same time, trade catalogues printed testimonials from and to physicians who invented, perfected, and endorsed medical instruments and devices. Sometimes the original publication of the inventor was reprinted and used to advertise the instrument.

A more effective argument for controlling the spread of information related to medical technology was a desire to protect the public from the incompetent and the quack who would make improper use of the facts and ideas obtained from popular and easily available publications. Quacks and charlatans had displayed a predilection for employing instruments and devices in their questionable treatments. Since antiquity, charlatans had advertised their special skills of being adept in manipulating a new device or applying a new drug. Physicians wary of these "specialists" found it difficult to accept any but the most modest claims for the virtues of instruments recommended by competent physicians and surgeons when these implements were introduced. Breaking down the physician's prejudices against a new instrument, which were made stronger by his desire not to appear to be a charlatan, became part of the medical instru-

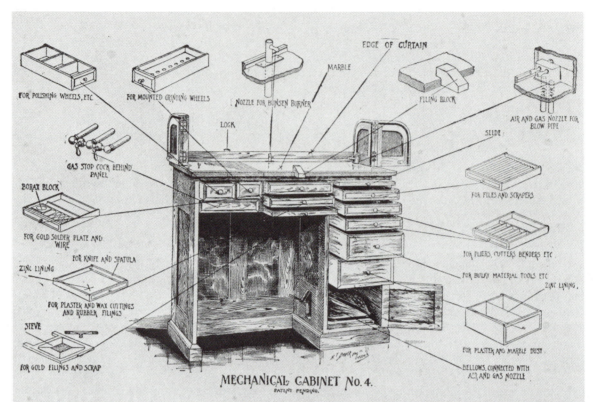

FOR POLISHING WHEELS, ETC

FOR MOUNTED GRINDING WHEELS

EDGE OF CURTAIN

MARBLE

NOZZLE FOR BUNSEN BURNER

FILING BLOCK

AIR AND GAS NOZZLE FOR BLOW PIPE

LOCK

GAS STOP COCK BEHIND PANEL

SLIDE

BORAX BLOCK

FOR FILES AND SCRAPERS

FOR GOLD SOLDER PLATE AND WIRE

FOR KNIFE AND SPATULA

FOR PLIERS, CUTTERS BENDERS ETC

ZINC LINING

FOR BULKY MATERIAL TOOLS ETC

ZINC LINING

FOR PLASTER AND WAX CUTTINGS AND RUBBER FILINGS

SIEVE

FOR PLASTER AND MARBLE DUST

FOR GOLD FILINGS AND SCRAP

BELLOWS, CONNECTED WITH AIR AND GAS NOZZLE

MECHANICAL CABINET No. 4.
PATENT PENDING.

This Cabinet is intended for use in the operating room. It is closed by a roll top, which follows the grooves in the upright sides above the bench top, at a height to clear any lathe heads or electric lathes on the market, and when closed every drawer, except two unimportant ones, is automatically locked. When open, the curtain is entirely concealed, and the ends fold back so as to leave no obstruction to the light.

Within the bench is a system of piping for carrying the gas through the concealed stop-cocks to the blow-pipe and Bunsen burner.

The bench is substantially built, with numerous dovetailed joints which render it rigid and strong.

The finish is of the highest grade, substantial and lasting. The back is paneled, and as well finished as the sides and front.

Dimensions—Height, over all, 3 feet 9½ inches; height of bench top, 3 feet; length, over all, 3 feet 8 inches; depth, over all, 1 foot 5¼ inches.

Prices Mahogany, $60.00   Quartered Oak, $50.00   Cock and Piping for Compressed
Walnut, - 55.00   Bellows, extra,   5.00   Air, extra, $2.50.

N. B.—The treadle used on the bellows in this bench is a special pattern, and will be furnished to those who wish to use bellows already on hand, at 50 cents.

Our catalogue, "Modern Office Furnishings," will tell you more about this Cabinet. Ask your Depot for one.

9

Figure 2.4. Dental cabinet circa 1910-1920 for implements used in dental surgery sold by Ransome and Randolph Co., of Toledo, Ohio. *Photo by author from catalogue.*

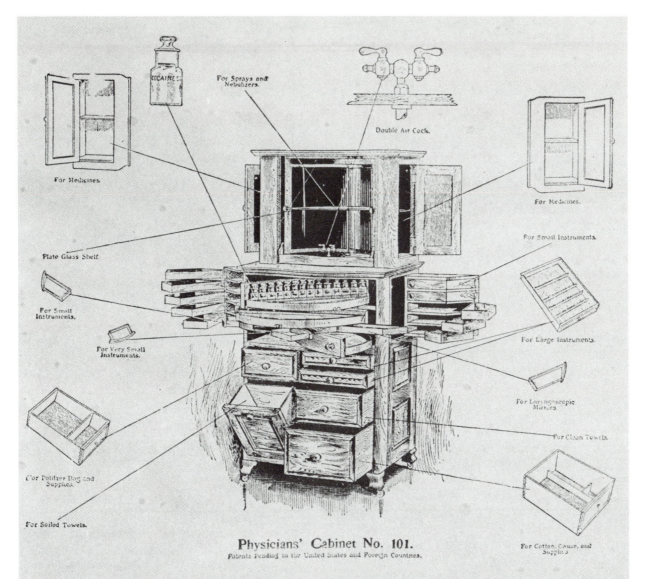

For Medicines.

For Sprays and Nebulizers.

Double Air Cock.

For Medicines.

For Small Instruments.

Plate Glass Shelf.

For Small Instruments.

For Large Instruments.

For Very Small Instruments.

For Laryngoscopic Mirrors.

For Clean Towels.

For Politzer Bag and Supplies.

For Soiled Towels.

For Cotton, Gauze, and Supplies.

Physicians' Cabinet No. 101.
Patents Pending in the United States and Foreign Countries.

This Cabinet is intended especially for the nose and throat specialist.

As far as we know there is no list of the names of those practicing this profession, so we cannot circularize them direct.

The Cabinet is a perfect one, ingeniously designed, conveniently arranged, attractive in appearance, beautifully finished, and is finding a ready market.

If you know a nose and throat specialist, will you kindly hand him this circular? Full description will be sent on application.

The Ransom & Randolph Co.
Toledo, Ohio.

Figure 2.5. Cabinet for Instruments of the nose and throat specialist, circa 1910-1920, made by the Ransome and Randolph Co. of Toledo, Ohio. *Photo by author from catalogue.*

ment inventor's responsibility. Instrument makers established the tradition of having physicians request technical details concerning advertised instruments on letterhead stationery. Instructions for the use of instruments were included with the implements at the time of purchase.

Medical instrument manufacturers had to understand the intellectual foundations of medical practice. In the regular physician's estimation, while an untutored practitioner might learn to apply some of the physical techniques of diagnosis and therapy, as long as he was unable to understand the theoretical basis for what he was doing and why it was being done, he remained unfit to practice medicine. Therefore, many physicians insisted that the full rationale for the use of all medical instruments be learned before they were applied. In the early period of the development of medical technology, physicians assumed that an individual capable of learning the facts and theories related to medicine would be able to master the manual skills required to diagnose and treat diseases with implements and devices. It became the manufacturer's task, in many instances, to alert the physician to his role as a physical diagnostician.

The engineering skill necessary for designing and, in part, for applying an instrument to the body differs from the types of skills required to learn the theoretical and scientific nature of anatomy, physiology, and pathology. Surgeons and dentists usually possessed a "feel" for instruments since mechanical manipulation was the focus of surgical treatment from its inception (see figure 2.6). A successful surgeon developed a mechanical sense and a delicate touch with implements. As surgeons and physicians became more aware of each other's functions and learned to use each other's methods, the mechanical "touch" became more common in medical practice with consequent appreciation of the fine details and functions of a medical instrument and surgical tool. After the medical practitioner became more technologically conscious, he demanded that manufacturers produce higher quality instruments with such properties as a high polish and fine details. Aspects of instrument design became more complex and required special knowledge to understand their intricacies, which made it more difficult to pass this technical information on to untutored individuals. The related literature grew more arcane and fragmented, being dispersed among trade catalogues and technical journals, as well as journals and texts. The medical technology literature became highly specialized and resulted in the fact that not only the layman was likely to be

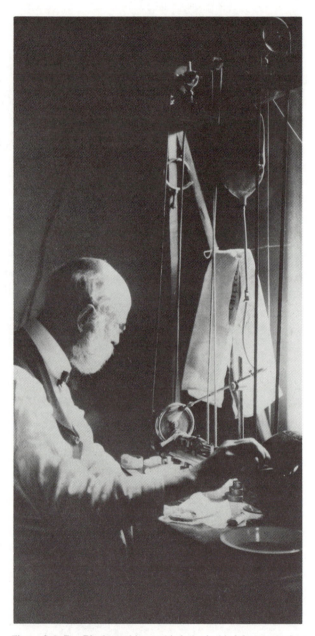

Figure 2.6. Dr. Black working at his lathe in his laboratory circa 1890. *Smithsonian Institution (SI) Photo No. 72-7911.*

bewildered by it but, too often, also the physicians who needed to learn the finer points about the use of medical instruments remained perplexed.

CATALOGUES OF COLLECTIONS:

MEDICAL INSTRUMENTS:

Considering the difficulties to be overcome in producing a catalogue will help to explain why there are so few published. One of the most obvious reasons for the neglect of the history of medical technology, the inability of museums with large collections to catalogue properly and publish information on their holdings which would bring medical equipment to the attention of the scholar, grows out of a number of factors. Cataloguing is expensive, requiring the skills of well-motivated historian-curators who must place in context many objects accumulated over a number of years, many with little documentation related to their dates of production, manufacturers, former owners, and uses. Accession records and catalogue cards on file in museums are notorious for providing a minimum of information, contributing to the lack of interest in objects as sources of data. G. L'E. Turner of the Museum of the History of Science of Oxford, who has provided some of the most useful and important studies of microscopes, stated in 1967: "Historians have long used manuscripts and books as their raw material. I hope I have suggested that collections of historic instruments can be just as useful. If the examination of collections develops as a new line of research, it will be necessary for accurate and detailed information to be more readily available than is the case at present.[58] Medical instrument collections that lack depth and range of objects, added to the difficulty in locating similar items in other collections, hamper the scholar in recognizing the full significance of an object and its application to medicine.

Among medical collections not described in a published catalogue is the one held by the University of Kansas Medical Center Museum in Kansas City, Kansas. This collection, as do others of its type, contains an assortment of interesting, partially unique but unrelated, objects and documents. Of approximately 600 items, there are diplomas; touch-pieces attributed to Edward IV, Elizabeth I, and other royalty; several dozen X-ray tubes; and surgical instruments. Microscopes, among which are several eighteenth-century models, particularly a Culpepper and a Nuremberg type; stethoscopes; obstetric forceps; and artifacts of national origin, such as Chinese,

Japanese, and Indian materials, are represented in the collection. The museum is not listed in the American Museums' Association Guide, and it appears to be one of the least known collections with a variety of medical items. The collection should be available to scholars through photographs and short descriptions of the objects in a published catalogue.[59]

Unlike most libraries, in which standard cataloguing systems such as the Dewey decimal and Library of Congress systems have been adopted, there are no major conventional cataloguing methods for history museum objects and particularly medical objects. After receiving an object, museums employ initial registration processes, called accessioning, in which objects are recorded by their class names. Additional information includes the details of how the objects came to the museum (donation, purchase, transfer), and each is assigned a number to distinguish it from all other objects in the museum. More information may be filed on each object, but usually the composition, dimensions, functions, and history of the items are left to be determined and described in the course of the cataloguing process. All too frequently this process is not completed or even initiated. The most important purpose in cataloguing an object is to retrieve information,[60] but the students' demands for facts may be so varied and unpredictable that the cataloguer is overwhelmed in making decisions on exactly what type of information to record in both the museum and printed catalogues. A book entering a library may not be catalogued immediately, but it never remains uncatalogued or it would be unretrievable. The information required to catalogue a book is defined in rules, which all librarians have adopted. Historical objects, on the other hand, are most often only partially catalogued and are usually located by the curator of a collection, who responds to specific requests. The greater difficulty in storing objects rather than books, the lack of adequate storage space, and ever-expanding collections are among the major causes of less well organized object collections. Personal service in locating objects to the extent provided by curators would never be possible in most libraries where the card catalogue is expected to lead readers to most of the books they are seeking.

History museums have devised various cataloguing systems over the past decades that are being entered into the computer. These systems attempt to arrange the documentation for an object or to prepare indexes to the documentation. To make the information as useful as possible, it must be cross-indexed in many ways but probably will never be adequately organized to meet the needs of all those asking specific questions of a museum historical collection.[61] According to Geoffrey Lewis, the ideal cataloguing system "appears to be a system which the smallest museum can afford to run (this means without mechanical aids) but which can also be used as computer-in-put for the larger collections, a national index and the research problem."[62]

It may not be economically sound to duplicate everything in the files of a museum in a computer format, but the cost rises in proportion as the "card catalogue syndrome" continues to be maintained. To expect printed copies of everything stored in a computer is one of the prevalent manifestations of this syndrome, which detracts from the creative functions of the computer.[63] Information stored in the computer should be significant and potentially useful for a variety of users.[64]

It is useful to take stock of existing medical instrument catalogues and the elements of their composition. Catalogues of medical collections are compiled from data found in patents, advertisements in journals, trade catalogues, trade cards, fair and exhibition lists and catalogues, testimonials of patients and physicians, and the monographs, articles, and manuscripts of inventors, physicians, surgeons, manufacturers, and occasionally, historians. Graphics, photographs, and drawings are essential supplements to these sources. To be able to read and interpret the information contained in such a diversity of sources demands an intense interest in the technicalities involved in the practice of medicine. Observing and maneuvering the objects under study adds a dimension difficult to acquire through the literature alone. In the process of analyzing the materials composing an object, which must usually be done with the help of experts in a conservation-analytical laboratory,[65] and arranging instruments to show their subtle aspects in a photograph or X-ray film, the historian may be presented with questions not apparent before examining the object. Studying the object through handling and comparing it with similar types, especially those produced over a span of centuries, brings to the surface some of the questions material cultural specialists grapple with routinely (see figure 2.7). The medical instrument cataloguer must emulate, in part, the techniques and studies of the material culture historian, combined with those of the anthropologist and archeologist. Some of the first descriptions of medical instruments were prepared by archeologists.

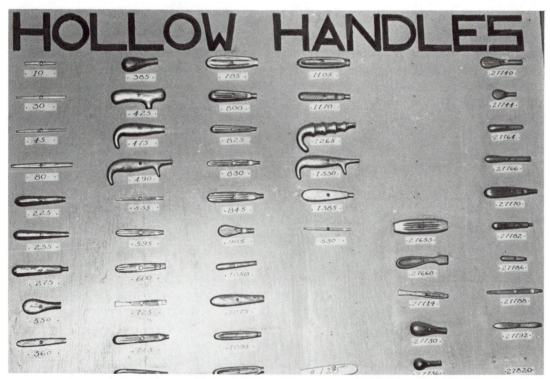

Figure 2.7. Assortment of handles for various surgical and diagnostic instruments made throughout the twentieth century by George P. Pilling Co. of Philadelphia. *Photo by author at the factory.*

MEDICAL OBJECTS:

As an example of material generally available in collections, the best documented and catalogued instrument of medical importance is the microscope. Microscopes have long been the most appealing items to collectors because of their instruments' intriguing shapes, the range of materials used in the constructions, and the decorations, which make them aesthetically appealing. The microscope's function and the existence of models representing at least several hundred years of evolution add even more luster to the instrument as a collectible item. Eighteenth- and nineteenth-century microscopes are being sold for increasingly large sums, thus straining the meager budgets of institutions and individuals wishing to enlarge and perfect the scope of their collections that were planned to be comprehensive. The basic microscope catalogue upon which American collectors may rely appeared in editions published in 1972 and 1974. The second edition was expanded to include ninety microscopes acquired since the first edition had appeared. The catalogue was prepared at the Armed Forces Institute of Pathology Museum and represents the long-term interest of Helen R. Purtle, museum specialist, now retired, who helped shape the collection and make it known through exhibitions, lectures, and publications. The catalogue contains succinct descriptions and photographic illustrations of about 700 microscopes. The collection was started by Lt. Col. George A. Otis in 1874, who preceded John Shaw Billings as curator of the collection. Billings enlarged the collection and provided an impetus that has resulted in its becoming the finest microscope collection in the United States. Thus, the collection bears the name, The Billings Microscope Collection.[66]

The other major collection in Washington, D.C., held by the Smithsonian Institution's National Museum of American History, consists of approximately 200 microscopes, primarily American made, dating from the nineteenth through the first half of the twentieth centuries. This group of microscopes has been catalogued in a computer format, incorporating information available from trade catalogues and direct study of the instrument: date of acquisition, donor or dealer, cost, age of instrument, size, major features of construction and composition, previous owner, use, and unusual attributes. More detailed research needs to be done on these instruments, especially on the nineteenth-century models. The categories of information provided for each instrument include those of interest to the scholar, collector,

registrar, and general student. An example of the method of cataloguing is represented by an early twentieth-century microscope manufactured by the Spencer Company. It was owned by Dr. Frederick Allen, who used the instrument in the course of his investigation of diabetes and cancer.[67]

Other collections of microscopes described in published catalogues include: the Utrecht University Museum Collection, Teyler Museum Collection, Union College (New York) Collection, and Sir Frank Crisp's collection of 3,000 microscopes, sold at auction in 1920, 1921, and 1925, a number of which are presently in the Wellcome Museum of the History of Medicine and the London Science Museum collection.[68] Among the excellent collections of microscopes are over a thousand specimens in the Wellcome Museum of the History of Medicine holdings transferred to the Science Museum of London, the Ashmolean and Science Museum specimens in Oxford, and several hundred important microscopes in medical museums in Cleveland, Ohio and Galveston, Texas.

In addition to this study of the microscope as object, there is the possibility of using the instrument in the manner of its original owner and user and reporting on these trials in a catalogue of the tested instruments. Microscopes are among the few medical instruments that the historian may set up and use in the manner described by their original owners and makers. Care must be taken in the type of information sought and the conclusions to be drawn, but the possibility remains for re-creating earlier observational and anatomic modes and verifying experimental evidence reported in the literature. Intriguing historical research has reported on the use of antique microscopes to observe organic structures described in seventeenth-, eighteenth-, and nineteenth-century publications, which appear questionable and unclear to the modern observer. Edwin Clarke has summarized the role of the microscope and a few other instruments in doing what he has termed "practical history"[69] in a book he edited in 1971.

Clarke's student, Brian Bracegirdle, curator of the medical collection at the Science Museum, has written an essay on the history of the microtome and microtechnique used in preparing specimens for viewing under the microscope. Bracegirdle has traced collections of prepared slides and the instruments used to make them, which were employed in historic histologic studies.[70] In a separately published survey of the sources for the study of histology, Bracegirdle discusses the history of specimen preparations and collections of slides and sliders. Sliders were made for amateur microscopists as a form of entertainment. Popular slider specimens observed with the microscope by the amateur included the Lord's Prayer engraved on the slides, single-cell animal and plant organisms, and unusual artistic designs made from natural materials, such as diatoms, which were sold by the thousands in the nineteenth and early twentieth centuries. Important slides of medical and scientific interest include William Hewson's preparations held by the Hunterian Museum of the Royal College of Surgeons of England. Made before 1774, they are "the earliest surviving histological slides in the world." Slides made by John Quekett and Joseph Hyrtl primarily before 1860 are also in the Hunterian Museum collection.[71]

Catalogues of other medical and surgical instruments are among the rarest items to be found partly because the publications often appeared in limited editions. One of the oldest medical object catalogues is the handwritten list of instruments owned by the Royal College of Surgeons in London. The folio-sized catalogue in several volumes was prepared by the retired surgeon Alban Doran and completed by C. J. S. Thompson. The collection, first assembled in the late eighteenth century, increased to over 2,000 specimens by the time Thompson published a *Guide to Surgical Instruments and Objects in the Historical Series with Their History and Development* in 1929.[72] The earliest attempt to organize the instruments owned by the college was made in 1871, followed by Walter Pye's efforts to list and number all the items in 1878. Doran began to classify, number, and measure every instrument in 1912 and had almost finished this process at the time of his death in 1927, when Thompson took over the responsibility for maintaining the collection and completing the guide. Doran, who wished to make publicly available segments of the collection as soon as they had been catalogued, published articles on those segments, as well as the *Descriptive Catalogue of the Obstetrical Instruments in the Museum of the Royal College of Surgeons* in 1921.[73]

The Royal College of Surgeons' collection was enriched in 1912 when Lord Lister's nephew, Rickman J. Godlee, gave his uncle's instruments to the college. The Lister collection, which is on display although not catalogued, consists of three groups of instruments: those devised, modified, and used by Lister; those used by his father-in-law, the surgeon Sir James Syme, consisting of about 2,000 objects; and finally, approximately forty items presented to Lister. The Wellcome Museum of the History of Medicine also includes over one hundred Lister items.[74]

Objects documenting Lister's application of the germ theory are complimented by a collection related to the other instrument of importance to surgery, which was used to apply anesthesia. Americans had successfully demonstrated through a much-heralded operation the soporific qualities of ether in 1847, following which the British wrote the early important texts and produced improved equipment for administering ether, chloroform, and other anesthetic gases. It is fitting, therefore, that the largest collection of historical anesthetic equipment should be located in Great Britain. On exhibit in the Faculty Research Department of Anesthesiology of the Royal College of Surgeons of England, the contents of the anesthesia collection has been made available to students through a published catalogue.[75]

The A. Charles King collection of anesthesia apparatus was inventoried, photographed, and brought together in a handsome volume by the late K. Bryan Thomas, who was an anesthesiologist at the Royal Berkshire Hospital in Reading, England.[76] Begun as an inventory published in 1970, the catalogue of the collection is supplemented with a historical essay, relying in part on Barbara M. Duncum's *The Development of Inhalation Anesthesia*.[77] The historical equipment is arranged in the catalogue according to the type of anesthetic substances these devices were designed to administer, including ether, chloroform, nitrous oxide, mixed vapors, and other analgesiacs. Anesthetic devices held by other museums are mentioned in the catalogue, especially those found in the important Geoffrey Kaye Museum of Anesthetic Apparatus in Melbourne, Australia. Thomas points out the value of medical theory in the design of a medical appliance by referring to John Snow's device for giving a low and precise amount of chloroform, which led his English followers to develop special inhalers that were not used in other countries. The King collection, which was amassed by a leading British manufacturer of medical supplies, has been increased by a substantial collection of twentieth-century devices presented by the British Oxygen Company. However, this collection was not received in time to be included in Thomas' catalogue. A fine American collection of anesthesia equipment is managed and displayed by the American Society of Anesthesiologists at their headquarters in Park Ridge, Illinois.

The Wellcome Museum of the History of Medicine at the Science Museum, the Armed Forces Institute of Pathology Medical Museum in Washington, D.C., the Howard Dittrick Museum of Historical Medicine in Cleveland, Ohio, and the Division of Medical Sciences of the National Museum of American History of the Smithsonian Institution, to mention some of the largest museums of medical objects, have most of their holdings recorded on catalogue cards filed on the museum's premises. Much of the catalogue information is nontechnical and needs to be supplemented with study of the literature, as well as the objects themselves. Published catalogues of parts of these collections and others are beginning to emerge, including those on ceramic pharmaceutical and therapeutic objects, mentioned earlier, diagnostic instruments, hearing aids, bloodletting equipment, and surgical tools.[78]

A well-illustrated book on medical instruments manufactured from the Renaissance period up to 1870 recently was published by Elisabeth Bennion of Simon Kaye, Ltd., a London antique dealer. Although the book is not a catalogue in the usual sense, Mrs. Bennion's book contains clear black and white photographs and color plates of a range of medical, pharmaceutical, dental, surgical, and veterinary instruments, as well as a listing of instrument makers based on the research of Raymond Russell and her own searches through British museums and town directories. A number of little-known museums were the sources of a number of the instruments illustrated in this text, which introduces these items to the medical collector.[79]

The collections that have garnered the most interest from physicians in the past because of their value as teaching aids were the anatomic and pathologic specimen collections stored in hospital and medical school museums. Specimens of healthy and diseased organs are essential in teaching the medical student to recognize the signs and effects of disease and the variations among organs at different ages, in all races, and in both sexes. Because of their direct relevance to the medical curriculum, catalogues and lists of specimens were prepared. These catalogues may not have been published and usually lack illustrations. They must be read by those familiar with anatomic terms, names of diseases, and surgical procedures. Catalogues of this type have long been appreciated by the medical profession. A reviewer of the St. George's Hospital Pathological Museum Catalogue in 1882 described the intellectual demands catalogues of this type made on their readers: "Catalogues in general, like dictionaries, are not regarded as interesting reading, and this criticism is just in most cases. They are devoid of plot of the time-honoured novel,

and the subject changes too frequently for a sustained interest."[80] However, another reviewer added: "Without a good descriptive catalogue a museum is of very little use; with one, it becomes an important means of study and instruction, more so, indeed, than is usually recognized. Any one who has attended a museum class at one of the London medical schools can appreciate the amount of practical information in medicine and surgery which can in this way be imparted."[81]

The first major United States catalogue of anatomic specimens was prepared under the direction of the Surgeon General Barnes in 1866-1867. His catalogue of the United States Army Medical Museum, presently located in Washington, D.C., contains a listing of 961 specimens. Three-fourths of the catalogue was devoted to surgical specimens and the remainder of the text to physiologic and pathologic anatomy specimens and photomicrography apparatus. The catalogue was described in 1867 as "something more than a catalogue, since the numbered specimens and name of contributor is invariably accompanied by a succinct description and history, calculated to satisfy any reasonable amount of curiosity regarding results. It can't be too highly appreciated."[82]

Anatomic and pathologic specimens were augmented and in some cases replaced by models of these body parts, thus introducing a form of technology to this aspect of medical science. Preserved specimens of human and animal organs possessed obvious limitations for students of anatomy, who wished to handle the specimens repeatedly. Modelers were encouraged to produce copies of body parts from wax, plaster, wood, papier-mâché, and other substantial materials. These models served as supplements to and replacements for preserved anatomic specimens.

Among the earliest types valued by modern physicians and surgeons for teaching purposes were the artistically appealing and anatomically authentic wax models.[83] Major collections of magnificent wax models were made by such talented European modelers as the eighteenth-century Italians Abate Gaetano, Guilio Zumbo, and Luigi Calamai, and the Frenchman Guillaume Desnoues.[84] An important project currently underway is a catalogue of the large ensemble of waxes of human anatomy, pathology, and comparative anatomy exhibited in the Specola Museum in Florence, Italy, some of which were prepared by Zumbo.[85] Calamai and the Italian, Felice Fontana, prepared the bulk of the collection consisting of 1,500 anatomic waxes, which originally were exhibited in the Florentine Museum that opened in 1775. At one time, the rich collection of Fontana models consisted of 2,800 specimens, which was the most illustrious anatomic collection of the eighteenth century.[86] Other good wax collections created in the eighteenth and nineteenth centuries are located at the Botany Institute of the University of Florence,[87] the Anatomical Institute of Bologna, and the Josephinium of Vienna, of which a catalogue appeared in 1965.[88] Fontana and Mascagni were commissioned by the Emporer Joseph II of Austria to provide the wax models for his intended Military Academy, which is now the Vienna Institute of Medicine.[89] Guy's Hospital in London possesses magnificently crafted waxes created by the talented Joseph Towne between 1826 and 1879. He produced more than ten thousand anatomic-pathologic models of all types in natural colors and to full scale.[90] The Hospital of St. Louis in Paris possessed more than 2,000 models made by Louis Baretta (d. 1894) in the same period.[91] Interesting wax specimens are preserved in the Wellcome Museum of the History of Medicine, which contains a series of half-sized models of waxes of the type held by the Specola in full size.[92] The Museum of American History possesses five wax embryologic views mounted in wooden panels, purchased in 1973, whose provenance is unknown. Collections of wax models of skin diseases remain and are recorded by Haviland and Parrish in their well-documented article on the subject published in 1970.[93]

Collections of anatomic models constructed out of other substances are scattered among several medical museums. These items testify to the great technological ingenuity of the nineteenth-century artisan. A catalogue of these objects is highly desirable because of the extensive teaching role these models played in medical schools, colleges, and secondary schools.

The era of using models to teach anatomy and physiology to the layman as well as to medical students blossomed when papier-mâché models became popular after being introduced in 1825 by the French physician, Louis Thomas Jerome Auzoux of Paris. Models made of wood and other materials, of course, had already been constructed, but none of these were satisfactory from the standpoint of accurate detail, color, and ability to be repeatedly manipulated by students.[94] As a medical student, Auzoux, who was frustrated by his inability to acquire sufficient anatomic specimens or to study them for long enough periods, experimented with various substances and techniques before he was able to produce models closely resembling actual human and animal bones, muscles, blood vessels, and other structures.[95] By adding clay to a basic papier-mâché mixture, he discovered how to create a very hard surface on a light-weight model, which could be easily shaped and painted with appropriate colors. The Auzoux models became self-teaching aids when numbers and letters were applied to each anatomic part, which were referenced to a key provided with each model. Printed arrows applied to the models indicated the order of assembling and disassembling the parts of the model, and hooks were fastened to the pieces to hold them together. Special models with parts made identifiable by touch were among the innovations Auzoux produced in response to requests to teach anatomy to special students such as those without vision.

Cheaper models made of plaster of Paris and other synthetic materials were introduced by the mid-nineteenth century by manufacturers in Europe and the United States. None of these models were equal to the Auzoux models in the accuracy of detail they displayed, but some were acceptable to teachers who only expected to teach the rudiments of body structure. As illustrations in textbooks improved through color printing and the use of overlays, models became less important in the classroom.[96]

Those aspiring to become medical specialists required enlarged and life-sized models of the body's structures they would be expected to examine and treat in their patients. Models for teaching medical specialists about the parts of the body of interest to them were incorporated into the medical school curriculum. Affording familiarity and dexterity in manipulating the hands and instruments with the model before meeting a patient was the goal of instruction by models. Most of those parts least accessible for reasons of modesty or lack of cooperation by patients were especially necessary. This is particularly well documented in the use of obstetrical models. Those made of chamois and soft leather were used to teach the student "to repair cervical lacerations, curette and pack the cavity."[97] Metal pelvic models, which could be manipulated to show deformities as well as normal positions, aided the lecturer in midwifery and obstetrics. Prof. J. Clifton Edgar of New York emphasized that "the rachitic pelvis, injuries to the pelvic floor, the relation of the uterus to surrounding parts are far better understood from casts and paper reproductions than from charts, however well executed. The models are particularly useful in the training of nurses. A further advantage in their use is the fact that they may be kept obstetrically clean and may be used at the bedside or in the obstetrical clinic."[98] Instrument manufacturers' catalogues of the late nineteenth and twentieth centuries provide illustrations of medical teaching models including the eyes, ears, head, and internal organs available to the medical professions.

Objects placed on display provide a visual catalogue for those able to visit the exhibit. The viewer usually sees the most significant items in a medical collection. Those who take the time to study an exhibit learn the basic information that might appear in an exhibit catalogue, even if the catalogue of the exhibit was not prepared for publication. It is difficult to display the richness and variety of medical collections today because available display space is usually much less than ten thousand square feet, which is the area provided in the Museum of American History of the Smithsonian Institution for display of pharmaceutical, dental, surgical, and medical objects. The Smithsonian Museum is able to exhibit about 5 percent of its collections. Approximately 50 percent of the Smithsonian medical object reserve collection is of equal significance to those objects placed on exhibition. One exceptional medical exhibition is provided by the Wellcome Historical Medical Museum in the Wellcome Building in London. The exhibit traces the development of medical objects from antiquity to the twentieth century in a variety of cultural settings. Temporary exhibits and those designed for special anniversaries, meetings, and conventions present opportunities to rotate new objects onto view, but the design, script writing, and production costs limit the frequency with which these featured exhibits can be mounted and, therefore, brought to public attention. Catalogues of the special exhibits presented by the Wellcome contain many treasures including rare books and objects.[99] However, exhibits do not provide the forum for a full understanding of a medical instrument collection.

Catalogues, guides, and articles supplement exhibits and sometimes discuss items remaining in storage. Typical medical museum guides include those of the Copenhagen, Rome, Semmelweis Medical Historical Museum and Library and Archives of Budapest, and Smithsonian museums.[100] The most comprehensive dental museum catalogue is the *Catalogue of the Menzies Campbell Collection of Dental Instruments, Pictures, Appliances, Ornaments, etc.* compiled by J. Menzies Campbell in 1966. *Triumph Over Disability* is an essay and exhibition catalogue tracing the history of American rehabilitation medicine and providing illustrations of the objects on display in an exhibit in the National Museum of American History. Historical photographs showing some of the devises in use supplement the actual objects on view. The catalogue was published in conjunction with the special exhibit of the same title, produced in 1973 to inaugurate the fiftieth year of the American Congress of Rehabilitation Medicine. The topical organization of the exhibit and catalogue was undertaken to portray the many dimensions of the hardware, procedures, and types of people served by this most socially oriented branch of medical practice.[101] If a catalogue or guide to an exhibit is not available, lists of items on exhibition, copies of exhibit scripts, and photographs of cases and objects that were displayed are usually on file in museums and remain the only documented source of information on an exhibit no longer on view. The time and expense required to publish exhibition catalogues often preclude their production, which is a major loss to historians and professionals, as well as numerous curious spectators.

OTHER LITERATURE:

The ability to see the consequences of relating the technological concerns of medicine to wider issues, both within and outside medicine generated an additional literature. The issues raised have been brought to public focus recently by the moral and economic discussions raised as a consequence of the spectacular achievements of modern medical technology including heart transplantation, installation of artificial kidneys, effective contraceptives, abortions, and the testing of the fetus for genetic defects. Stanley Reiser has discussed, from an historical viewpoint, some of the issues raised by nineteenth- and twentieth-century medical technology, which has challenged the use of medical instruments. He stresses those aspects of the debate opposing the use of medical instruments. In another publication growing out of a Harvard symposium on recent technologically based medical practices and the questions these procedures have elicited, it is related that almost every technological advance in any industry, institution, or area affects medical practice to some degree.[102] Victor Seidel, a contributor to this symposium, concluded that the greatest impact of technology on medicine in reaching its goals through the use of mechanical methods was to amplify problems that might have remained hidden except for the qualities of these techniques and devices to magnify the dimensions of the physiological, emotional, and social problems accompanying disease. He cites the confusion between cause and effect that sometimes emerges when technology is applied to medicine. Technology is blamed for creating the problem, rather than serving as a springboard for identifying and exploring the underlying causes of an issue that is due to deeper societal forces. Ethical dilemmas change in quantity and quality along with the change in medical technology for both the physician and the patient.[103] These topics, while requiring immediate response, deserve a full historical assessment of their rise and the social, economic, and technological positions to which they led. Such topics might be explored in a social history of medical technology, which would require access to data on the responses of patients as well as physicians to different medical instruments, devices, and procedures.

Another segment of the medical literature that relates to technology is that devoted to the implications of medical instruments in producing harm to the patient. The harm produced by medical instruments had to be shared by medical instrument manufacturers and physicians. Patients are most aware of the medical errors or accidents resulting from the application of medical and surgical instruments, since the evidence for the accident is less ambiguous than if it had resulted from misdiagnosis or the improper dose of a drug. The function and placement of instruments can be more accurately understood and attested to by medical experts than can unaided treatments, and therefore, the technique and skill of the physician in applying an instrument can be more easily assessed by all concerned (see figure 2.8).

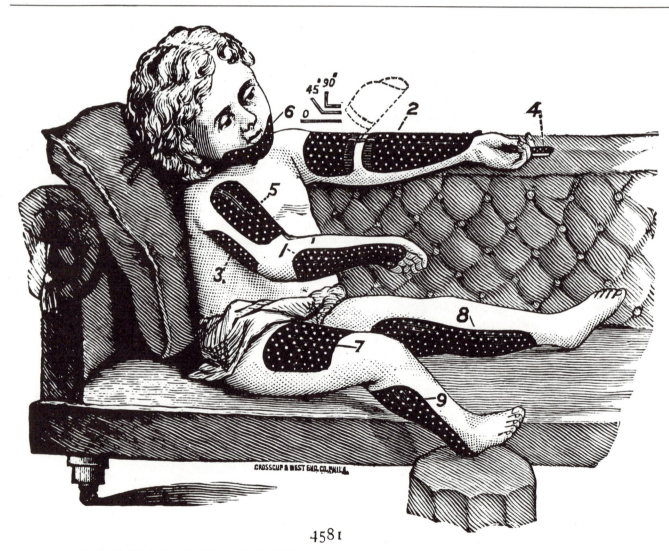

Figure 2.8. Illustration of splints applied in 1893 to various body sites and sold by A. S. Aloe Co. *SI Photo from 1893 catalogue.*

Accidents involving surgical instruments and diagnostic procedures with instruments are discussed in the medical literature and provide a guide to the nature of some of the problems and their solutions. A few documented instances are presented here, but a volume on the causes and consequences of technologically related incidents might well be prepared. One conclusion that is likely to be demonstrated is that problems related to medical instrumentation are repetitive, even though the construction and functions of instruments have changed. The displacement, testing, repair, and removal of living tissues with instruments made up of substances such as wood, metal, rubber, plastic, and others have presented continued challenges to the medical instrument designer and the physician.

Among the accident accounts published in the nineteenth century, some ascribe the blame to defective or poorly constructed implements and others to improper techniques in their use. In one incident recorded in 1891, the shaft of a lithotrite was broken off when placed inside the bladder. Another report concerned the perforation of the uterus by an implement used to inspect and apply medication to it.[104] A common accident before the introduction of diphtheria vaccine cured many victims of this disease was the perforation of the trachea by the tube introduced into the throat of a child with diphtheria to clear out the breathing passage. Perforation of other internal organs with a tube introduced for the purpose of observing their tissues has occurred in the esophagus, stomach, intestines, and ear, among others. One of the most dangerous tubes to insert was the laparoscope, which was used to drain fluid from the abdomen and chest. Injection of fluids and drugs with syringes always presented the danger of accidental introduction of air into the blood vessels. When an instrument was constructed of different substances or modified in design, the physician or surgeon had to respond by adjusting his techniques, but he may not always have been successful. Subtle changes in materials and workmanship sometimes deceived the unsuspecting surgeon and contributed to the bending, twisting, and breaking of an instrument at points where the stress was too great because of faulty engineering or the application of poor technique or both.

The most difficult and yet fairly common problem faced by the nineteenth- and twentieth-century surgeon was one created by leaving an instrument or accessory in the patient's body after an operation. Negebauer of Warsaw in 1900 published an account of 101 instances in which a foreign body was left in the patient who had undergone an operation. In thirty-eight of these patients, the object was found during the postmortem examination. The most frequently misplaced object was the sponge.[105] Patient acceptance of this type of accident and the surgeons' chagrined view of a problem they were responsible for extend back to the time when instruments were first introduced into the body. The quality of the instrument was among the first objectives of investigations of all accidents. A study of the legal decisions related to accidents in which medical and surgical instruments played a part would reveal the extent of society's awareness of the practitioners' responsibilities to their patients and the patients' acceptance of the medical treatment they received involving the use of medical instruments.

3

COLLECTIONS OF MEDICAL INSTRUMENTS

The raw material used in studying the history of medical technology consists of printed descriptions and the instruments themselves that have survived. This chapter concerns the instruments available for study in museums and private collections and the development of major medical instrument collections.

Artisans and craftsmen who employed instruments used distinctive terms for these implements. A tool usually signified a useful and necessary thing. Instrument is the word that was applied by the early surgeons to their tools, since the word implied an instructional role, in addition to its specific connotation as an extension of the hand and arm used to remove foreign objects and diseased body tissues.[1] Among surgical instruments were the scalpel, knife, saw, trephine, and others that the surgeon used to move and remove tissues and to make adjustments in diseased parts (see figure 3.1).

In addition to surgical instruments in the last two centuries, medical instruments have grown to include apparatus, hardware, machines, tools, utensils, devices, aids, and artificial body parts (see figure 3.2). Some of these items were made in earlier periods, such as rudimentary artificial limbs, but these items were rare and often were designated surgical accessories. A drug is not usually defined as a medical instrument, although instruments may be applied with drugs or be essential to introduce drugs into the body. The efficacy or use of an instrument may also depend on a drug. Chemicals such as barium compounds, which are ingested to explore the digestive system through X-ray analysis, function in much the same way as a diagnostic instrument.

In a discussion of those instruments that have found their way into museums, exhibits, and private collections, the word *artifact*, described by the noted

American archeologist, Ivor Nöel-Hume, as "a three-dimensional addition to the pages of history,"[2] is appropriately applied. Artifact and object are basic terms, which delineate the central three-dimensional documents of the historian of medical instruments. Artifacts and objects supplement information contained in published and manuscript accounts and offer opportunities for the scholar to discover meanings not fully suggested or substantiated by the literature related to medical technology. Throughout this chapter, I will discuss all types of medical instruments, whether used for diagnostic or therapeutic purposes. Museums and private holders have tended to be eclectic in assembling medical instrument collections and were guided in selecting the objects to be saved not only by the perspective of the physician or surgeon who used them, but also by the collector's own aesthetic and collecting instincts.

HISTORY OF EARLY COLLECTIONS:

Collecting medical instruments and artifacts for the purpose of preserving them has been customary, albeit not systematic, since antiquity. Archeologists in the nineteenth century were among the earliest systematic collectors to search for and save artifacts of primitive and ancient cultures, which included medically related items of all types. In antiquity, some of the largest medical collections were formed in response to an early belief in the efficacy of supplicating and honoring the healing gods with carved stone replicas of the diseased body parts that had been healed. Patients who had been cured of diseases presented to the temple of Asclepius in Greece, in which their treatment was undertaken, likenesses of the organs or body parts in which their diseases were located. These replicas, known as votives, were dis-

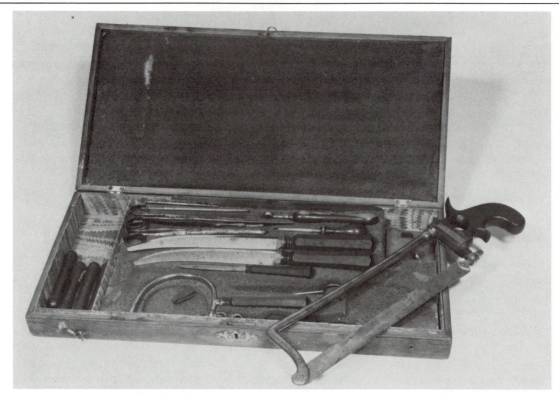

Figure 3.1. Revolutionary War surgical set of Dr. Charles McKnight. *NMAH No. 79.0264.01, SI Photo No. 79-10775.*

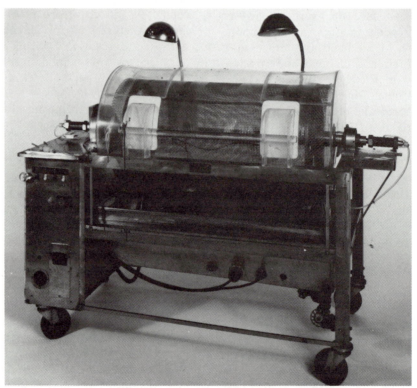

Figure 3.2. Kolff-Brigham kidney machine circa 1949. *NMAH No. M 3132, SI Photo No. 77-10382.*

played for future patients to see, and in hope that the individuals who placed them there would not be afflicted with the same diseases in the future. Many of these votives are preserved in the National Museum of Athens.[3] Medical artifacts were included among the broader collections of natural and scientific objects made in antiquity. In the museum at Alexandria, formed by Ptolemy in the third century B.C., statues, votive offerings, and surgical instruments were among the items collected for consultation by the scholars working in this research institute.[4]

In a unique study, "The Evolution of Science Museums," Silvio Bedini has traced the history of science collections "to the great private libraries and cabinets of curiosities of Renaissance princes, scholars and wealthy amateurs. In fact, some of the scientific memorabilia included in the Renaissance cabinets have survived through the centuries to form the nucleus around which some of the modern science museums have grown."[5] Some medical items were included in the cabinets of curiosities, but the most prized health and medically related objects to be collected up to the Renaissance were those believed to possess magical and supernatural powers controlling life and health. Varying among different cultures in their application, these objects were thought to heal, extend life, increase fertility, and extend sexual power.[6] Among the actual instruments applied by a physician or surgeon that have been discovered are the ancient bronze surgical instruments buried at Pompei and other European sites, which remained underground until archeologists began to excavate them in the nineteenth century or they were accidentally unearthed in the course of another excavation project. The best preserved of these objects provide the most reliable examples of the earliest surgical instruments, which often were incompletely described in the ancient literature.

The durability and attractiveness of ancient tools have prompted collectors to seek them out and preserve them. Their simple and functional design contrasts with the detailed workmanship, tooling, and design displayed in instruments used by Renaissance surgeons, bone setters, bloodletters, midwives, dentists, and other healers, making these objects also valuable to collectors, especially those interested in the development of craftsmanship as applied to science and medicine. Scholars, interested in the tools as well as the surgical texts in which they were illustrated and described, urged that surgical instruments be added to natural curiosity collections, containing rocks, fossils, minerals, plants, anatomic specimens,

and stuffed animals.[7] Occasionally, the tools used to dissect and preserve the biological specimens were included in these collections. Medical and surgical instruments were also collected as part of the "artificial curiosities"[8] representing the technological craftsmanship of a period. The skilled workers who produced these implements were organized into guilds in European countries. As members of a craft society, they kept specimens of their labor on display to mark the history of their craft and to inspire apprentices.

Science museums holding instruments that had been used to make observations and perform experiments were formed in the seventeenth century, primarily in England, Germany, and Italy. These institutions grew out of the general scholarly movement to study all aspects of nature. The term *museum*, while already applied to centers of research with collections in ancient Greece, began to be generally used in the late sixteenth century. Bedini explains that the word *museum* "was first revived to describe the great Medici collection in Florence which combined art objects and natural and artificial curiosities with one of the earliest collections related to the physical sciences and technology."[9] In museums, scientific collections appear to be more extensive and better preserved then medical instruments, although perhaps as many or more medical instruments and devices have survived because more medical instruments were produced to be used by a profession with more practitioners.

Another reason for the survival of Medieval and Renaissance medical objects is the apothecary shop. A large catalogue of the Museum of Francis Calcari, published in 1622, reveals the similarities between the seventeenth-century public museum and the apothecary shop in which animal, vegetable, and mineral sources of all types were displayed.[10] Apothecary shops as display centers were preserved and even restored as early as the seventeenth century, illustrated in the instance of a Dresden shop and laboratory.[11]

Bedini has listed over fifty major science collections in the Western world, brought together through the nineteenth century, some of which are still extant.[12] Most of the significant medical object collections made over the last three centuries were gathered without regard to specific and rationalized collecting policies. The preferences of the physician and surgeon collector and the vagaries of antique dealers and others, hoping to make a profit by trading in old objects, shaped many medical collections. Some eighteenth- and nineteenth-century medical collections were dispersed in the twentieth century and became the nuclei of presently existing and admired collections. Occasionally, important medical instruments were passed down to successive generations, especially in families that spawned medical practitioners in each generation. In other instances, the tools and inventions of notable physicians and surgeons have been preserved by the institutions, including hospitals, medical schools, and medical societies, with which they had been associated or to which these items were donated after their deaths. Some of these small collections formed the display motifs of private medical museums and were permanently exhibited as a monument to the advance of medicine and its distinguished medical leaders.

In the nineteenth century, medical instruments also were stored in closets, basements, and attics of hospitals, doctors' offices, and private homes and often regarded as evidence of the failures or discredited and obsolete practices of earlier physicians and surgeons. E. Andrews of Mercy Hospital, who delivered a poignant lecture entitled "Fossil Trusses," described the sources and value of these old medical devices to his practitioner colleagues in 1885.

In every hospital there is apt to be some dark closet which becomes by degrees a sort of museum of rejected apparatus. It slowly grows to a small mountain of old instrumental fossils, full of all sorts of broken and discarded trusses, aborted splints, deceased galvanic batteries whose dry cells no longer throb, and patent wooden legs, whose inventors died in poverty because the legs would not run under the patients, nor the patients run after the legs.

My learned friend, Prof. D. R. V. Cobwebs, has been excavating with great enthusiasm in our mountain. He declares that these fossils are arranged in regular decennial strata, with the ideas expanded horizontally, and that by the aid of his wonderful new science of comparative instrumentology he can tell the age of every specimen, from the primeval implements of Brainard up to the quaternary appliances of Andrews, Hollister and Dudley. He goes still further and maintains that there is evolution here, that our mountain has been developed by a kind of unnatural selection and the survival of the unfittest, so that in its deposits he can find relics of the pet hobbies and cranky experiments of all the surgeons within a hundred miles of this place. . . . Our Prof. Cobwebs claims that from a few pads of old fossil trusses, with here a screw and there a buckle, he can depict the progress of past surgical thought as well as Cuvier did—or didn't—restore the Paleotherium.[13]

Andrews reviewed the major forms of trusses and ended his talk by providing five principles for selecting an effective truss to support a hernia. His discourse on the collection and significance of fracture, rupture, and amputation devices could be applied to a variety of other instruments and appliances.

Medical libraries were, and continue to be, likely to acquire medical instruments and objects. Not all librarians were enthusiastic about medical objects or equipped to supervise them, either when kept in storage or put on display. One exception was W. B. McDaniel, who as librarian of the College of Physicians Library of Philadelphia, found developing a medical museum as an integral part of the library to be a lifelong process. He emphasized that the objects most treasured in a library-centered medical collection were those that appealed to the human instincts, such as memorabilia and personal items that belonged to noted physicians or historic patients and may not have possessed scientific or technological significance.[14] Today, medical instruments are interspersed in public and private collections in many countries, representing the medical specialties and forms of medical research and practice of all periods. The American Museums' Association Guide to Museums or Museum Directory has listed some of the medical museums in the United States open to the public since 1965. The 1977 edition lists forty-five museums under the heading "Medical, Dental, Health, Pharmacology, Apothecary and Psychiatry Museums." The Smithsonian Institution's medical exhibit is not listed in this directory nor are other museums that only permit professionals to view their exhibits. Medical museums in the United States that restrict their visitors or display their objects on an irregular schedule are not found in any guide. In seeking public instrument collections, it is useful to contact the medical society or medical library of the state, city, region, or country to be visited.

INTERNATIONAL FAIRS AND EXHIBITIONS:

Nineteenth-century medical technology exhibitions introduced to a wide spectrum of the public some of the technology formerly only known to the medical community. The earliest exhibitions displaying medical instruments and devices appeared in large cities for a short period, often during a medical convention, and were not generally opened to the public. More popular because they welcomed all visitors and were often part of a broad industrial exhibition were health or hygiene exhibitions, which featured public health-preserving systems, including drainage, sewerage, water supply, and other technology. These exhibitions attracted large audiences in London, Paris, Vienna, and a number of German and American cities during the last half of the nineteenth century. Most large exhibitions were modeled on the famous 1851 International Exhibition and the Fisheries Exhibition of 1883, both of which were held in London.[15] Only in the last quarter of the nineteenth century were a sizable number of medically related items displayed in any international exhibition (see figure 3.3). In the 1851 exhibition, there were only three dozen surgical instruments and a few medical items on display, which were grouped into class ten under the heading "Philosophical, Musical, Horological and Surgical Instruments."[16] However, the overall impact of the 1851 exhibition on the formation of museums was tremendous. It spawned six museums, including the Victoria and Albert, nine teaching institutions, and other communal meeting places like the Royal Albert Hall in London.[17] The British Parliament also was prompted to encourage the foundation of museums of Arts and Sciences in towns with populations greater than ten thousand people, by permitting the town councils to levy a small tax on each resident to pay for these museums.[18]

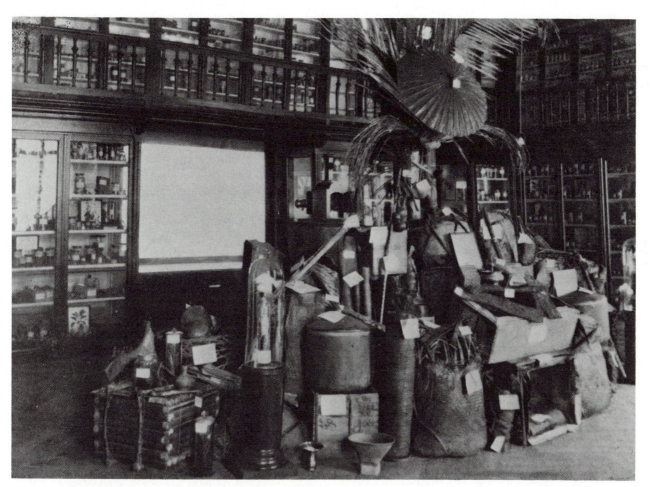

Figure 3.3 Crude drugs on exhibit circa 1880 at the Pharmacy Institute in Bern, Switzerland. *American Pharmaceutical Association Collections. SI Photo No. 78-18713.*

Commercial trade fairs provided the earliest setting for exhibitions of manufactured and crafted items. Fairs in market places had appeared as early as the fifteenth century, such as the "messe" held in Leipzig in 1497[19] and others in Frankfurt am Main and Lyons. The earliest industrial exhibition appears to have been sponsored by the British Society of Arts in April 1761. The society placed on display all machines or models of machines that had been awarded a prize in past competitions. National fairs commenced on the continent after the French Revolution, when the French mounted an exposition in 1798, to celebrate the freedom of trades and professions.

In the United States, the first large medical exhibition was the medical and sanitary exhibit sponsored by the federal government at the 1876 Centennial held in Philadelphia. The medical department of the army under Assistant Surgeon General J. J. Woodward erected a model of a military hospital and scale models of five hospital railroad cars employed during the Civil War.

Arranged in cases erected around the wall [were] numerous pathological specimens from the Army Medical Museum, and some beautiful microphotographs, made by Dr. Woodward [which adorned] the window panes. The other rooms of the hospital were devoted to the exhibition of medicines, medical and chemical stores, and surgical instruments, medical books, blanks, chemical apparatus, mess furniture and utensils, and kitchen utensils, which are issued to medical officers on requisition. In the second story [were] exhibited artificial limbs, such as [were] issued gratuitously to those who lost their limbs in the service, litters and stretchers, medical panniers, army medical chests, etc. In the office [were] also to be seen specimen copies of the various valuable publications . . . [issued] from the Surgeon General's Office.[20]

The medical technology of foreign nations also was represented. Extensive reports of these exhibits appeared in the medical journals in 1876 and 1877. Photographs of the exhibits were made.[21] Later, exhibitions in the United States, such as the Columbian Exposition in Chicago in 1893, emphasized the public health-related appliances, techniques and methods developed to improve sanitation in the home, school, factory, and streets. Models of sanitary dwellings, schools, public lavatories, and crematories were displayed.[22]

Authors of exposition catalogues and guides published in Europe expressed the hope that attractive fairs would lead to the formation of permanent medical museums and exhibitions of the most important objects, which had been placed on temporary display.

G. E. Mergier in commenting on the medically related displays in the World Exposition held in Paris in 1889 opined that this exposition should become the basis of a medical science museum similar to the museum of the Conservatory of Arts and Measures in Paris.[23] Mergier's wish was not fulfilled. Dr. Ganther had similar aspirations for the formation of a biological museum in London. He believed that the art museum that grew out of the South Kensington Exhibition had produced an English population that rivaled, and perhaps, even surpassed the French in art appreciation; he expected the same educational goals would be reached in the biological and medical sciences if a large museum could be erected in England. He also expected the English to surpass the Germans in their scientific acumen[24] with the resources of the national science museum. A number of health museums and science museums with health displays have appeared in the twentieth century in Europe and the United States. These will not be discussed here, but the reader is referred to the publications of Bruno Gebhard, one of the outstanding architects of the modern health museum.[25]

MEDICAL SOCIETY EXHIBITIONS:

Medical societies proudly evolved the practice of exhibiting examples of their distinguished members' achievements. These exhibits contained mostly anatomic-pathologic specimens carefully prepared and mounted to show an unusual disease and the exquisite dissecting and preserving talents of the preparator. The Pathological Society of London, founded in 1846, adopted as its first objective for holding meetings, to present specimens, drawings, models, and casts for its members' examination.[26] Pathologic specimens also were the first objects exhibited at medical society conferences. The attention these exhibits garnered paved the way for the exhibition of books, charts, instruments, appliances, and devices at professional medical meetings. The medical exhibit customarily lasted for the length of the meetings—one to several days—which were held once or occasionally twice a year, except for those of local societies, which were held regularly once every month or so.

BRITISH MEDICAL ASSOCIATION:

The annual medical exhibit with the most distinguished heritage was sponsored by the British Medical Association. Named the Annual Museum, the first exhibition was mounted in 1868 in conjunction with the thirty-sixth annual meeting of the association in Oxford. The first exhibit was hurriedly organized in response to Jonathan Hutchinson's proposal published in the *British Medical Journal* several months before the annual meeting. Hutchinson suggested that all new inventions of instruments, mechanical apparatus, casts, wax models, photographs, drawings, and pathologic specimens of unusual interest or rarity be included in the exhibit.[27] He wanted the exhibit to be open throughout the meeting and a catalogue of the objects on display to be prepared. The *BMJ* strongly supported this proposal.

Hutchinson envisioned that "should the plan be successful, I feel sure that a busy man might learn more in such a museum in an hour than he could by far longer and much more wearisome attendance in the section rooms. Here he would find the cream of the year's progress, and with perfect liberty to select what interested him. . . ."[28] One advantage to the professional would be the opportunity to see specimens prepared in provincial hospitals that warranted wide publicity for their unusual teaching value. Hutchinson commented on the tremendous impact of exposing selected specimens to the profession at the Annual Museum. He added: "If Dr. Addison could have placed under the investigation of the whole profession, the drawings, specimens, etc. by which his great discovery [adrenal disease] was illustrated, how much more readily would it have gained general attention, and how many misconceptions would have been avoided."[29]

The items were exhibited at Oxford in the lecture room of the University Museum and were organized in four groups: (1) pathologic drawings, preparations, wax models, and similar items; (2) new instruments and appliances in medicine and surgery; (3) drugs and articles of medical diet; and (4) new English and foreign medical works.[30] Hutchinson's own pathologic drawings were a highlight of the exhibit. The first Annual Museum was a success, although the space provided for it was not adequate, it was located too far from the general sessions, and of course, with so little time to prepare it, a catalogue could not be published. In addition to overcoming these impediments to a successful exhibit, Hutchinson suggested that one or two museum-related lectures, perhaps given by the exhibitors, be incorporated into the next Annual Museum program.[31]

The second Annual Museum at Leeds was also placed too far away from the general sessions, but a list of the items displayed was included with the program of the sessions.[32] At the third meeting in Newcastle in 1870, the items exhibited fell into seven categories: (1) new instruments and appliances in medi-

cine, surgery, and midwifery; (2) new drugs and preparations; (3) new books in English and foreign languages; (4) pathologic, physiologic, anatomic, and microscopic specimens; (5) models of new instruments relating to public health; and (7) new preparations of foods and other items.[33] The exhibition was disappointing, for attendance was poor. The museum's location, away from the general sessions, appeared to be the major cause for the small number of visitors.[34] This problem continued with later exhibits until an exhibit space closer to the sessions was obtained. However, the Annual Museum continued to be mounted and to gain sponsors among medical instrument manufacturers.

The first catalogue of an Annual Museum was prepared by Warren Tay for the sixth Annual Museum (1874) in London, held at King's College. The catalogue was sold for six pence.[35] The following year the catalogue listed 556 instruments exhibited in Edinburgh.[36] Two thousand copies of the catalogue were distributed to BMA members at the Manchester Meeting in 1902.[37] Exhibitors were charged for any advertisements that they placed in the catalogue to defray the cost of mounting their exhibits.

The Annual Museum was organized each year by a local arrangements committee with an honorary secretary appointed for each section. The exhibit settled into a pattern of four sections for a period (1) food and drugs; (2) recent books, instruments, appliances, ambulances, and supplies in medicine, surgery, and electricity; (3) anatomic and pathologic specimens, drawings, microscopic and macroscopic preparations; and (4) hygiene and sanitary appliances, including equipment of houses, public institutions, and hospitals, improvement in drainage, water supply, ventilation, illumination, and clothing. Five sections were established when the anatomic and physiologic specimens were separated from the pathologic specimens in 1888. Preferred items were those not previously exhibited and those displaying innovative qualities. By the turn of the century, a separate section was added for exhibiting carriages, automobiles, and ambulances.[38] In 1890, increasing costs forced a tax to be placed on exhibitors who were not members of the association. They were charged for the space they occupied at the rate of two shillings per square foot of table space, and six pence per square foot of floor space. Four thousand square feet of floor space was provided for exhibits in 1881 at the sixteenth Annual Museum.

In 1901 the building provided for the exhibit in Cheltenham was newly renovated, with good ventilation and lighting.[39] In 1902, at the meeting in Manchester, gas and electricity were offered to exhibitors who requested them. Medical electric devices and appliances were featured in this museum.[40] Local museums and collectors provided each Annual Museum with distinctive display opportunities.

Arnold and Sons, Allen and Hanburys, Krohne and Seseman, Schall, Salt and Son, Harvey and Reynolds, and a variety of drug manufacturers were among the steady and outstanding producers of medical equipment and supplies exhibiting their products at the Annual Museum into the twentieth century.

AMERICAN MEDICAL ASSOCIATION:

A review of the growth of the American Medical Association's Annual Meeting exhibit program shows the general pattern of increasing sophistication in exhibits, beginning at the turn of the twentieth century. In the last quarter of the nineteenth century, state medical societies, such as the New Jersey Medical Society, occasionally sponsored health exhibits at state fairs.[41] The editor of *JAMA* published a short notice in 1892, which originally appeared in the *Medical Review* of St. Louis, on the increasing value of an annual exhibit that would include pathologic specimens, instruments, appliances, and other novel and interesting items produced during the preceding year.[42] Echoing the comments of Hutchinson, who had supported the idea of annual museums a few decades earlier, the editor envisioned that the competition spurred by those attempting to put on the best exhibit would benefit the entire medical profession. "It is only for the Association to determine that it will have such a museum, and much of the work is done,"[43] claimed the editor of the *JAMA*. Earlier notices to exhibitors were published in the *JAMA* requesting cooperation to organize the exhibit.[44]

Bruno Gebhard has summarized the crucial stages in the evolution of the temporary American medical exhibit, which first appeared in 1899 when a small assortment of pathologic specimens were exhibited in Columbus, Ohio. From this modest beginning, medical exhibits grew to include pathologic specimens, scientific apparatus, medical instruments, books, and other literature. These items continue to be displayed during the annual AMA convention and at some of the individual meetings of its constituent specialty sections. Gebhard's summary of the development of these exhibitions parallels the historical sketch provided by Thomas G. Hull in his chapter "Bureau of Exhibits" in Morris Fishbein's *A History of the American Medical Association 1847 to 1949.*[45]

Hull described the first exhibit "in 1899, which members of the Indiana State Medical Society presented at their annual meeting that included a large exhibit of pathological specimens. Pathology had but recently come into its own as a specialty of medicine and the exhibit created great interest. It was decided to show it at the next meeting of the American Medical Association held the following week in Columbus, Ohio. Much favorable comment resulted."[46] The success of the pathologic exhibit was expressed in these contemporary remarks: "the most instructive feature of the meeting" and "worth more than a thousand papers."[47] In conjunction with these exhibits as a place to mount objects received for the temporary exhibits, it was proposed to build a medical museum as "a lasting monument to the work of the Association." The plan for this museum never materialized.[48]

Beginning in 1908, medals were awarded for the best annual exhibits, a practice that has continued ever since. All winners of exhibition medals up to 1946 are listed in Fishbein's history.[49] The exhibit categories established by 1916 included: (1) institution exhibits; (2) research exhibits; (3) exhibits relating to methods of laboratory diagnosis; (4) public health exhibits; (5) medical society exhibits; and (6) practical exhibits.[50]

The most successful annual exhibits were brought to the AMA headquarters in Chicago, a practice continued until 1934, when space could no longer be provided for this purpose.[51] The AMA began a concerted effort in 1930 to meet some of the demands for health exhibits in the areas of physiology, anatomy, medical economics, patent medicines, self-diagnosis, communicable diseases, nutrition, posture, and medical and hospital practice. Exhibits were prepared for state and county medical societies and other organizations requesting them. Among the international expositions for which the AMA provided health exhibits were the San Francisco Exhibition of 1915, Chicago 1933-1934, California Pacific International Exposition at San Diego in 1936, Texas Centennial Exposition at Dallas in 1936-1937, Great Lakes Exposition in Cleveland, Ohio in 1937, the Golden Gate International Exposition at San Francisco in 1939, and the New York World's Fair in 1939-1940.[52]

SPECIALTY ASSOCIATIONS:

Dental Association meetings also prompted some of its members to prepare exhibits (see figure 3.4). For the meeting of the National Dental Association in 1918, held in Chicago, a large exhibition was mounted containing the reconstructed offices, original manuscripts, instruments, and personal items of

Greene Vardiman Black, who had died in 1915. Black invented a number of instruments, including the first dental engine with a cord-driven foot pedal (1870), a bracket table, crown and bridge bench, and numerous hand tools.[53] Some of Black's equipment, displayed in a reduced version of his office, may be viewed in the National Museum of American History of the Smithsonian Institution.

Encouraged by the successful displays at British and American medical meetings, specialty medical groups in other countries also planned museums on a temporary or permanent basis. Among the lesser known of these endeavors is the museum established

to commemorate the thirtieth anniversary of the psychiatric clinic in St. Petersburg. A psychiatric museum was proposed to include

plans, photographs, models etc. of asylums for the insane; models of dress for the insane; work done by the insane; photographs of the insane at different periods of their disease; the apparatus used in examining the insane; skulls and brains of the insane; microscopical preparations; documents relating to the care of the insane. At the same time there will be established a neurological museum to contain normal brains of men and the lower animals, and microscopical preparations of the nerve tissues, preparations of pathological brains; instruments for weighing and methods

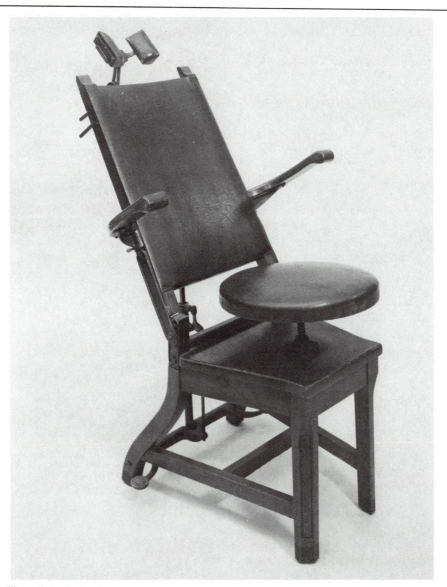

Figure 3.4. Nineteenth-century (1860) dental chair, one of the earliest to have an adjustable seat. American made, used aboard ship. Gift of Bethesda Naval Dental School. *NMAH No. 263973, SI Photo No. 72-10331.*

of preserving the brain; photographs and representations of pathological processes; the different forms of apparatus employed in treatment, plans and photographs of neurological institutions.[54]

An appeal to students in all nations to send in appropriate objects and to visit the museum appeared in the *Medical Record* of 1898. Exhibits with special interest for nurses appeared in the same year at the International Health Exposition in New York City. Examples of modern medical instruments and surgical appliances, together with their older counterparts, were displayed in an operating room setting at this exposition.[55]

SIGNIFICANT MODERN COLLECTIONS:

WELLCOME MUSEUM OF THE HISTORY OF MEDICINE

The largest and most important collection of medical instruments and artifacts was assembled by the pharmacist, Sir Henry Wellcome, who began to collect in the last decade of the nineteenth century. He collected everything, including graphics, books, paintings, trade catalogues, advertisements, sculpture, objects and instruments, that shed light on attitudes toward diseases and the professional and nonprofessional efforts to maintain and restore health.[56] The strength of Wellcome's collection is in its pharmaceutical jars and fixtures and drugs, as well as surgical implements and diagnostic instruments of the nineteenth century. Several well-illustrated catalogues of the ceramic and glass components of this collection have been published by John Crellin (see figure 3.5).[57] The most comprehensive array of military and civilian surgical implements, chests, and kits are found in the Wellcome collection. Almost every aspect of medical technology is represented in the collection, including models and replicas of the ancient bronze instruments found at Pompei and preserved in the National Museum in Naples. The most poorly represented objects in the Wellcome collection are dental artifacts and instruments. Nevertheless, London is host to the fine Smith-Turner dental museum, which is maintained by the British Dental Association in its headquarters and may have been a factor in Wellcome's decision to ignore dentistry in his own collecting forays. During the last decades, in an attempt to rationalize the collection and reduce its size, some of the ethnographic, military, and cultural objects have been given to museums that collect and display in these areas.[58]

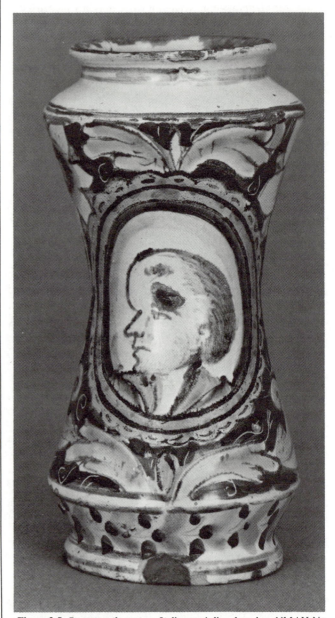

Figure 3.5. Seventeenth-century Italian majolica drug jar. *NMAH No. M-5763, SI Photo No. 61-794a*

Wellcome's pharmaceutical business provided the money for his omnivorous collecting and enabled him to purchase entire collections, such as the important one brought together in the nineteenth century by the French physician, Pierre Hamonic.[59] Purchased for over $5,000 in 1928 from Hamonic's son Nöel, the collection included a wealth of unique items including: from the fifteenth century, speculums; from the sixteenth century, an artificial hand and arm; from the seventeenth century, orthopedic devices, dental instruments, circumcision knives, and artificial eyes; from the eighteenth century, pewter syringes, trocars, midwifery forceps, medicine spoons, and tongue depressors; bloodletting equipment from the seventeenth through nineteenth centuries; several early microscopes; seventeenth- and eighteenth-century amputation, trepanning, lithotomy, and surgical sets; and a variety of Greek, Roman, and Japanese surgical instruments, some of which were excavated at Peronne in Somma, along the Tiber River, at Canea in Crete, in Syria, in Treves, Germany, in Ephesus in Asia Minor, and in Pereia, Greece.

At the suggestion of Sir William Osler, Sir Norman Moore, and Dr. J. F. Payne, a small fraction of the quarter of a million objects of the Wellcome collection was exhibited for the first time in 1913 to members of the International Congress of Medicine convening in London. This successful display of medical objects eventually led to the opening of the Wellcome Historical Medical Museum on Wigmore Street. After a period of being in storage during World War I, the collection was taken to another location on Euston Road. Halls of modern design were mounted in the 1960s.[60] There four museum galleries, with an approximate total of 17,000 sq. ft. of exhibit space, in which forty-one cases were mounted, in addition to associated workrooms, a lecture room, offices, and storage spaces, were used to display and maintain much of the collection.[61] In 1968, the museum and library was renamed the Wellcome Institute of the History of Medicine.[62]

A few museum leaders in the twentieth century realized that the medical museum had to be restructured to meet the changing needs of the twentieth-century medical student by including both the physiologic and pathologic specimens and the new tools of medicine in its collections. The most outstanding of these planners was S. H. Daukes, Director of the Wellcome Museum of Medical Science in London (not to be confused with the Wellcome Museum of the History of Medicine), who recognized the fact that the museum was flagging as a supplement to the medical school in presenting both the medical student and the practitioner with a "centre where he can view the subject as a whole and fit the various sections of the puzzle together." Daukes proposed that the museum "cease being a pathological collection and become a compendium of medical knowledge,"[63] which would educate the student and layman and provide material for the research specialist. The methods, appliances, and apparatus for obtaining physiologic and pathologic information together with the results they revealed were to be part of the revitalized museum collection and its display. The pathology museum was to be enlarged into a museum representing all phases of medical knowledge and application. It would display the technology used on the body as well as the body parts. Exhibiting the processes of gaining medical knowledge through the methods and materials used in laboratory experimentation offered opportunities for the medical museum to regain its function as a "workshop for scientific study."

Daukes emphasized the absolute need for strict organization within the museum, an approach stemming from his admiration for the Deutsches Museum of Science and Industry in Munich.[64] He arranged the pathologic sections of the museum on an etiologic basis—grouping together the diseases caused by similar types of agents. These exhibits were arranged according to the causes of diseases, including metazoa, protozoa, spirochaetes, bacteria, food deficiencies, metabolic dysfunctions, and unknown causes.[65] The Wellcome Museum of Medical Sciences remains a model of the type of museum planned and begun by Daukes and is a rich source of technical information to the physician who visits the Wellcome collections in London.

All the medical objects and instruments of the Wellcome Museum have been transferred to the Science Museum in London, where a curator and staff supervise, maintain, and exhibit selected items in medical history exhibits covering about 30,000 sq. ft. It is expected that a larger segment of the public will have an opportunity to view these objects along with the great variety of other technological and scientific objects displayed in this famous science museum. The separation of the objects and the medical books, which will remain in the Wellcome building, has been looked upon by some researchers with disfavor, but except for a few students, no great hardship is expected to result for those studying both the Wellcome object and book collections. If the instrument collection can be better housed, studied, and brought to the attention of more people, it seems that the decision to tranfer the medical objects to the Science Museum is wise. The medical collection will be joined to other historical technological collections, a policy comparable to the collecting policy of the National Museum of American History of the Smithsonian Institution.

SMITHSONIAN INSTITUTION:

The other major medical collection, which also sprang from a pharmacy base, is the Division of Medical Sciences of the National Museum of American History of the Smithsonian Institution. The section of Materia Medica was established in the United States National Museum of the Smithsonian Institution when the museum building was completed in 1881. The first items collected for the museum consisted of crude drugs exhibited in the 1876 Centennial Exhibition in Philadelphia,[66] other drugs and plants transferred from the Department of Agriculture, and those contributed by the pharmaceutical manufacturers, Parke, Davis & Co. of Detroit, Michigan; Wallace Brothers of Statesville, North Carolina; and Schieffelin & Co. of New York.[67] The first catalogue of the Smithsonian collection was prepared in 1883 by Dr. James Flint, the first honorary curator, who was an assistant surgeon of the United States Navy. The catalogue remained unpublished. The folio volumes, containing neat handwritten entries, are in the possession of the Archives of the Smithsonian Institution.

In 1898 the title of the medical section was changed to reflect its broader scope and became the Division of Medicine.[68] The division sponsored exhibits on magical, psychical, physical, external, and internal, as well as preventive medicine (see figure 3.6). Over the next fifty years, pharmaceutical products, including synthetic, chemical, and crude drugs, constituted the primary specimens added to the collection under the supervision of curators, of which the pharmacist, Charles Whitebread, remained in charge from 1918 to 1948. When the United States National Museum was reorganized in 1957 into the United States Museum of Natural History and the Museum of History and Technology, the division was given its present name, Division of Medical Sciences, and subdivided into a section of Pharmaceutical History and Public Health, and a section of Medical and Dental History. Important medical items began to be collected the same year, when John Blake, currently chief of the History of Medicine Division of the Na-

tional Library of Medicine in Bethesda, Maryland, was appointed the first curator of the Section of Medical and Dental History. Some of these items include portable X-ray machines, the Lindbergh-Carrel perfusion pump, designed in 1935, the Sewell heart pump, designed in 1950, the Universities of Pennsylvania and Illinois dental collections, and various significant pieces of physiologic apparatus. The first catalogue of any part of the collection to be published is entitled *Bloodletting Instruments in the National Museum of History and Technology.*[69]

In the last several decades, many significant medical objects, representing the contributions of noted American physicians such as Chevalier Jackson and Rudolf Schindler, the heart surgeons, Adrian Kantrowitz and Denton Cooley, and the pioneering dentists, G. V. Black and Edward Angle, and other prominent specialists have been added to the Smithsonian Museum's collections. (See figures 3.7, 3.8, and 3.9).

The dental collection, which ranks among the finest in the world, had been gathered with the assistance of dental organizations headed by the American Association of the History of Dentistry, dental schools of the Universities of Maryland, Columbia, Northwestern, and Pennsylvania, and noted dentists such as the late Admiral Alfred Chandler, Robert Nelson (inventor of the high-speed drill), and the late dental historian J. Ben Robinson. In the collection are represented an extensive and intensive array of dental tools, including drills, extractors, scalers, mallets, pluggers, toothbrushes, toothpicks, and about thirty-five dental chairs, representing nineteenth- and twentieth-century models. Many fine ivory and pearl handle sets of instruments produced in the nineteenth century illustrate the fine craftsmanship applied to these items and the pride of the dentist in his implements. Items manufactured by the S. S. White Co. of Philadelphia, one of the oldest dental instrument firms, which had and continues to have a great impact on American dental technology, are found in the collection in abundance. Samples of artificial teeth, in the form of plates and single teeth show the evolution of the materials used to make these prosthetic appliances throughout the past several centuries.[70]

Modern instruments and hospital aids, including heart pacemakers, plastic heart valves, disposable scalpels and needles, operating room utensils, furniture, and surgical staplers are constantly being evaluated for inclusion into the Smithsonian collection. Some modern medical objects must be added to com-

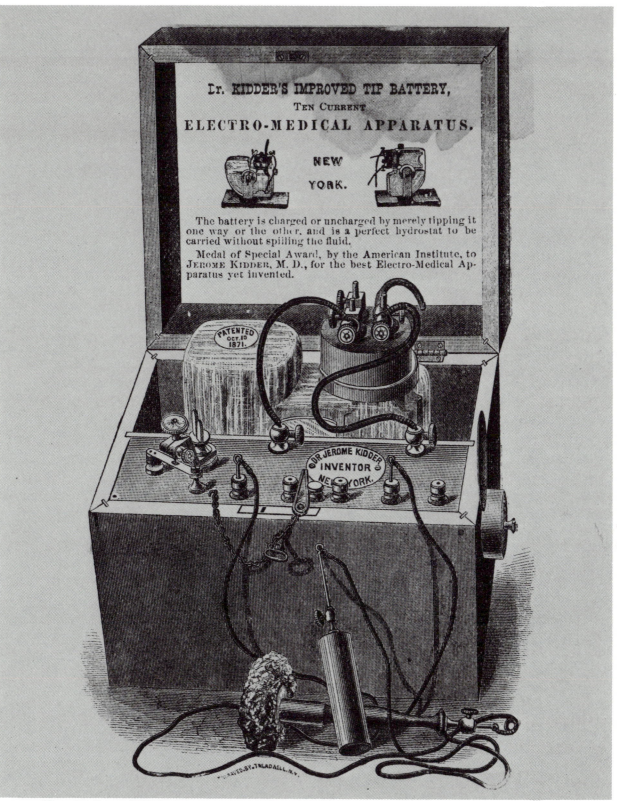

Figure 3.6. Jerome Kidder's tip battery, patented 1871. One of the common types of battery used by physicians in the nineteenth and twentieth centuries. *SI Photo No. 73-6258.*

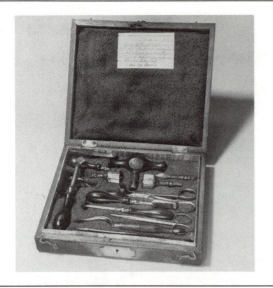

Figure 3.7. Trepanning set of Dr. Charles McKnight *NMAH No. 79.0264.02, SI Photo No. 79-10774.*

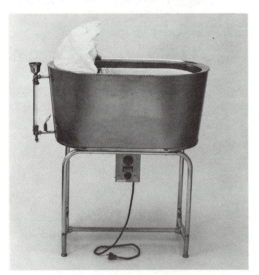

Figure 3.8. 1933 incubator for premature infants designed by Dr. Julius H. Hess. Donated by the Michael Reese Hospital. Pat. 7 Nov. 1933 No. 1, 933,733. *NMAH No. M-12230, SI Photo No. 62919.*

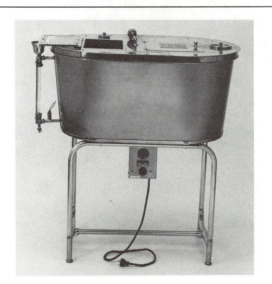

Figure 3.9. Another photograph of the 1933 incubator for premature infants designed by Dr. Julius. *SI Photo No. 62918.*

prehensive collections if they are properly to represent the development of twentieth-century American medical technology and techniques. (See figures 3.10, 3.11, and 3.12). The United States began to produce medical instruments in earnest to compete with and replace imported items after World War I, although some instruments are still imported from Europe and Japan. Examples of all these changes in production and the style of medical practice they represent belong in a complete medical collection.

MUETTER MUSEUM:

Two American medical museums, whose heritage traces back to the nineteenth century and which contain collections of both anatomic specimens and instruments, illustrate the dual functions of medical collections. The Muetter Museum of the College of Physicians in Philadelphia and the Medical Museum of the Armed Forces Institute of Pathology in Washington, D.C. have evolved from institutions set up for physicians and surgeons into museums exhibiting

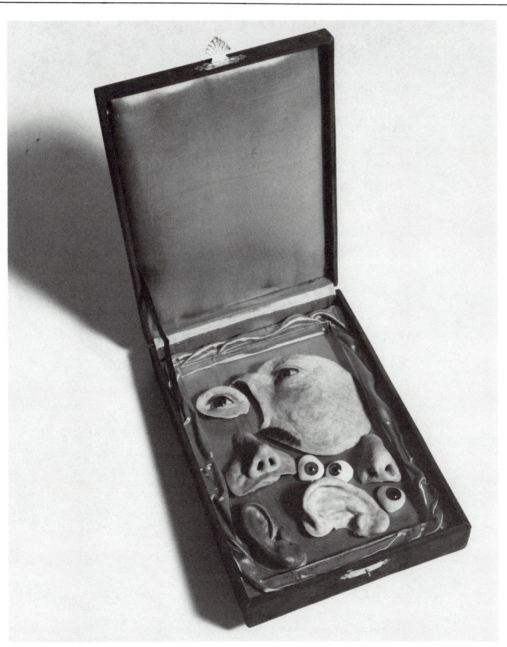

Figure 3.10. Facial prosthetics in case. *NMAH No. 306965.01-.09, SI Photo No. 73-9441.*

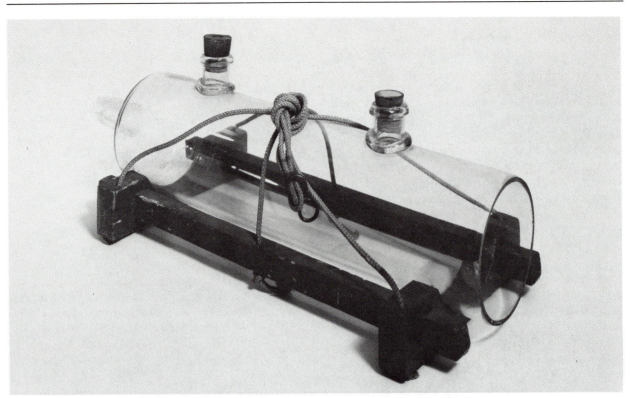

Figure 3.11. Plethysmograph *NMAH No. M-2383, SI Photo No. 72-754.*

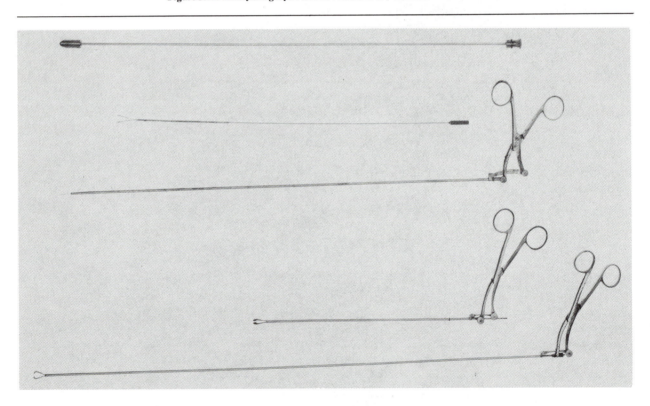

Figure 3.12. Bronchoscope and accessories circa 1925 of Chavalier Jackson. *SI Photo No. 72-8121.*

objects for a wider audience. The Museum of Pathological Anatomy was founded in 1849 at the College of Physicians in Philadelphia when fifty dollars was appropriated for the erection of exhibit cases and the preparation and arrangement of anatomic specimens.[71] This budget reflects the minimal amount of financial support given to the museum of the College of Physicians throughout its history. Consequently, the museum has not fared nearly as well as the library, which ranks as one of the richest medical libraries in the United States. The value of the museum to the college was discussed in 1887, with little enthusiasm being expressed for the museum's importance.[72]

The name of the Anatomical Museum was changed to the Muetter Museum in 1863 in honor of Dr. Thomas Dent Muetter, who donated his collection of over 1,200 specimens (anatomic, wax, papier-mâché models, casts, and other items) and $30,000 to maintain the museum.[73] The Muetter Museum was provided with a building in 1863, but presently, it is located in one corner of the College of Physicians' building and is open to visitors.

Among the earliest objects bought for the collection was a series of pathologic models purchased in Europe for nine hundred and ninety-eight dollars in 1878. Among the significant items still held by the museum are a collection of one hundred and thirty-nine human skulls bought from Dr. Joseph Hyrtl of Vienna in 1874 and a series of ossicles and labyrinths of the ear of all stages of development, which were prepared by Hyrtl over a period of fourteen years. Also in the museum are one hundred intricate wax models displaying eye diseases and deformities labeled in French, the unique Matthew H. Cryer collection of skulls and cranial segments illustrating the anatomy of the jaws and paranasal sinuses, the Adam Politzer series of tympanic membranes that were exhibited at the Centennial Exhibition in 1876, and the casts taken from bones passed off as the remains of the Piltdown man, purported in 1933 to be three-fourths to one million years old. Many of these well-preserved and carefully organized specimens are extremely valuable for the specialist and nonspecialist, who wishes to learn the intricacies of body structures and understand the impact of individual variations.

As part of a major center of American medical education and practice that existed for two hundred years, the Muetter Museum amassed a significant collection of medical inventions and equipment associated with leading Philadelphia practitioners. Among the notable items are a medicine chest used by Benjamin Rush, a Laennec stethoscope reported to be an original model, a Pond sphygmograph, a MacKenzie polygraph, a modified Helmholtz ophthalmoscope, a Loring ophthalmoscope, one of Lister's carbolic acid spray apparatuses, Madame Curie's piezoelectrometer, several early hypodermic syringes, clinical thermometers, hearing aids, surgical instruments, early Auzoux papier-mâché anatomic models, and a collection of 25,000 foreign bodies which the Philadelphia bronchoscopist, Chevalier Jackson, extracted from the throats, bronchi, and lungs of his patients.[74]

ARMY MEDICAL MUSEUM:

Philadelphia physicians contributed to the formation of another medical museum in 1862, which is known as the Army Medical Museum of Washington, D.C. The first specimens collected for this museum were the result of a directive from Surgeon-General William A. Hammond of Philadelphia that all medical officers serving in the Civil War send him all valuable anatomic and pathologic specimens at their disposal. As we have noted earlier, the first catalogue of these specimens appeared in 1866-1867, attesting to the rapidity with which museum staffs functioned in this period. Presently, the museum is attached to the Armed Forces Institute of Pathology (AFIP), a research institution sponsoring a range of disease studies. These investigations are facilitated by having on call army physicians and surgeons all over the world to contribute information and specimens required for any investigation.

The medical instrument part of the museum's collections was inaugurated by the efforts of John Shaw Billings, also of Philadelphia. Placed in charge of the museum in 1883, Billings encouraged physicians and surgeons to send in specimens of the instruments they had devised or discovered in order to build up a national reference collection of technologic aids to medicine, the first project of its kind in the United States. Important desiderata for Billings were objects used in research, like kymographs, anthropometric measuring aids, and constant temperature devices.[75]

The legacy of Billings to the study of medical technology bears no comparison to his legacy to American medical book collecting. Unfortunately, many of the collected medical objects have not survived, which is particularly disappointing since no other museum has been able to build a satisfactory collection of these early examples of American medical technology (see figure 3.13). The Division of Medical Sciences in collaboration with the Division of Mathematics of the National Museum of American His-

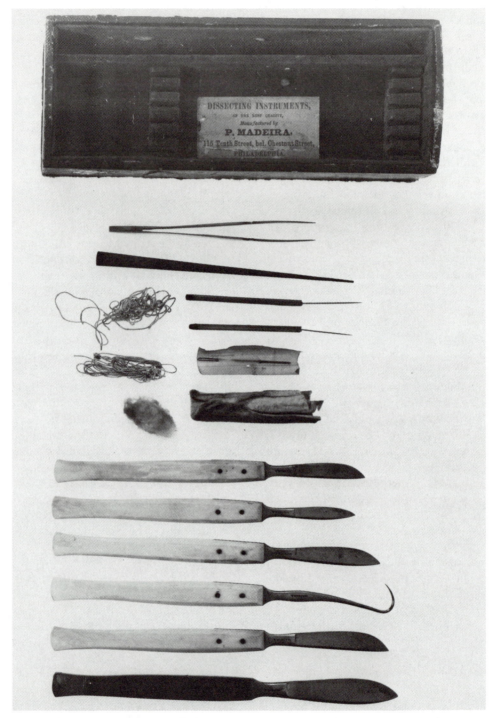

Figure 3.13. Dissecting Instruments (Madeira) from top to bottom: 1. case for dissecting instruments, 2. dissecting forceps, 3. blow pipe, 4. surgical probe w/wooden handle, 5. surgical probe w/wooden handle, 6. probe (straight-silver), 7. bloodletting lancets (2), 8. medium scalpel, 9. small scalpel, 10. medium scalpel, 11. tenaculum, 12. large scalpel, 13. cartilage knife (steel handle), 14. twisted silk cord, 15. absorbant stopping material. *SI Photo No. 74-10321.*

tory of the Smithsonian Institution has collected the instruments remaining from the late nineteenth and early twentieth centuries in several important experimental psychology departments, which employed equipment similar to the items Billings collected. A search through trade catalogues, however, reveals that much delicate and specialized equipment has not been saved or come to the attention of the collectors who have made a concerted effort to locate it.

Billings was alert to the educational and other effects a medical museum might have on its visitors. He noted the emotional impact of a medical museum that displayed the anatomic parts of famous and infamous personalities and the natural but self-conscious curiosity of some museum visitors, particularly women, who wanted to learn about the sexual organs and their diseases. To Billings it seemed that the museum should provide the proper setting for these visitors.[76] The AFIP museum was admirably successful in this role. Visitors to the Smithsonian Institution frequently ask to see the AFIP anatomic specimens. The Army Medical Museum was located on the Mall until 1969 when the building was torn down and the medical museum moved to its present location on the grounds of the Walter Reed Army Hospital.

Evaluations of the Army Medical Museum were more favorable than those of the Muetter Museum. D. L. Huntington, the curator in charge of the museum in 1896 described the goals of the library and museum. He explained that "in fact, we desire by this museum to effect through object teaching that which is secured in the library by written books and treatises, viz. a thorough illustration of the science of medicine as it is found at the present day."[77] His request for objects to expand the collection included dental specimens and equpiment. In the same year, the American Dental Association designated the museum as the national repository of historic dental instruments developed by its members.

In 1901, the American Ophthalmological Society, and shortly thereafter, the American Urological Society designated the medical museum as the repository of instruments employed by their members. These societies encouraged inventors and practitioners to donate samples of their equipment to the museum. With the stimulus of their professional associations, American physicians and surgeons developed a pride in the museum, which expressed itself in the donation of notable pieces of equipment. For instance, in 1950 Harry Friedenwald of Baltimore, Maryland presented one of the first ophthalmoscopes made from the drawings of the inventor, Hermann von Helmholtz.[78]

The microscope collection discussed earlier is the most famous instrumental segment of the museum's collections. Unique microscopes include the electron microscope reportedly used by Adolf Hitler's physician and some rare seventeenth-century elaborately tooled specimens made by the Italian artisan, Giuseppi Campani, and the English craftsman, John Marshall.

The Army Medical Museum expanded its collections during each war. Medical records of the army including pathologic specimens and exhibits documenting special techniques developed in surgery, orthopedics, and dentistry to cope with battle-incurred wounds and disabilities were displayed in the museum to teach medical students, physicians, and interested laymen. Induced by the socializing influence of world wars and the ascending interest in health and disease throughout the twentieth century, the medical museum enlarged the scope of its collections and its functions to the general public, thus taking on more of the characteristics of the public health museum.[79]

HOWARD DITTRICK MUSEUM:

Medical museums that collect and display items formerly owned by local physicians are intriguing for the valuable information pertaining to the use and function of the artifacts and objects they preserve and the charm with which these items are usually displayed in the museum. The Howard Dittrick Museum of Historical Medicine, originally the Museum of Historical and Cultural Medicine, provides an excellent example of the growth of a collection that includes mementoes and items used since the eighteenth century to practice medicine in the Western Reserve region centered in Cleveland, Ohio. Additional object materials depicting medicine among other cultures and in other periods is also represented to provide a more complete picture of the history of medicine and to place local medical history in a broader context.

The museum is located in the Allen Library building, erected in 1926. A third-generation physician, Dr. Dudley P. Allen, who had practiced in the area, deposited instruments and equipment used by his father, an Oberlin practitioner, and his grandfather, who settled in Kinsman, Ohio.[80] Through gifts from descendants of physicians, some of whom began to practice in the late eighteenth century, a composite doctor's office was reconstructed and placed on exhibit. The one-room office includes medical items used by five generations of physicians, all of whom were named Adam Benjamin Denison.[81] This reconstruction is one of the few doctor's offices on exhibit in the United States. More commonly exhibited are pharmacies and, occasionally, a dentist's office. Friends and supporters of the Dittrick Museum over the past fifty years have donated a spectrum of objects including ivory-, bone-, and wood-handled dental instruments; a sixteenth-century artificial arm; obstetrical forceps; microscopes, including an early Martin type (1740-1750); stethoscopes; tourniquets; splints; amputation sets; saddle bags; bleeding instruments; pharmacy objects; votives; military medicine items used in the Civil, Spanish American, and World Wars; photographs and replicas, including thirty-three Pompeian surgical instruments; the Chamberlen obstetrical instruments; and the wooden Smellie forceps.[82] Some of the equipment, including one pair of obstetrical forceps, was forged in a local blacksmith shop for Dr. John B. Harmon of Warren, Ohio. Another pair of forceps was forged by Dr. Theodatus Garlick himself.[83]

The museum also holds "nursing appliances chiefly hot water bottles of pewter or copper, cold water coils of lead, and bedpans of pewter, tin and pottery. A special collection called the Wykoff collection of nursing bottles comprises many designs in glass. Two replicas in terra cotta illustrate Roman Carthaginian examples."[84]

OTHER COLLECTIONS:

The medical museum at the Knoxville Academy of Medicine was established from medical instrument and book collections gathered by Dr. Samuel Joseph Platt, who has published an illustrated catalogue of the collection and exhibitions. The illustrations present overall views of the museum but do not reveal the details of instruments. The exhibit includes a doctor's office and treatment room containing instruments and furniture from fifty to one hundred years old, over 2,000 instruments, and 250 leather-bound books dating from 1798 to 1870. All the instruments are displayed, although only a small proportion are listed in the catalogue. The rationale for assembling this medical collection is summed up in a statement appearing on the door of the museum. It reads: "The entire idea of the museum was to accept not only old instruments but also those which are no longer being manufactured, are becoming scarce, are increasing in value as collector's items, or, for simply memorializing some particular physician."[85] Instruments and objects were collected with the proviso that, if the museum should be dismantled, all items would be returned to their donors.

The Society of Anesthesiologists maintains a collection of primarily twentieth-century anesthesia devices and equipment, as well as a library in the Wood Memorial Library and Museum located in Park Ridge, Illinois, a suburb of Chicago. Mr. Patrick Sim, who manages the collections, has prepared a typescript listing of this equipment.

Individuals with specific educational missions have set up and promoted medical museums to carry their messages to the public. One of these unusual museums displays the damage caused when electricity strikes the human body and other objects. Stephen Jellinek founded the Electropathological Museum in Vienna in 1936. Jellinek devoted his career to understanding the physical and biological effects of electricity. The Jellinek Museum made its founder's discoveries widely known among those outside the medical profession. All types of items struck by lightning are featured in the museum, along with methods of avoiding this type of disaster; or if someone is struck by lightning or electrocuted, the display indicates what steps to take in resuscitating the victim.[86]

In the last decade, a museum dedicated to the collection of books and objects related to the use of electricity for medical purposes was founded under the auspices of Earl Bakken, a pioneer American manufacturer of heart pacemakers under the trade name Medtronic. The Museum of Electricity and Life in Minneapolis, Minnesota contains important eighteenth- and nineteenth-century electrical machines, as well as a number of pieces used by prominent nineteenth-century experimentalists, who studied the nervous system and revealed some of its characteristics. A catalogue of the collections is being prepared by Dennis Stillings, the curator and major organizer of the collection.

Medical pioneers have provided the raison d'être for museums displaying the medical objects these individuals employed, together with personal and family memorabilia. The Semmelweis Medical Historical Museum, Library, and Archives in Budapest contains medical and pharmaceutical objects, pictures of distinguished physicians and of the locale, family, and memorabilia related to Ignaz Semmelweis, who improved the care of postpartum patients to avoid infection and death by puerperal fever. The Semmelweis items are arranged in one room of the museum and other parts of the collection are exhibited in other rooms. These include several Czermak laryngoscopes, a full-sized female wax anatomic model, and a metal midwives set. An illustrated catalogue of the museum was published in 1972.[87]

The value of medical museums has increased to the extent that, in spite of the vast cost of creating and maintaining a museum, medical museums continue to be established by medical societies and supported with private funds. For instance, the Historical Museum of Medicine and Dentistry of the Hartford Medical Society and Hartford Dental Society was opened in 1974. Encompassing eight wooden cabinets of medical instruments and three rooms of exhibits, this collection includes the memorabilia and manuscripts of prominent local figures, such as Horace Wells and Gershom Bulkeley (1635-1713), and an assortment of surgical and medical instruments.[88]

PART II

SIGNIFICANT INSTRUMENTATION

4

MEDICAL THERMOMETRY

INTRODUCTION:

The thermometer is the most convenient of instruments to apply among those diagnostic instruments selected for more intensive discussion. Although it had a heritage older than the stethoscope and as old as the microscope, the thermometer was absorbed into the spectrum of physical diagnostic equipment as late as or later than both these instruments. In 1866, F. W. Gibson wrote "the day is not, I think, very far distant when the physician will consider the thermometer not less indispensable to him than the stethoscope and microscope, and when the surgeon will not neglect the observations of the temperature."[1] Even though it did not require any more special education to apply it, the thermometer was overshadowed in medical practice by other more elaborate and specialized instruments.

Reasons for the delayed acceptance of thermometry in medicine include that its use did not contribute to the prevailing diagnostic pattern established in part with the stethoscope and microscope and that the information it revealed could not be directly related to pathologic anatomy. In the nineteenth century, local alterations of body structure and function were beginning to be considered the ultimate foci of disease and were increasingly uncovered with the aid of specialized instruments and laboratory tests. The local disease concept could not readily be related to overall body heat, even when measured.[2] In an age when intensive interest in specific parts of the body and methods of studying them blossomed, an instrument that provided information about a general phenomenon such as body temperature seemed less important, although it was understood by those who used the thermometer regularly in their practices that temperature variations could be ascribed to both

organic and functional local disorders "either by producing local variations of temperature or by affecting that of the system at large."[3] Other objections to the use of the thermometer were similar to those advanced against the stethoscope and other instruments involving the time required to master them and the need to carry the instruments and keep them from being broken.[4] To balance resistance to the thermometer on these grounds, it was practical and convenient to have hospital attendants regularly take the temperatures of patients. Commentators, in admitting that thermometry had failed to become part of clinical practice, continued to stress, as J. F. Goodhart did in 1869, the similarity between Laennec's forecast that stethoscopy would become a hospital-based practice, and the fact that recording the body temperature would prove adaptable to hospital medicine.[5] Research-oriented physicians saw the limitations of subjectively derived information available to them in the diagnosis of disease, and therefore, welcomed all objective measurements, including body temperature. The establishment of body heat as a physiologic constant especially appealed to teachers and those who could call on a regular staff of students and assistants to take repeated temperature recordings of their patients.

Repeated and systematic temperature records provided insights into a variety of disease processes. Carl Wunderlich, whose monograph on clinical thermometry in 1868 provided the most systematic analysis of the procedure, demonstrated the relationship between changes in body temperature and the courses a number of diseases followed. Soon others related body heat to other bodily impairments. For instance, J. W. Stickler in 1882, while a house surgeon to the Presbyterian Hospital in New York, took the temperature twice daily of patients with simple long bone fractures and noted that a maximum temperature of approximately 101-102 degrees Fahrenheit was reached by the third day. He attributed the increase to "the period of inflammation."[6]

Into the fourth quarter of the nineteenth century, using the thermometer in clinical practice was complicated by undependable instruments and an uncertain mode of observation. Major impetus to persevere was provided by German and British clinical investigators from whom the French and American physicians learned the importance of the thermometer.[7] Nineteenth-century British and German medical journals included discussion of the salient points for deciding how often and when to take the temperature, in what body part or parts temperature was of diagnostic value, what were the limits of normal body temperature, how temperature related to other diagnostic signs, and which instruments to employ. Wunderlich, leading nineteenth-century medical spokesman for thermometry, stated the fundamental axiom, which claimed that only a narrow difference existed between body temperature in health and disease. This was demonstrated both during the onset and progress of diseases and in the regular daily fluctuations in healthy individuals. It was impossible in theory or practice to indicate the exact thermometric point between health and disease,[8] and yet it was claimed by some that the body temperature in disease is more readily and rapidly changed than either the pulse or the respiration.

Nevertheless, recording the temperature of normal and abnormal individuals was important to build up the record upon which a standard of body temperature could be based. The pattern of normal daily temperature variations was studied by clinicians, including William Carter of the Royal Southern Hospital, Liverpool. After taking the temperatures of six nurses, who worked the night shift, he reported

that a daily depression of temperature takes place in the healthy during night and early morning; that such a change of habit as turns night into day, so far as employment is concerned, does not permanently affect the character of this depression; that a daily range of from two to three degrees Fahr. may take place consistently with health; that an axillary [under the arm] temperature of 96 degrees, or even lower, at some period of the night, is consistent with health, and that the character of the daily oscillation is not markedly affected by food.[9]

Physicians who were convinced of the thermometer's value to medical diagnosis persisted in its use in spite of their own ineffective application of the instrument. One example is provided by the divergence

between the thought and practice of the instrument-promoting physician Pierre Adolph Piorry. A decade after popularizing the technique of percussion with a pleximeter, he encouraged use of the thermometer, which transcended the local disease concept he had helped generate. His belief in the facilitating function of medical instruments inspired him to rhapsodize about the thermometer: "When one sees such results obtained by the sole aid of a little bit of iron suspended on a pivot, surely nothing which can supplement or perfect the operation of our senses should be held in slight estimation."[10] Piorry's enthusiasm did not carry over into his practice. He carried his thermometer conveniently within his stethoscope and used it to make temperature readings that were considered inaccurate for the period.

By the 1880s, the value of measuring body temperature was recognized by many physicians. Regardless of the difficulties in using the thermometer, John B. Bradbury argued in an address on "Modern Scientific Medicine" before the British Medical Association in 1880 that

The Thermometer had done more than the microscope to place medicine on a scientific basis. Owing to it we are able to diagnosticate diseases which before, at an early stage, were confounded as tuberculosis and typhoid fever. We can make more confident prognoses, and use our drugs with more precision. It has led to the antipyretic treatment of fevers.[11]

Before the technological development of the clinical thermometer is discussed, a brief review is useful of how physicians viewed abnormal body heat or fever and how they recognized different fevers before the clinical thermometer was available. The introduction of a new technique or instrument for investigating body heat raises basic issues concerning the assimilation of technology into medical practice. Among them is the shift in emphasis from the cause and mechanism of a disease to the signs and symptoms, which provide clues to effective treatment.

THE THERMOMETER AND THEORIES OF FEVER:

Hippocrates and Galen defined fever (pyrexia in Greek), as the elevation of body heat, or "calor praetor naturam," a view that remained unchallenged until the Renaissance.[12] Primarily as a disease entity in itself, which produced other symptoms such as weakness, rapid pulse, and vomiting, but also as a sign of other diseases, the rise in body heat was described according to the impression revealed by touching the feverish patient. When it became feasible to measure body heat on a numerical scale, fever as a disease and as a symptom was placed in another context along with the signs provided by other instruments. Treatment consisted of lowering excessively high fevers by applying cooling liquids externally and prescribing special fever-reducing drugs or febrifuges.

Wunderlich realized that the importance of body heat as the source or as a type of disease had diminished in the period when body heat fluctuations could be defined more accurately with the thermometer.[13] He explained the delay in accepting the thermometer in the clinic as a consequence of the preoccupation with the mechanical explanations related to the circulation.[14] The link between the circulation of the body and the concept of fever originated in the seventeenth century. Iatro-chemists and iatro-mechanists, exemplified by Thomas Willis and Hermann Boerhaave in the eighteenth century, attributed the rise in body heat to the circulation of the blood.[15] Concentration on circulatory changes, especially accompanying a fever, which Willis defined as a fermentation or "an intestine motion of the blood,"[16] changed the pattern established in antiquity of using the change in body heat as a primary diagnostic sign of fever. Abnormal body heat began to be recognized as a secondary symptom of basic changes within the blood's circulation which, in turn, required treatment with drugs directed to the regulation of the circulation. The circulation of the blood might have been expected to propel heat to all the tissues; however, eighteenth-century physicians believed that the thermometer measured the heat of the external parts of the body and was not a good guide to the internal body temperature. Boerhaave, for instance, preferred to gauge internal body heat by inspection of the urine. A red color indicated a higher body heat.[17] Later, in the eighteenth century, physicians including John Hunter in 1773-1774 argued against the view that body temperature was produced by the blood's circulation. In this period, Antoine Lavoisier and Adair Crawford derived a chemical explanation for body heat[18] based on laboratory experiments with small animals. According to their conception of body heat as a form of combustion, they placed the center of heat control in the tissues. Not all tissues produced heat equally. They noted that "the glandular organs, the great nervous centers, and the muscular tissue might well be assumed to take a prominent part in the production of heat."[19]

When the mechanical view of fever in which the role of the circulation was stressed began to lose favor, theories of fever centered on the role of the nervous system. John Parkes in 1855 in his Gulstonian lectures on pyrexia explained the general rise in temperature on the basis of the accepted theory of Virchow, who placed the control of body heat in the nervous center.[20] Parkes, working at King's College Hospital, demonstrated with the thermometer that when nervous control was altered, undue heat or cold was produced in the body. One example of a loss of nervous control resulted from an injury to the spinal cord at the cervical level, which was demonstrated by Wood of Philadelphia. "He found . . . that at a low external temperature, after section of the cervical cord, there was increased evolution, with diminished production of heat; while at high external temperature, both the production and evolution of heat were diminished."[21] Claude Bernard experimentally verified a number of theories of heat production involving the nervous system. As a British observer explained: "Indeed, there is not a modern theory of fever that has been set, unless it absolutely excludes the nervous system from all place in it, in which Bernard's work is not the very key-stone of the arch."[22]

The thermotaxic heat centers in the brain and spinal cord were discovered in the 1870s by the Americans Horatio C. Wood and Isaac Ott. They concluded that the deeper structures of the brain "act both as exciting and inhibitory centers according to the form of stimulus they receive."[23]

The discussion of the direct cause of fever centered on two main concepts: (1) the continual additional production of heat by the body beyond its normal requirements and (2) a lack of sufficient evaporation of the body heat, which allowed it to build up within the body and resulted in a temperature rise. Louis Traube, mentor of Wunderlich, supported the second view.

One characteristic of fever revealed by the thermometer and previously unproven by other methods of observation was the continuous elevation of temperature throughout the course of a disease. Traube showed in 1851 that a fever, whether accompanied by chills, a damp skin, or other seemingly contrary symptoms, expressed an elevation in temperature throughout its course.[24] Parkes' studies also revealed this relationship.

A thermometer for measuring the temperatures of the superficial and deeper tissues of the body simultaneously, called a thermopile, provided data relevant to the pattern and control of body temperature in different regions of the body. Clifford Allbutt described a thermopile in 1873, in use since 1868,[25] for measuring the surface and deeper tissue temperatures. Etienne Marey devised a thermopile with a mechanism for recording the temperature on a paper dial (thermograph), which consisted of a small Bourdon tube with a curve that changed in response to the expansion of the oil filling the apparatus. The thermometer was a cylindrical brass reservoir, six millimeters in diameter and three millimeters long, ending in a capillary tube of copper that opened into the tube, to which the dial was attached for marking the temperature. Marey's thermograph revealed that in vasomotor disturbances, temperature changes in the interior and peripheral parts of the body were unequal, and in vasomotor paralysis, the surface temperature rose, while the interior temperature remained constant.[26]

After the thermometer had been adopted in the clinic, medical investigators concentrated on the course, rather than mechanism, of fevers.[27] Henry Goodridge of England remarked in 1885 that "the etiological aspect of certain specific fevers and febrile processes has so engrossed attention of late, and such encouraging results have attended the study of the same, that inquiries into the essential nature and mechanism of fever in general, pyrexia as it is called, seem in danger of slipping into the background."[28] The discovery of bacteria and their implication in generating many fevers shifted emphasis from the origin of body heat to these disease-producing organisms and how to rid the body of them.

Another investigation entailed the effect of antipyretic drugs on the control of fevers, undertaken by among others, Carl Emil Buss of Basel, who was among the first to treat acute rheumatism with salicylic acid or aspirin.[29] His aim was to measure the amount of carbonic acid excreted as a crucial factor in the heat production of the body. To do this, he placed the subject in a small chamber, based on the chamber of Liebermeister, but more complex to ensure greater accuracy. Buss administered the heat-reducing drugs including sulfate of quinine, salicylate of soda, and creosotate of soda.

The object was to ascertain what alterations the heat production undergoes when the febrile regulation of heat passes into the normal, that is, when heat regulation of the fever patient is set to that of the healthy person. The result was quite unexpected; viz, whereas under the influence of quinine a considerable diminution of the carbonic acid production occurred after the administration of salicylate of soda or of the creosotate, the carbonic acid production continued unaltered and as it was before. . . . [This result] carries with it a positive conclusion of pathological importance; viz., that by heat discharge alone and without diminished heat production, the resetting of the heat regulation to the normal temperature can be effected.[30]

It was also discovered that fever does not result from excess heat production alone. Studies on the regulation of fever in tetanus provided evidence for this conclusion. "By fever then, according to Buss, we are to understand that pathological modification of the regulation of heat of the body, in which with increased heat production there is relatively diminished heat discharge, whereby the temperature is elevated above the normal standard."[31] These conclusions, carefully supported by the experiments with antipyretic drugs, still left the basic question unanswered: "Yet, what is fever? Is it not the most common morbid condition of the organism? And, again, though it may sometimes be only a trivial disorder, is it not very apt to be as formidable as any we have to deal with, carrying off its victims from all classes of society?"[32] While the mechanism of fever remained inscrutable, the fact that fevers could be delineated by differing causal agents was a source of pride to the nineteenth-century British physician. For example, Richard Quain, who delivered a lecture in London entitled "On the History and Progress of Medicine" in 1885, concluded that there had been no medical discovery greater than the differentiation of some fevers.[33]

Without solving the problem of the nature of a fever, the self-registering thermometer permitted precise measurements of the body temperature that led to rational treatment. The thermometer had the most profound effect of all diagnostic instruments on therapeutics in this period, which led Thomas Brunton to cite the control of fever as the greatest advance in medicine during the quarter century before 1891. When the thermometer revealed a dangerously rising body temperature, immediate action could be taken. He explained that

the use of the thermometer enables the merest tyro to recognize . . . a case of . . . hyperpyrexia. . . . The constant employment of the instrument shows everyone, nurses as well as doctors, when the temperature of a patient is rising so high as to be dangerous, and allows them . . . in most cases, to prevent a further rise by the use of antithermic measures, such as cradling, cold sponging, cold affusion, cold baths, or by the administration of antipyretic remedies.[34]

Some drugs, such as quinine and salicylic acid, appeared to have a double curative effect: to reduce fever and to remove the disease (malaria) that may have brought on the fever. American physicians preferred treatment with drugs for most patients, while the Germans promoted cold baths especially among their more hardy patients.[35]

Measuring Body Temperature Before the Thermometer:

When Galen introduced the idea of "degrees of heat and cold"[36] as part of his theory of elements and their relationship to human physiology, he provided the basis for the concept of a fixed point or standard of temperature, which was essential to the concept of the thermometer. His scale, employed without reference to an instrument, placed a neutral point midway between four degrees leading to the hottest point on one end and four degrees to the coldest point at the opposite end. The neutral point consisted of equal quantities of ice and boiling water without a specification of their volumes or weights. Interest in the fourteenth century in quantifying all of the qualities including heat was followed in the late sixteenth and early seventeenth centuries by attempts to measure body temperature while recognizing some of the physiologic conditions under which it should change. Johannis Hasler in *De logistica medica* (1578) hoped to find the natural temperature of each man, "as determined by his age, the time of the year, the elevation of the pole [latitude], etc."[37] Hasler accepted the medieval belief that the temperature of individuals, foods, drugs, and other items in the tropics was higher than in other latitudes.[38] In his scale, Hasler displayed side by side the relationship between the nine degrees of heat and the eight degrees of quality specified by Galen and how they related to the degrees of latitude. The physician thus was provided with a scale with which to compare his patient's degree of heat and determine its expected normality for the latitude in which he lived. Upon this information was based the doctor's selection of drugs to bring the temperature to its normal level,[39] according to the original schema of Galen and the formulas worked out in the Middle Ages by the Arab, Alkindi, the Spaniard, Arnold of Villanova, and others.[40]

Before an instrument to measure the body temperature was designed, the patient's temperature was compared to the temperature of the person applying the treatment. Nurses and midwives estimated the temperature of bathing water by immersing their feet, elbows, and hands into it and regulating it to their sense of warmth before putting their patients into the water. An illustration of 1513 on the title page of Eucharius Roslin Rosengarten depicts this practice.[41]

Thermometry Instruments:

The concept of temperature as the property of a body to heat other bodies led to the design of an instrument to measure this transfer of energy. Physicians were among the seventeenth-century pioneers who became aware of the possibility of recording temperature by transferring heat to a glass tube with a bulb placed in the patient's mouth or hand. The air or fluid contained within the bulb expanded in proportion to the amount of heat within the body with which the tube was placed in contact.[42]

EARLY THERMOMETERS:

Debate over who designed the earliest thermometer began in the seventeenth century. W. E. Knowles Middleton, who investigated the history of the thermometer, refined the issue of the invention of the instrument by distinguishing the thermoscope or instrument without a scale from the thermometer, which contained a scale. Both of these instruments were arranged to display visibly the changes brought about by heat transfer. The term *thermoscope* appears first in 1617 in *Sphaera mundi* by Guiseppe Bianci, who also provided an illustration of it.[43] The term *thermometer* first appears in 1626 in H. Van Etten's *Récreation mathématique*.[44] Without providing a correct account of its functions, Bartholomew Telioux of Rome depicted a thermometer in a manuscript of 1611,[45] which led historians to suspect that the thermometer was more widely known in 1611 than the extant literature indicates.[46] Santorio introduced the thermometer to his students to measure both air temperature and the temperature of the human body. In 1612 Santorio in his *Commentaria in artem medicinalem Galeni*, part three explained "I wish to tell you about a marvellous way in which I am accustomed to measure, with a certain glass instrument, the cold and hot temperature of the air of all regions and places, and of all parts of the body; and so exactly, that we can measure with the compass the degrees and ultimate limits of heat and cold at any time of day."[47] He also promised to give an illustration of the instrument and describe its construction and uses in another book. Thirteen years later in *Commentaria in primam fen primi libri canonis Avicennae*, he described several thermometers. All the instruments with scales have a bulb at the top and a tube dipping into an open vessel, which are the most well known of Santorio's instruments. The rate of change of the patient's temperature was measured by observing the change in the reading during ten beats of the small pendulum[48] or pulsilogium while the instrument remained in the patient's mouth or hand.

Three types of thermometers were introduced in

the seventeenth century. These three types differed in their fluid content, containing either air, spirit or alcohol, or mercury. Seventeenth-century thermometers were based on the expansion of air in narrow glass tubes, some of which were coiled and curved. These served until it was realized that air responds as quickly to pressure as to heat. Spirit or alcohol in glass thermometers were constructed in 1654. The mercury thermometer was tried in 1660 and abandoned for a while since its rate of expansion was low.[49] Until the bore of the thermometer tube could be made considerably smaller and uniform, mercury could not be used to indicate temperature changes precisely and quickly.

In the last decades of the seventeenth century (1679), two end points based on the physical changes in water were chosen: the levels reached at the lower end by the formation of ice and snow and at the higher end by boiling water.[50]

A major difficulty in constructing a universal scale for a thermometer rested on the fact that most substances change their volumes unevenly over the range of a complete temperature scale between the freezing and boiling points of the substance. A linear scale would only be possible when a substance that expanded evenly was placed in the thermometer.[51] The problem of constructing a thermometer that contained alcohol or mercury, substances which expanded more evenly than any others when heated, was solved by Daniel Gabriel Fahrenheit and Anders Celsius. Fahrenheit described his 212-degree scale thermometer in 1724 and Celsius his 100-degree scale instrument in 1742. Fahrenheit's original scale was fixed at two points: the melting point of ice (32) and blood temperature (96). Shortly after his death, by 1740, the boiling point of water was fixed at 212 degrees, which brought the blood heat point to 98.6 degrees.[52] Celsius divided his scale into one hundred degrees, but it remained for the botanist, Carl von Linné, a close friend, to reverse the original scale so that zero became the freezing point and one hundred became the boiling point of water on the Celsius scale. The equivalent for 98.6 degrees Fahrenheit is 37 degrees on the Celsius or Centigrade scale. The Fahrenheit and Celsius scales became the most popular for clinical and meteorologic purposes and continue to be used to the present. A third scale was Réaumur's containing eighty degrees, which was popular in France and Germany in the nineteenth century. Standardization to one unique thermometric scale for medical use was encouraged by 1876.

Seventeenth-century thermometers were also barometers because they were open at one end. Those used by physicians were marked by tieing a string at the level of the water reached in the tube. In these thermometers, as the bulb was warmed, the water descended, in contrast to the flow of liquid in the closed thermometer.[53] By 1630 Santorio had determined the limits of his air thermometer by applying snow to it to find out how high the water would ascend in the tube, and the flame of a candle for the lowest limit to which it would descend. When these extremes were known, it was possible to determine how the temperature of any other substances, including the human body, departed from these points. The heat of the body was not a fixed point for Santorio.[54]

The first proposed thermometer scale to include the body temperature or body heat as one of its reference points was attributed to Isaac Newton. An account of this scale was published anonymously in the *Philosophical Transactions* of 1701.[55] Roger Cotes established in 1738 that he learned from Newton that the description of this linseed oil thermometer had been suggested by Newton. The zero degree point was "the heat of the air in water when water begins to freeze" and the second point was placed at twelve degrees or "the maximum heat that the thermometer can attain by contact with the human body."[56] Rapidly boiling water was thirty-four degrees on this scale.

The medical thermometer, like other medical devices with scales, had to be correlated with the limits of the physiologic function it recorded. A number of investigators discovered by trial and error which parts of the scale and what differences between numbers contributed to an evaluation of the type, progress, and cure of disease. Conversion of the changes in body heat to a numerical sequence for the physician did not depend on a full understanding of the concepts of heat and temperature but on a correlation between the number marked on the instrument and the symptoms of each disease, as well as normal bodily functions.

The clinical thermometer, first described in England at the Ashmolean School of Natural History at a meeting of the Oxford Philosophical Society on 13 May 1684, contained mercury. This model invented by du Val of Paris was three inches long, four to five lines in diameter, and half a line in the diameter of the mercury column.[57] Many details of the development of the medical thermometer are given in several well-documented sources including a chapter of Wunderlich's text,[58] a series of five articles in the *Lancet* of 1916 by G. Sims Woodhead and P. C. Varrier-Jones of the University of Cambridge, and also Erich Ebstein's "Die Entwicklung der Klinischen

Thermometrie.''[59] Ebstein provides a twenty-four-page bibliography emphasizing non-English sources. Therefore, it is not imperative that I provide a comprehensive review of the numerous changes in the thermometer and the various attempts to employ it in the practice of medicine between the early seventeenth century and the nineteenth century.

The shape of the clinical thermometer was determined by the part of the body to which it was applied. In the seventeenth century, thermometers were strapped to the wrist of a fever patient. A typical one was designed by the Grand Duke, Ferdinand II, who improved upon Galileo's thermometer. Some of these types were displayed in 1876 in the South Kensington Exhibition of scientific instruments in London.[60] A thermometer in the shape of a frog contained balls of different densities and colors, which descended as the fluid within the instruments increased in temperature and consequently diminished in density.[61]

A popular site for taking the body temperature in the eighteenth and nineteenth centuries was in the armpit or axilla. Thermometers placed in the armpit bore scales printed on attached strips of ivory or bone with tips two inches or more long, bent at right angles to the stem, which was three or four inches long. This shape permitted the instrument to be read while it remained in place under the arm, which was essential for an accurate reading before the introduction of the index thermometer in the mid-nineteenth century (see figure 4.1).

Before a discussion is presented of some of the important changes in thermometer design made in the nineteenth century, several questions raised by Boerhaave's biographer, G. A. Lindeboom,[62] concerning Boerhaave's use of the thermometer and the state of the art in this period should be addressed. Boerhaave provided an important impetus to the use of the instrument among physicians, particularly the Fahrenheit scale designed by his countryman. A

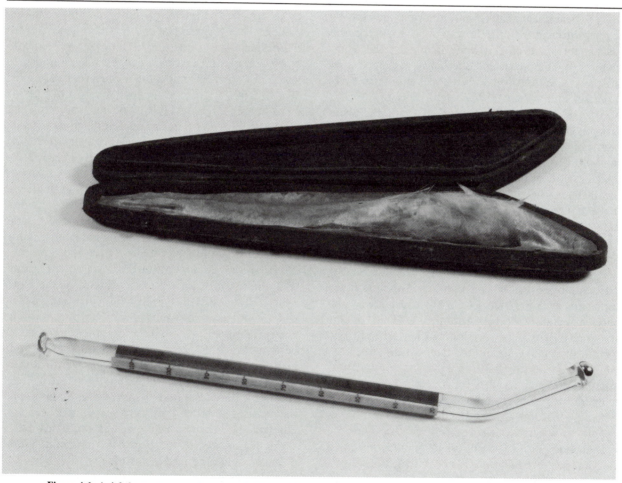

Figure 4.1. Axial thermometer and case. *NMAH No. 316528.01, SI Photo No. 78-695.* The ivory scale is placed on the outside of the glass tube.

letter from Fahrenheit to Boerhaave remains the best evidence for the documentation of Fahrenheit's improvement of his own thermometer.[63] Boerhaave used the thermometer astutely. In comparing Fahrenheit's mercurial and alcoholic thermometers, Boerhaave noted discrepancies in their readings. In reply to Boerhaave, as to the reason for the unequal readings, Fahrenheit stated that the different types of glass in the thermometers was the source of the problem; however, the differences in the expansion rates of mercury and alcohol were the most likely cause of the dissimilar readings.[64] Boerhaave used alcohol thermometers until 1718 when Fahrenheit began to make mercury-filled thermometers commercially, and from that time Boerhaave preferred the mercury type of instrument. Lindeboom was perplexed about the lack of temperature records in Boerhaave's publications.[65] It should be understood that in his period numerical relationships to denote bodily functions were not usually applied by physicians. The Santorian method of recording body temperatures, by comparing a patient's temperature with a normal individual's temperature and noting how long it took for the instrument to reach this limit, remained the usual method for the physician. Boerhaave explained how this was accomplished: "With a Fahrenheit thermometer let the heat of the healthy person be first measured, and the degree marked upon the scale affixed, and then, this being known, if the same thermometer is held in the hand of a febrile patient, or the bulb of it put into his mouth, or applied to the naked breast, or under the armpit for a few minutes, the different height of the ascending mercury will make it appear how much the febrile exceeds the natural and healthy heat."[66] In this manner, each thermometer was standardized at the time of application. It was not important to publish temperature records of different patients when the thermometer was employed in this fashion since the numbers found for each individual were not considered to be necessary or comparable. Antonius de Haen, one of Boerhaave's students, was among the earliest to systematically make accurate temperature records, which he began to publish in 1757 and continued to amass for several decades. He concluded that human temperature varies from 95 to 99 degrees Fahrenheit but that "natural warmth has the same value in all people, irrespective of age and sex."[67]

Lindeboom called attention to an illustration in Boerhaave's text *Elementa Chemia*, which displays a thermometer with a scale ending at ninety-six degrees, but failed to account for the discrepancy between this illustrated thermometer and later Fahrenheit models.

According to Middleton, this was the last version of Fahrenheit's thermometer produced before his death. Fahrenheit stated that the boiling point of water was 212 degrees, which when it was applied to his thermometer after his death, raised the blood point to 98.6 degrees to conform to the boiling point of 212 degrees.

Fahrenheit thermometers continued to be used by English and American physicians, even though medical leaders regretted the instruments' use because they were not compatible with the Celsius scale. Some instruments were marked with both scales, which sometimes confused the physician.[68]

A French physician who emigrated to America in 1848 hoped to abandon use of both these scales in favor of one he had designed especially for measuring body heat. Following in the tradition of J. B. Bouillard's unique human body thermometer, Eduoard Seguin placed the point of normal body temperature at zero and proposed six degrees above and five degrees below, each of which was described by a term to indicate the type of pathology taking place or "the thermal status of man."[69] One of these thermometers was manufactured by George Tiemann of New York and marked with the following degree levels: 5-6 degrees or death, 4-5 degrees or almost always fatal, 3.5 degrees or high fever, 3 degrees or considerably high fever, 2.5 degrees or moderate fever, zero degrees norm of health equivalent to 37 degrees Celsius and 98.6 degrees Fahrenheit, 0.5 degrees of subnormal, 1 degree or depression, 2 degrees or collapse, and 3 degrees or algide collapse.[70] In the second edition of his book, Seguin increased the scale to include one more degree at each extreme.

Employing words as well as numbers to mark the clinical thermometer was not original with Seguin. Eighteenth-century barometers and thermometers displayed the Latin word for the heat marked numerically on the instrument.[71] One example is the Fahrenheit thermometer supplied to Christian Wolff, which contained a twenty-four-degree scale. The ancient descriptions used before the thermometer became available to indicate the stages of fevers included terms such as mildly hot and warm. Robert Fludd was one of the early writers to depict in chart form how the pulse, body temperature, humors, and the diseases to which they were subject were related. His scale was divided in the center and extended to seven degrees above and below the midpoint. Fludd did not equate the numbers with specific body temperatures as measured with a thermometer but with the pulse, which he described according to the Galenic system with terms like slow and strong. The heat-pulse index was linked to the seasons as well as the diseases they produced.[72]

Seguin defended the idea of a special human body thermometer claiming that it belonged in the same class of instruments as the lactometer for measuring breast milk, the saccharmometer for measuring blood sugar, the acetometer for measuring vinegar and alcohol, and the urinometer for measuring urine, all of which had unique scales.[73] Seguin recommended that to be completely equipped a physician carry an additional thermometer, known as the Walfardin thermometer, which was calibrated into four hundred degrees and marked in one-fifth-degree separations. The zero level of this instrument could be set at any point along the immense scale which made it convenient to conceal the actual body temperature from the patient.[74] Two decades later, Mercier reported to the Zurich Medical Society that he had devised a thermometer without a scale for the same purpose. After the instrument was taken from the patient, a case marked with a scale could be slipped over it and the temperature recorded.[75]

NINETEENTH-CENTURY THERMOMETERS:

Because of its uniform expansion, mercury was reintroduced commercially as the preferred liquid for thermometers in 1822.[76] The slow rise in the zero point of mercury thermometers, previously noted by Angelo Bellini in 1808,[77] but not acted upon in the design of thermometers, was rediscovered by L. Gourdon. He explained this shift as due to the release of a small amount of air from the mercury. The ability of a small amount of air to move mercury inspired Prof. John Phillips, a geologist in Oxford, to incorporate this property into his design of the first self-registering thermometer in 1832. The mercury thermometer became important in clinical medicine a quarter of a century later and was reinvented in 1855 by the French civil servant Francois Hippolyte Walfardin.[78] It consisted of a half-inch portion of mercury manuevered so that it was detached from the remainder of the mercury column by an air space. As the column of mercury expanded and rose when exposed to heat, the detached portion was carried along with it. When the column receded upon being cooled and contracted, the separated portion remained at the point to which it had been propelled. Noyes explained,

The mercury squeezing through the narrowest part of the constriction tends to take that shape which has a minimum surface—that is, a sphere. The globules then rush through the contraction in small drops . . ., and the mercury above

the contraction is never in contact with the mercury in the bulb. The only way to get the mercury from above the contraction is to shake it down by means of centrifugal force. Unfortunately, all clinical thermometers do not act as they are supposed to act, and in some of them the mercury above the contraction tends to run back into the bulb and will run back unless the bulb is cooled so rapidly that it cannot run through fast enough and so breaks.[79]

Louis P. Casella, instrument maker to the Admiralty, reported on 19 October 1869 in the *Medical Times and Gazette* that Phillips exhibited his thermometer for the first time at the Great Exhibition in 1851. Number 3745 of section 5 of the catalogue lists "Thermometric apparatus used in Physiological Research" in which are included clinical thermometers made according to Dr. Phillips' principle by Francis Pastorelli.[80] John Welch adapted the self-registering thermometer for meteorologic use by detaching a larger portion of mercury to make the index. The index thermometer received no notice from physicians until William Aitkin of the Royal Victoria Hospital in Netley looked for a more suitable thermometer to use in carrying on his studies of fevers in the mid-1850s (see figure 4.2). Aitkin arranged to have Casella produce a self-registering instrument about ten inches long. The length was increased to expand the distance between the degree markings and also to keep the graduations a sufficient distance from the bulb.[81] Aitkin believed that inexperienced individuals needed the extra separation between the bulb and the graduations to prevent them from shaking the index down into the bulb.[82] The elongation acted as a supplementary reservoir to catch the index before it entered the bulb.

Among a number of similar improvements to the instrument was the insertion of a slight enlargement of the thermometer bore a short distance above the bulb, which was produced by the American firm of F. G. Otto and Son of New York. In 1855 a method was found to permit the mercury column to be trapped at its foot, and yet, when partially shaken into the bulb, allow it to rise again during its next use (see figure 4.3). For those who had difficulty in shaking the mercury back into the bulb, Aitkin of Belfast suggested a device permitting the thermometer to be swung freely, thus using centrifugal force to reset the index. Fannin and Co. of Ireland manufactured a small band with eyelet holes for a cord with a knot at each end to be fastened to each instrument for this purpose.[83] To ensure greater visibility of the mercury column, Harvey and Reynolds of Leeds applied a convex lens in front of the index.[84] However, it re-

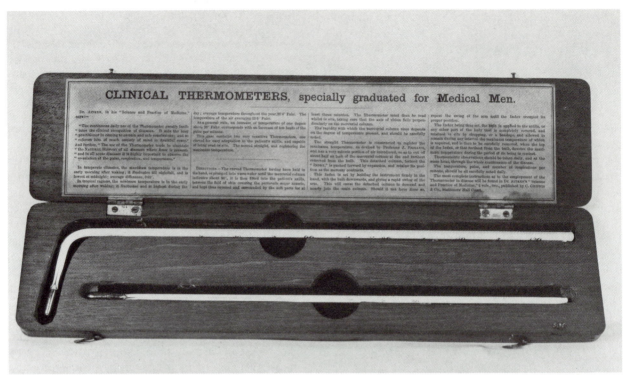

Figure 4.2. 1865 thermometer of the type recommended by William Aitkin. Anon., no date. *Wellcome No. R 2075/1936, Wellcome Photo No. M 11464.*

quired good eyesight to distinguish the mercury column within the glass tube, which has a diameter about the size of the human hair.[85]

Ten years later, the thermometer was strengthened at the constriction of the index to minimize breakage when it was dropped or bitten into (see figure 4.4). Hospitals were concerned over the cost of replacing broken thermometers. One estimate of the financial loss in London each year was that it was equal to the cost of two hospital beds.[86] An American practitioner in Shreveport, Louisiana suggested that the gutta percha thermometer cases be lined with velvet to minimize breakage while carrying them, especially when riding in a horse and buggy.[87] Other suggestions for preserving the thermometer while transporting it included securing the instrument in a case with wads of cotton or by wrapping rubberbands about it, or using a case molded to the shape of the instrument which would hold the thermometer securely in place.[88]

By registering the highest point reached by the thermometer when placed in or on the body and maintaining the point until it was shaken down, the mercury index presented wider opportunities for the physician to use the thermometer. He could, as

James Finlayson did, leave several self-registering thermometers with a patient and instruct someone in the household to take the patient's temperature at specific times of the day, and then set the thermometer aside to be read by the physician upon his return the next day.[89] Edwyn Andrew Shrewsbury had a case of two thermometers, one marked morning and the other marked night, which he left for the same purpose. These instruments were carried in a case seven inches long and one inch wide and they were made by Harvey and Reynolds of Leeds.[90] Clifford Allbutt had called upon these instrument makers for his own thermometers and praised their skill in his widely influential publications directed to the value of temperature recording in medicine (see figure 4.5).[91] The direct benefit to the physician using the self-registering thermometer was that he did not have to bend over the patient to read it, which was especially important when the patient had a contagious disease such as typhus fever.[92] For those who were learning to use the thermometer, it was recommended that they not use the self-registering type until they had studied the changes in temperature visible with the regular thermometer and had learned to appreciate the significance of these changes. It was possible

CLINICAL THERMOMETERS.

Please Read and Carefully Observe these Directions.

Thermometers are in working order, and always ready for application when the top part of the small bit of mercury that forms the Index is below the arrow point. After using it, and in order to bring the Index again below the arrow point and ready for use, take the top part of the stem of the Thermometer (near the 105) between the thumb and first finger, with the bulb turned downward, or inclined toward the floor. In this position quietly swing from you (like a pendulum) from the elbow down, leave wrist hang as loose as possible. Always look at the position of your Index after each swing, until you again see the top part of it below the arrow point, and it is again ready for application. If it be found that one or two quiet swings is not sufficient to bring the top part of the Index below the arrow point let your swing be somewhat forcible. Don't shake the Index lower than is necessary.

One or more separations of the column does not put the instrument out of order. Always take the top part of the top separation for a reading, and so long as any separation remains the instrument is good for years.

By observing these directions you will have no trouble with your Thermometer.

FIG.		
*2892	Sharp & Smith's Self-Registering Indestructible Index Thermometer..	$1 25
2893	Sharp & Smith's Self-Registering Indestructible Index Thermometer, black....................................	1 50
*2894	Sharp & Smith's (Gilt Case and Chain) Self-Registering Indestructible Index Thermometer....................	1 75
*2895	Sharp & Smith's (one minute) Self-Registering Indestructible Index Thermometer.............................	1 50
*2896	Hicks' Self-Registering Indestructible Index Thermometer.	1 50
2897	" Lens front " " " "	2 75
*2898	Spiral " " " " "	1 25
*2899	T. & Co.'s Syphon " " " " "	2 50
*2900	Spiral Surface Self-Registering Thermometer ....$6 00 to	7 50
2900A	Surface " " .... 2 50 to	7 50
*2901	Seguin's Surface " "	2 00

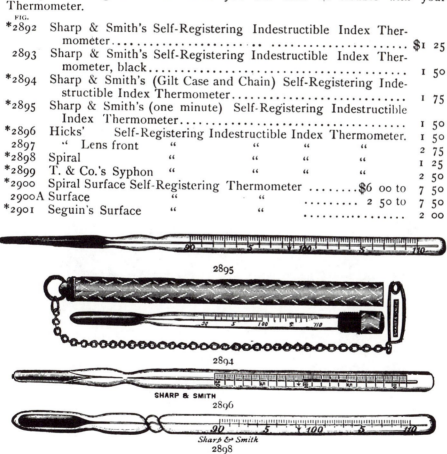

Figure 4.3. **Four types of clinical thermometers in 1889 advertisement** of Sharp and Smith Catalogue, p. 534. *SI Photo No. 79-5036*

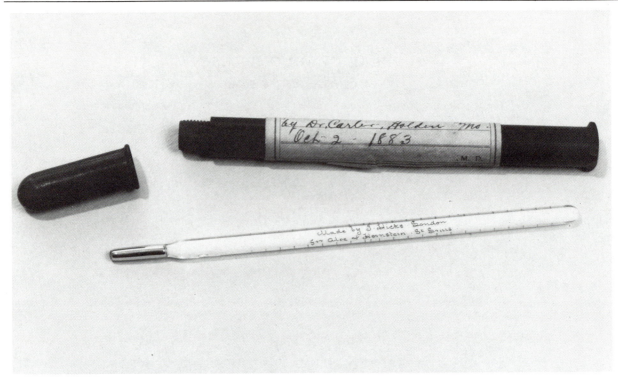

Figure 4.4. Clinical thermometer owned in 1883 by Dr. Carter Holden and donated by Dr. Paul Johnstone to the History and Philosophy of Medicine Department of the University of Kansas Medical Center, Kansas City, Kansas. *Kansas No. 36372.*

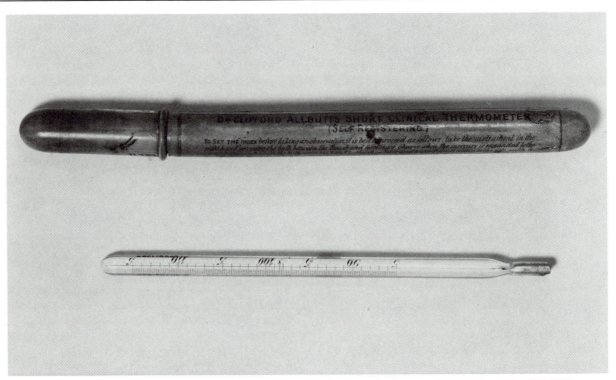

Figure 4.5. Dr. Clifford Allbutt's short clinical thermometer (self-registering), anon., no date. *Wellcome No. 2038/1936 Wellcome Photo No. M 18985.*

to notice the slight slippage of the mercury in thermometers without an index, which then needed to be recalibrated.[93]

PROBLEMS WITH THERMOMETERS:

CALIBRATION:

One problem persisted with all thermometers: to sustain their calibration. Engraving or etching the scale directly on the thermometer tube was essential for clinical applications. Thermometers appear to have first been etched at the end of the eighteenth century, since several by the maker Crichton, who worked in this period, remain in Paris.[94] Thermometers etched in glass graduations to one-fifth degree Fahrenheit and one-tenth degree Celsius were called for by Finlayson in 1874 and Curtis in 1872, whereas accuracy to one-half degree was generally considered ample at this time. Accuracy remained a transient quality unobtainable until the end of the century.

When it was realized that it was not the enclosed air but the changes within the glass that altered the thermometer scale, annealed glass thermometers required recalibration.[95] In England thermometers were checked for accuracy at the Kew Observatory in London.[96] One way for manufacturers to compensate for the fluctuation of the zero point of mercury thermometers due to the expansion of glass was to store newly manufactured thermometers at least several months before calibrating them.[97] The problem of the expansion of glass was solved when Frederick Otto Schoot of Jena discovered a special stable glass for making thermometers in 1891.[98] Known as "Jena Normal," this glass expanded and contracted one-tenth as much as regular glass.[99] Meanwhile, physicians who used the thermometer were cautioned about its main deficiency. Allbutt recommended that every clinical thermometer be checked for accuracy six to twelve months after its purchase.[100] The best clinical thermometer available was manufactured by Mr. Hawksley, who formerly was a foreman in the shop of Baker and Holborn of London. It was six inches long, of which five inches were marked in twenty Fahrenheit degrees, providing one quarter of an inch for each degree, which was further divided into five parts.[101] The glass of the bulb was "dulled" to make it more heat absorbent. Three minutes was the recommended time required to hold the thermometer in the mouth and record the temperature accurately. On the cover of its wooden case, the Centigrade and Fahrenheit scales were marked so that

they could be easily interconverted. The case was made square so that it would not roll off a surface.[102] Fox recommended that a physician purchase a thermometer that was two to three years old, designed on the Phillip's principle, calibrated from 90 to 112 degrees Fahrenheit, and certified by an observatory.[103] A clinical thermometer that could be calibrated at the time of its use with an attached scale or timed according to how fast the index reached its maximum after exposure to the body was made by Eduoard Seguin in 1875. He called his instrument a clinical thermoscope, which was modeled after the differential thermometer of Rumford and Leslie in 1804.[104] It consisted of a glass tube with a one-quarter line bore seven inches long, closed at one end by a bulb nine lines in diameter and open at the other end. The water index was prepared by heating the bulb to dilate the air and quickly plunging the open end into one inch of cold water so that a drop or two would be taken into the tube. If the water stopped near the bulb, it became the index, since the air behind the water index became isothermal to ambient temperature. The bulb was then put into the patient's hand and within five to ten seconds, the index reached its maximum height or descent. The starting point and the time it took to reach the other point were recorded. If a scale was attached it was lined up with the index and the level it reached read off the scale directly; therefore, the thermoscope was always correctly calibrated, a quality Seguin noted, not possessed by other clinical thermometers at this time.[105]

American thermometer manufacturers were at a disadvantage with their European competitors until a calibration center was established in the United States. In 1880 the Thermometric Bureau of the Yale College of New Haven, Connecticut, at the recommendation of the Board of Managers of Winchester Observatory, began to verify the calibration of thermometers and issue certificates of accuracy.[106] Certificates stating the amount of correction needed at each degree were returned with the thermometer. To obviate the necessity of keeping a separate paper with corrections with the instrument, James Hicks of London patented a device for etching the corrected point on the glass tube. It was manufactured by Shepard and Dudley of New York.[107] The observatory also provided a few standardized thermometers for use by the manufacturers. Until the Yale standards center opened, manufacturers approached whomever they could find to acquire a standard to check the calibration of their newly manufactured thermometers.[108]

A brochure was prepared to explain the service

provided by the Thermometric Bureau. Leonard Waldo, astronomer in charge of the Bureau, stipulated that all thermometers sent into the observatory for calibration must have the name of the owner and the serial number of the manufacturer etched on the glass. Instruments with graduations engraved on the glass were preferred and only those scales, printed or stamped on the thermometer mount, that were of good quality workmanship would be accepted. Charges for his service varied from fifty cents per clinical thermometer to one dollar for a standard meteorologic thermometer. It was necessary to recalibrate the self-registering thermometer as well, since it would perform erratically if too much air separated the index from the mercury column. Any air lodged above the index would force the index down after the thermometer had cooled, thus losing its value as a marker.[109]

One request that the observatory could not meet was to record on the thermometer the time it took for the thermometer to reach its maximum level. E. R. Squibb in 1882 asked for this service since thermometers varied a good deal in this respect. However, the observatory was not able to devise a simple test for approximating the conditions that would prevail during use with the patient, and therefore, could not measure this factor. Depending on the thickness and shape of the glass, the thermometer had to remain in contact with the body from three, five, fifteen up to thirty minutes.[110] Thermometers that would reach the maximum temperature in one minute or less were advertised widely in the 1890s (see figure 4.6). Charles Truax of Chicago advertised a one-minute thermometer in 1893. In 1897 Fannin and Co. of Dublin sold an instrument which they claimed reached its maximum level in half a minute.[111]

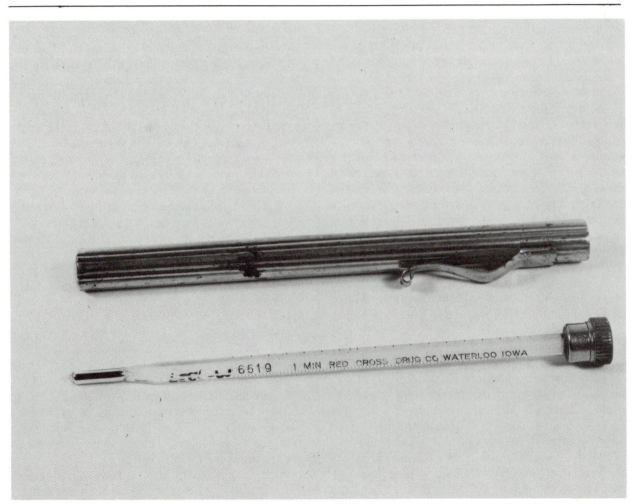

Figure 4.6. One-minute thermometer. Red Cross Drug Co. of Waterloo, Iowa. *NMAH, No. M 7337, SI Photo No. 78-705.*

In the first few years, physicians took increasing advantage of the observatory's calibration service. In 1880 and 1881, physicians sent in 1,637 thermometers, in the following year 3,811 thermometers, and two years later 6,321 instruments were turned over for calibration.[112] The Kew Observatory received 3,400 thermometers for calibration from British physicians in 1876.[113] American physicians imported fewer than fifty thermometers from England in 1867, but more than 3,000 instruments by 1876.[114] The increasing use of thermometers by the medical profession over the next decades was testified to by Orran T. Sherman of Baltimore, Maryland, who examined thirty to forty thousand thermometers for the Yale Observatory up to his retirement in 1893.[115] In 1901 the National Bureau of Standards was established in Washington, D.C., and one of its initial services to American industries was to check the calibration of thermometers.

Under the direction of C. W. Waidner, a thermometric testing station was inaugurated to which American manufacturers sent their instruments for calibration. The thermometers the Bureau used as its standards were graduated according to the international hydrogen scale adopted by the International Committee of Weights and Measures in 1887. To compare newly manufactured thermometers with the standard

the thermometers are immersed in a tank of water whose temperature can be controlled by means of hot and cold water and a system of heating coils through which current can be passed at the will of the observer, who thus is enabled to secure with accuracy any desired temperature. The thermometers are read by means of the small microscope through the glass window in the cylinder, while an electrically driven agitator keeps the water in constant circulation. Such an instrument enables a direct comparison to be made between a standard and other thermometers for all points between the boiling and freezing points of water. The first practical result of this activity . . . was to bring to the same standard scale of temperature all the makes of clinical thermometers in the United States, and this was immediately shown in a highly improved grade of thermometers.[116]

Lots of twenty-four instruments, each one separately numbered, were placed in a rack to be whirled for throwing the index down, and then, to be compared with the standard. Equipment was installed to test six hundred thermometers in half an hour.[117] For an instrument to merit certification, the difference at any point in the two tests given to each instrument could not be greater than 0.15 degree Fahrenheit. At

the end of the year 1904, of the thermometers submitted for testing to the bureau, 88.2 percent were certified.[118]

One of the largest American manufacturers of thermometers in the nineteenth and twentieth centuries, the Taylor Instrument Company of Rochester, New York, made the equivalent of "Jena Normal" known as "Corning Normal" glass thermometers (see figure 4.7). Although this glass was the least subject to shrinkage, to ensure complete safety from change, the blank glass tubes were laid aside for four months before the scales were engraved on them.[119] As a result of suggestions by physicians like W. B. Kesteven and Eduoard Seguin[120] that thermometers not be marked until the glass had seasoned or had contracted completely, sealed and numbered ungraded thermometers were sent to the Yale Observatory for aging before being calibrated.

SIZE:

The length of the thermometer was important to the clinician, who often preferred a short instrument. Short instruments had been described since the seventeenth century. The first clinical thermometer, which was designed by du Val of Paris, as we have noted above was three inches long, four or five lines in diameter, and contained a mercury column half a line in diameter.[121] In 1800, the London chemists, Allen and Howard, advertised a portable thermometer five inches long and one-quarter inch in diameter. The scale extended from 80 to 112 degrees and was attached to the tube enclosed in a cylindrical case. It was advertised as sensitive enough to record the maximum temperature in ten seconds.[122] The English instrument maker Casella recalled that in 1839 he had seen a small clinical thermometer which contained a round bore, and although not graduated on its stem, he thought it was accurate.[123] Even though smaller clinical thermometers were known since the seventeenth century until the last quarter of the nineteenth century, clinical thermometers were often as long as one foot. In 1867, Clifford Allbutt recommended that they be made shorter, so that more physicians would use them. A small chamber in the bulb was designed to collect the mercury when the reading was low, thereby shortening the instrument. By 1895, it was generally accepted that a scale of ten degrees provided a sufficient range of markings on a clinical thermometer, specifically from 97 degrees Fahrenheit to 107 degrees Fahrenheit. C. Fahrney of Harrisburg, Pennsylvania, recommended that clinical thermometers be manufactured within

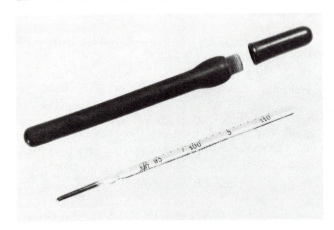

Figure 4.7. Taylor Instrument Company medical thermometer and case circa 1900. *SI Photo No. 74-4397.*

this range of degrees, so that the degree markings could be spaced further apart for easier reading, and the thermometer made smaller so that it could be carried on a watch chain.[125] The scales for thermometers usually were printed in black until the noted British manufacturer, Arnold and Sons, patented a clinical thermometer with red indelible numbers in 1875.[126]

By the twentieth century, the most useful medical thermometer remained, as described in 1869 by an American reviewer of Wunderlich's text, "the ordinary mercurial thermometer with such modifications only as are necessitated by an application to the person, by the limited range of bodily temperature, and for accuracy of observation."[127] The manufacturers of these instruments were concentrated in a few Western European countries until the turn of the century. A brief review of the instruments sold by a number of these producers indicates the range of thermometers available to medical practitioners and the types of instruments medical instrument collections might contain (see figure 4.8).

STATE OF THE INDUSTRY:

England produced the most accurate and finely crafted medical thermometers in the nineteenth century. The firm of Casella, which supplied thermometers for meteorologic observations and scientific research throughout the century, provided the most valued clinical thermometers to many practitioners. Etched graduations on the glass tubes of various sizes in a range of scales, with or without an index, were among the finer details perfected by Casella. He claimed in an advertisement that "The only real improvements which have been made in these instruments were accomplished by the *Originator* who first

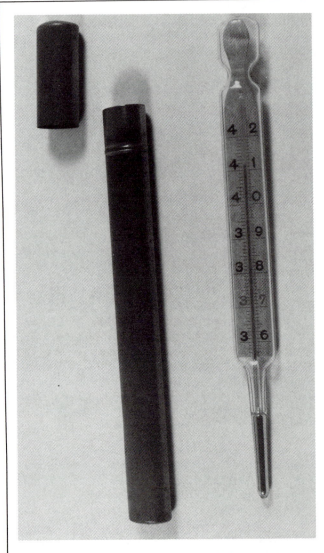

Figure 4.8 Clinical thermometer in centigrade degrees with wooden scale and Red Cross symbol. *NMAH No. M 10725, SI Photo No. 78-704.*

designed them, and now has much pleasure in introducing his *NEW PATENT PROTECTED INSTRUMENT*, which he guarantees cannot be disarranged by any amount of violence, either in the hands of the physician or the most inexperienced person."[128] Negretti and Zambra, Smith and Beck,[129] and Hawksley of London were competitors in producing quality thermometers. Harvey and Reynolds of Leeds[130] manufactured thermometers under the guidance of the physicians William Aitkin and Clifford Allbutt.[131] By the 1880s, Ferris and Evan's and Wormull also manufactured thermometers.[132] F. Darton and Company of West Smithfield regularly exhibited their thermometers, which ranged from two to six inches in length, at the annual museum of the British Medical Association and the seventh International Congress of Hygiene and Demography in London.[133] Primavesi Brothers of Bournemouth sold recording thermometers.[134] Dr. Alfred Eddons of Market Drayton, Salop designed and sold a thermophant, which was reported to be a thermometer for indicating and controlling the temperature within desired limits.[135] Griffin imported German thermometers.[136] In the last decades of the century, a number of medical and surgical instrument makers, including Arnold and Sons of London, George Tiemann of New York, and Codman and Shurtleff of Boston[137] were selling thermometers, which they manufactured or sold for the major producers as a service to their customers. In the *Journal of the American Medical Association* (JAMA) in the last decades of the nineteenth century, Codman and Shurtleff advertised English thermometers as the most correct and reliable, especially those made by James J. Hicks of London.[138]

Self-registering thermometers were manufactured in the United States from 1872 (see figure 4.9). Weinhagen of New York, established in 1885, advertised proudly in 1893 that they were continuing to deserve their fine reputation by producing the finest grade thermometers in the world.[139] *JAMA* carried advertisements for Weinhagen thermometers beginning in the mid-1880s when the first issues of this journal appeared. Some of these advertisements featured an instrument mounted on a black surface and containing a broad mercury column for use in a darkened room.[140]

German manufacturers included Charles F. Giessler and Son of Berlin and William Hack of Thueringen.[141] Thermometers manufactured in Germany, where some of the earliest and most convincing medical evidence for using the thermometer in the clinic was gathered, frequently contained scales detached from the body of the thermometer instead of being etched on the glass. The thermometer was inserted into a tube into which the paper scale was placed. These thermometers were less expensive but also less accurate and more difficult to read.[142] By 1895 Hicks refined this arrangement by placing a transparent scale within the body of the thermometer. His motivation was to provide a smooth, unetched surface on the thermometer, so that it could be kept sterilized and not retain bacteria in the small crevices of the etching. A second result was to preserve the scale from wearing away in the process of wiping the instrument to keep it clean. The tube could also be made of magnifying glass to enlarge the scale.[143]

A special thermometer was designed by Immisch, who received a patent for it on 3 January 1882 (see figure 4.10). Shaped like a pocket watch, one inch in

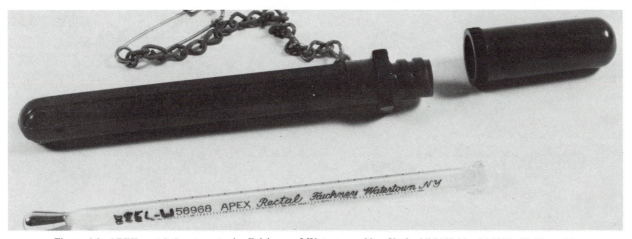

Figure 4.9. APEX rectal thermometer by Faichney of Watertown, New York. *NMAH No. M 7338, SI Photo No. 78-711.*

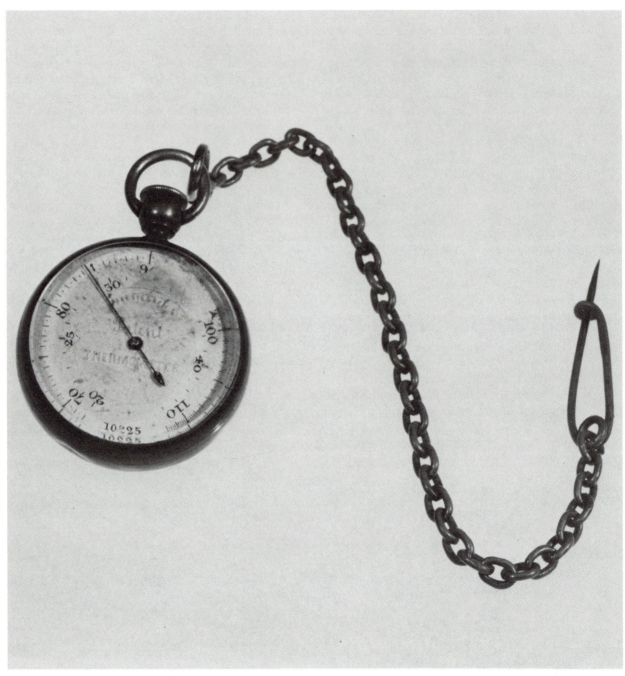

Figure 4.10. 1882 Immisch thermometer advertised in A. S. Aloe Surgical Instruments and Supplies Catalogue circa 1893, Patent 1882, p. 577. *SI Photo No. 81-2539.*

diameter, "the action of the instrument depended upon the opening and closing of a metallic tube which is filled with highly expansive liquids, . . ."[144] therefore, it is not subject to barometric pressure changes. It was designed for measuring the body surface temperature. With a stop button placed on top, the temperature recorded could be locked into place and reset without shaking the instrument. Easy to apply, safe, small, and accurate even with age, this thermometer received the first-class award at the International Medical Congress in 1881 and three silver medals in 1885 and 1886. Alfred L. Loomis of New York endorsed it in advertisements placed in *JAMA* by Sardy, Coles and Co. of New York, who were owners of the American patent.[145]

Not all improvements in the design of thermometers were suggested by manufacturers. A professor of chemistry at Union College, Schenectady, New York suggested in 1877 that thermometer scales could be restored by painting the instrument with an alcohol solution of an aniline dye. The aniline was not soluble in water, which ensured that the marks would remain intact a long while even after frequent use.[146]

The manufacturer, J. Gall of New York, improved the thermometer by fusing a glass convex cylinder of very short focus on the outer surface of the stem to magnify the index, which could be read in the horizontal position.[147] Block's thermometer with a sliding magnifying glass appeared in the early twentieth century.[148]

A thermometer with a flattened back to prevent it from rolling off a surface was introduced by Arnold and Sons in 1896. The numbers were marked on the back of the instrument, so that they would not obscure the column of mercury.[149]

The Surgeon General of the United States, Walter Reed, directed the manufacture of a self-sterilizing thermometer case, patented in 1895. It was tested repeatedly and found to kill disease germs placed on it within twenty-five minutes or less. In the bottom of the hard rubber case was placed a pledget of cotton soaked in glyceraldehyde, a formaldehyde-based substance, which volatilized, allowing the fumes to course over the instrument when placed in the case after each use.[150]

Hicks designed a broader and flatter thermometer bulb by joining two parallel tubes of mercury, encased in glass and brought together at the index. This bulb was expected to be more sensitive, easier to place in the body, and more resistant to breakage.[151]

By the end of the century, English thermometers continued to be ranked among the best produced. One proof of their excellence rests in the great number of instruments, sent by manufacturers and certified at Kew Observatory, that were found not to require recalibration.[152] An issue of the *Boston Medical and Surgical Journal* in 1893 carried a notice that, because of the excessive cost, few American-made thermometers were being sent to the Yale Observatory. Of those sent in, which were carefully selected, sometimes 25 percent up to 75 percent were rejected. The editorialist speculated that when manufacturers thought that their instruments would not be checked at the observatory, their workers slackened off and produced less accurate instruments.[153] The most popular American clinical thermometer in the last decade of the century was one constructed with an indestructible register, formed by a small contraction near the bulb that permitted the mercury column to rise, but to break when contracting or cooling, thus leaving the column above it as a stationary register until shaken down by the operator. Most clinical thermometers were provided with this constriction.[154]

The thermometer lacked the physical appeal of other medical instruments, especially the microscope and stethoscope. Instruments with wider applications, as in the microscope used to explore plant as well as animal tissues, led to the design of a greater variety of models. The pride of owning a brass microscope surpassed the pride in owning a thermometer. As an instrument with popular appeal, the microscope held greater fascination for a large group of people throughout its history. Although possessed of less glamor, the accuracy and convenience of the thermometer provided producers with the prospect of continuing sales to the medical profession and to every household after body temperature became a common denominator for detecting and following the course of a variety of illnesses, a topic to which we shall return below.

THE THERMOMETER AND SPECIALISM:

With the advent of the specialized clinical thermometer in mid-century, data that led to the development and revision of medical theories as well as practices emerged. The historian of medical thermometry, Erich Ebstein, concluded that "since this time, not only the practical but also the theoretical areas of medicine have been influenced by thermometrical methods."[155] The local disease concept soon led to specialized uses of the thermometer.

In keeping with the physician's emphasis on locating and treating disease in specific body parts, the thermometer was applied to selected organs and tissues. In 1878 American specialists, including the neurologist L. C. Gray and the physiologist J. S. Lombard, hoped to obtain more facts about the brain by measuring the temperature of the skull. Gray arranged Seguin's surface thermometers on a belt, which he tied around the skull so that the instruments were placed over the thinnest portions of the bone. Gray regarded a temperature elevation of two to two and a half degrees or more as indicative of a possible abnormality of the brain.[156] The findings of Paul Broca of Paris and Gray were confirmed and extended by Edoardo Maragliano and Guiseppe Seppili of Reggio-Emilia, Italy. They successfully measured the temperature by Gray's method of using a water-filled skull.[157] Another challenge came from François Frank of Paris in 1880. His experiments were repeated by R. W. Avidon of New York with the assistance of Seguin, who proved that heat can be transmitted through "dead human cerebral envelopes in appreciable quantities."[158] George F. Shrady, editor of the *Medical Record*, which reported all phases of research on cerebral thermometric studies, wrote with a touch of cynicism in 1879: "When it is established, as it is hoped it may be, that the value of a thought is to be measured by the amount of cerebral tissue consumed and heat evolved, everyman's intellectual calibre can be definitely established in degrees Fahrenheit, the problems of life will then be greatly simplified."[159] Nevertheless, he predicted that fundamental physiologic correlations would be found with the thermometer. J. S. Lombard of Harvard in 1879 meticulously recorded 60,000 observations to discover the normal range of surface temperatures on the head, the effect of voluntary muscular contractions on the temperature of the skull, and the influence of the surrounding air temperature on the temperature of the head.[160]

J. T. Eskridge, the prolific neurologist, a few years later, showed that variations of head temperature in diseases of the brain appear slowly. Brain lesions combined with congestion and inflammation have a higher local temperature than is the effect of general suppuration within the cranium. The temperature of the scalp and of the brain within is a physiologic, rather than a physical, relationship that is due to the function of the nervous system. Cerebral temperature could provide only limited assistance in diagnosis, but when the brain was organically disturbed, the thermometric variations could be of value.[161]

In the meantime, M. Peter of Paris was investigating the relationship of surface temperature to lung disease and concluded that with careful measure-ments, slight changes in temperature could be detected over the area of internal congestion of inflammatory foci in lung tissues. Few physicians applied or refuted Peter's thermometric method of diagnosis, but he proceeded to adapt the method of thermometric diagnosis of disease to other visceral organs including the stomach. He found an increase of one to two degrees Centigrade in some ailments of this organ.[162]

Diagnosis of internal ear disease was another application of the thermometer. Bogdan Flitner of Russia in 1882 measured the temperature of the external auditory meatus in health and disease.[163] He found that the temperature in the ear bore a uniform relationship to the temperature of the system at large. *JAMA*, reporting on this research, foresaw the possibility of using ear temperature as "a reliable method of detecting, at their outset, obscure inflammatory processes within the cranial cavity."[164] Joseph Edwards of Toronto in 1891 reported a rise of from one-eighth to one degree in temperature when the thermometer was inserted into the ear canal of an inflamed middle ear. A colleague, Birkitt, had applied the thermometer to the mastoid bone to detect deep-seated ear disease and expected the method to become an important diagnostic technique.[165]

Specially designed thermometers for specialists who wanted to know the body temperature of a patient were exemplified by the one recommended to gynecologists. It displayed unusual ingenuity. Otto Kuestner of Jena in 1879 described the thermometer, which was inserted into a silver female catheter for recording the temperature of the urine. He explained:

The catheter tapers sharply below the point to which the bulb of the thermometer reaches, [and] . . . near the external end provides for the escape of the urine. . . . The thermometer is firmly soldered to a silver top which fits closely into the outer end of the catheter. . . . The space left between the thermometer and the wall of the catheter [allows] the urine [to] pass freely, bathing the thermometer in its course. . . . When the instrument is introduced into a moderately filled bladder, the column of mercury in the thermometer attains its maximum point in from eight to fifteen seconds according to the rapidity with which the urine escapes. . . . The average quantity of urine that escapes through the instrument in fifteen seconds is about sixty centimeters [about two ounces].[166]

Its advantage was to record the temperature in a much shorter period, than the usual five minutes required if the instrument was placed in the vagina or under the arm. Oertman of Germany had been the first to suggest measuring the temperature of the urine to determine body temperature. He proposed having the patient urinate on the bulb of the thermometer, which "was intended only for the use of men, and moreover only for men who pass larger streams of urine."[167]

The first clinical maximal thermometer was devised by Karl Ehrle in 1886 and displayed a ten-degree spread between thirty-three to forty-three degrees Centigrade. It could be applied to specific parts of the body. Another suggestion by Oertman in 1904-1905 was to insert a thermometer into a hemorrhoidal pessary.[168] The glassblowers Frank of Halle, Geissler of Bonn, and C. Erbe of Tuebingen made these instruments.

THE THERMOMETER AND SOCIETY:

Moving the diagnostic signs of disease to an earlier stage in the disease process reinforced the search for the stage at which it would be possible to prevent disease. Prevention with concomitant social and economic benefits became the theme for a number of authors who promoted the use of instruments in diagnosis. The thermometer offered maximum opportunities for use in preventive disease programs. The most imaginative medical exponent of the thermometer and its implications for social change was Eduoard Seguin, who appended his lengthy views to an abridged translation of Wunderlich's 1868 volume on thermometry in 1871 and an expanded second edition in 1876.[169]

Seguin captured the enthusiasm of Émile Littré, the noted translator of Hippocrates and member of the Institute of France, who prophesied: "Human thermometry will render such services in families, in schools, and in society, that we must not tire of preaching it until public opinion will be fully aware of its usefulness."[170] Seguin, who had spent his career between 1837 and 1866 organizing schools for subnormal children in France and the United States, set up the first school for idiots in 1839.[171] After 1848, he found it politically expedient to come to the United States, where he spent his first decade in Cleveland. Finally, settling in New York, he spent the last decade of his life promoting the thermometer and the metric system in medicine.[172] Seguin provided the most effective English language assessment of medical thermometry. Wunderlich inspired Seguin to publish his wide-ranging views and to design a special clinical thermometer discussed earlier. Seguin's success lay in making American physicians aware of the value of the thermometer in medical diagnosis

and encouraging them to understand the social forces its use could unleash.

Seguin's statements on the thermometer and other medical instruments, explaining how they enriched life, are the most explicit on these points and demonstrate how it was possible to envision that medical technology would contribute to social advancement. In a lyrical and exuberant style, he described the potential health improving and health guidance aspects of taking body temperature on a regular schedule.

But who knows what medical . . . thermometry could do, when the simplicity of its procedures, the adaptability of its instruments, the number of its devotees will permit its applications, not only to the treatment, but to the prevention of disease, and especially to the high supervision of the training of youth, in reference to the dosing of air, moisture, heat, light, food, exercise, studies, in the sickly conditions of the growing stages. Then we can understand that for physicians thermometry is not only knowledge, but social power.[173]

To reach these goals Seguin emphasized that thermometry was a simple procedure, so that individuals other than physicians could be expected to record the temperature accurately. The main criterion was to provide a simple thermometer that everyone could learn to apply.[174] By amassing temperature data on a wide scale, Seguin recognized the possibility of being able to detect health changes correlated with such characteristics as age, location, and occupation, which might then be corrected before serious problems developed. He believed the thermometer could become an instrument for the control of disease on a community-wide basis, making medicine the arbiter of social actions.[175] In replacing the pulse as the cornerstone of diagnosis, thermometry could play a role in the family, school, insurance office, workshop, prison, army, navy, and hospital.[176]

Seguin's statistical approach to classification of health and disease expressed itself in his call for the compilation of numerous records of all patients, regardless of the severity or unusual nature of their diseases. He pointed out that the greatest medical observers, such as Sydenham, Andral, Louis, and Wunderlich "have demonstrated that the most ordinary diseases and most plain cases are the most fruitful subjects of observation which are useful for the progress of theory and practice of medicine."[177] Therefore, he recommended that all physicians send the records they collected to their county or state medical society, which would, in turn, compile them with the records of their colleagues. Publishing studies containing temperature records was hailed as an effective method of

inducing some of the excellent practitioners of medicine in the South, U.S.A. who have not yet adopted the use of the clinical thermometer, to resort to it, not only for their own satisfaction, and in the interest of their patients, but for furnishing additional graphic delineations of the course of yellow fever. And also, of the various forms of malarial fevers, which have not yet been sufficiently investigated by this method.[178]

Seguin predicted that in the next fifteen years the thermometer would be the source of the next milestone in medical progress.

To distinguish between graduated instruments including the thermometer, the microscope, aesthesiometer, dynamometer, sphygmograph, and others applied to physical diagnosis, he called the former numerically based devices, instruments of "positive diagnosis." Through positive diagnosis, he believed "we will soon be able to settle, like mathematical affairs, all questions relating not only to disease, but to vitality, longevity, training studies, sports, indulgences, labors, individual and social fitness."[179]

Since these instruments provided immediate information that did not depend on the judgment of the individual applying them, Seguin encouraged the widest use of them. He wanted the public to be educated, to understand fully the "individual, commercial and social value of the 'predictions' founded upon the signs of health and vitality given out by the physical, chemical, microscopic and thermometeric methods of diagnosis."[180] The main function of the physician in society was "to advise not the sick, but those who being well or apparently well, may become exposed [and lose] vitality by the straining of the exigencies of modern life."[181] These strains could come from jobs, business, and social arrangements in which people engaged. To understand the impact on health of the various exposures to contemporary social conditions was a novel element in Seguin's program of disease prevention and health preservation through medical examination with special devices. Emphasis on the inception and earliest stages of disease, rather than on the cure of existing disease permeated Seguin's plans. At the core of this advance in his view was "thermometry, which will find new laws of disease, new relations of temperature to the various modes of vitality, new standards of observation and new means of communicating them among physicians."[182] One means to achieve his goals was to

have a thermometer placed in every home and have it used regularly.[183]

Seguin's plans for accumulating voluminous temperature records led him to investigate the main sources of diagnostic records of normal individuals—the life insurance policy applicant records and to recommend how these records could be improved. He was critical of the usual physical diagnostic methods employed because they did not provide sufficient information for making the diagnosis of future terminal diseases. The applicant who might feel the earliest symptoms of diseases was among those more inclined to buy life insurance. It was all too readily granted to him by the company, which accepted the doctor's favorable prognosis based on a physical examination consisting of superficial tests like auscultation and percussion, which could not, in isolation, readily detect the earliest signs of dangerous diseases. However, it was possible to detect those signs, Seguin believed, if a physician applied the various modes of positive diagnosis, thereby advising the company against insuring poor health risk applicants. Tuberculosis, the greatest disease threat of the age, could be more effectively diagnosed early with the aid of the thermometer. By saving lives, preventing serious disorders through early detection, and revealing the best methods of educating children, "thermometry—without ceasing to be 'medical,' becomes 'human.' It fulfills the prophesy of Descartes *"if it is possible to improve mankind, physic will give us the means thereof."*[184]

Public reaction to the thermometer in the nineteenth century is reflected in some comments made by hospitalized patients. Patients both understood and misunderstood the purpose of the instrument. Hospital attendants in 1876 reported that one woman attributed her relapse in recovering from a fever to "no glass under her arm for a week," while a man with rheumatism refused to have his temperature taken because "it took too much out of him." Other patients assumed the purpose of the thermometer was to discover when one of them had consumed unauthorized food, a misconception encouraged by nurses anxious to control the patient's diet.[185] Patients or relatives of patients occasionally expected the thermometer to provide convincing evidence of their diseases and their progress in being cured. They tolerated the abuse of the instrument such as that cited by L. M. Powers of Los Angeles, who was shocked to witness colleagues carrying mucus-encrusted instruments to their patients. He insisted that the instrument be cleaned after each use.[186]

CONCLUSION:

Clinicians, manufacturers, and society all shared in the benefits of thermometry. Charles Wilson Ingraham in 1895 described the effect of the thermometer on medical diagnosis and treatment in this way:

Not a day passes but that the fever-thermometer gives additional evidence of its being one of the most accurate and scientific diagnostic instruments. . . . Though the thermometer is but a piece of glass containing mercury, yet it diffuses information that sways the opinions of physicians in council; it indicates the best course of treatment to pursue, it decides doubtful points, and brings order, and method out of confusion and uncertainty. In the practice of every physician, many lives are annually saved by what the fever thermometer had detected and brought forth for consideration. Fatal complications are averted, and unfavorable changes, particularly in the course of acute disease, are, by its use, detected sufficiently early to allow of prompt treatment. We cannot but wonder how our ancestors could have intelligently practiced medicine and surgery without the aid of the thermometer.[187]

Of particular value for the diagnosis of tuberculosis in the nineteenth century, "the fever thermometer approaches more nearly the zenith of its perfection and utility in cases of suspected tuberculosis."[188]

Requiring a minimal amount of skill to apply it, and yet providing objective diagnostic evidence, the thermometer linked the old and new concepts of disease. (See figures 4.11, 4.12, 4.13, and 4.14.) The thermometer indicated the general physiologic state of the body and could be applied selectively to indicate diseases in specific organs and bodily parts, thus supporting belief in the localized nature of many diseases. Investigators recorded their temperature data gathered from all parts of the body—often from the surface over an internal organ—and frequently noted a difference in temperature when an organ such as the ear, brain, or stomach was diseased. The precision and ease with which the body temperature could be measured encouraged physicians to make and compile records based on hundreds of thousands of individuals. The vast number of records suggested the need and value of describing physiologic and pathologic constants to be classified within the terms or standards derived from many clinical observations. Recognition of the small numerical differences measured by the clinical thermometer in distinguishing health and disease evolved as the instrument was refined.

The design of thermometers contributed to their adoption by the medical community. Until the index

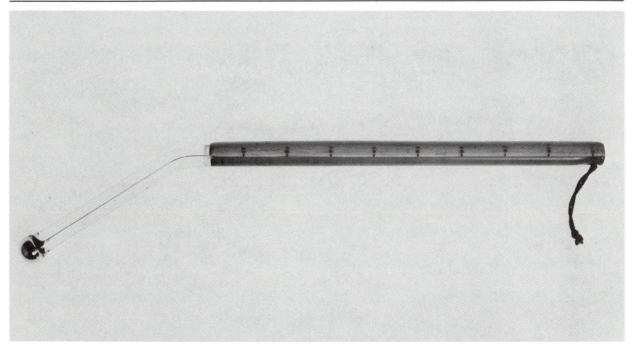

Figure 4.11. Thermometer circa 1800 of the type described by James Currie, anon., no date. *Wellcome No. R 2080/1936, Wellcome Photo No. L 12323.*

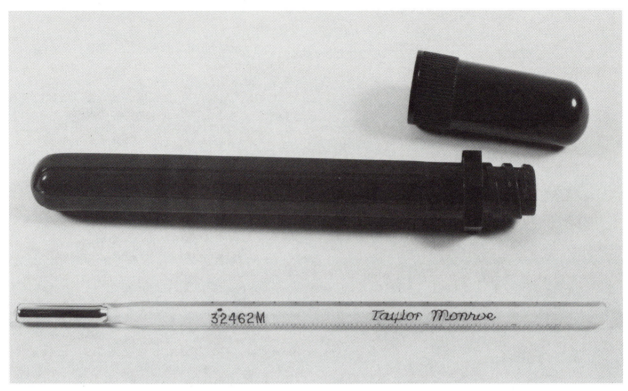

Figure 4.12. Taylor Monroe thermometer. *NMAH No. 11135. SI Photo No. 78-710.*

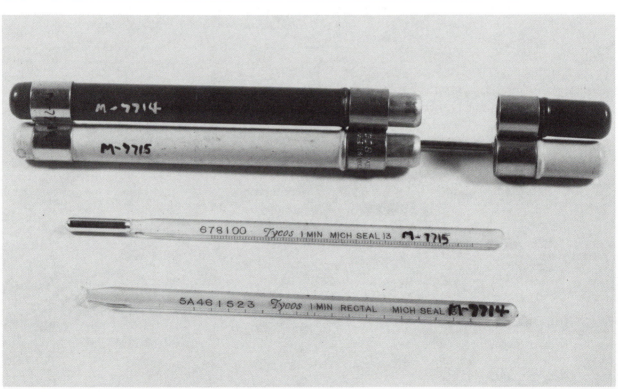

Figure 4.13. Two Tycos thermometers. *NMAH Nos. M 7714 and M 7715, SI Photo No. 78-708.*

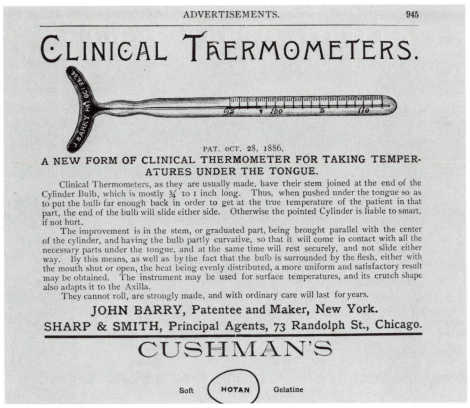

Figure 4.14 1889 John Barry's clinical thermometer sold by Sharp and Smith Surgical Instruments, Chicago. *SI Photo No. 79-5030.*

thermometer appeared, accurate recording of the body temperature was difficult and required immediate attention to the instrument as it was removed or even while it remained in place. This constraint limited its use to those who could be trusted to record the results accurately. With the introduction of the index thermometer, more individuals could give the thermometer to the patient, and if necessary, leave the instrument to be read by the physician when he next visited the patient.

The fever thermometer was the earliest of diagnostic instruments to be supplied in large quantities and to be produced according to rigid standards. The nineteenth-century physician turned to a specialized industry for his clinical thermometers. Because of the instrument's general use in other areas of science and commerce, the thermometer industry was one of the earliest to provide sufficient instruments at low cost and with the high standards demanded by physicians.

The thermometer, more than other diagnostic and surgical instruments of the nineteenth century, convinced physicians that physiologic and pathologic data gathered directly from the body could be quantified in a meaningful way. When combined with similar information collected by the physician's predecessors and colleagues, there ensued a refinement of physiology and pathology not previously imagined or anticipated.

The conceptions of the physician as clinician and that of the physician as scientific investigator were drawn closer in both theory and practice. The use of instruments to provide numerical data initiated the nineteenth-century physician into some of the complexities of precision diagnosis. In the mid-nineteenth century, physicians needed to be reminded of the patience required to use the thermometer,[189] but by the end of the century they were quite familiar with its benefits and limitations. Other diagnostic instruments, not as widely employed because of their sophistication, were developed to record the functions of the circulatory system, introducing another level of precision into medicine. These instruments introduced standards and raised questions that will be discussed in the following chapters.

5

THE STETHOSCOPE

INTRODUCTION:

Customarily, historical precedents have been brought forth to justify the use of a number of nineteenth-century physical diagnostic techniques and instruments. Foremost among the instruments that appealed to the medical historian was the stethoscope (from the Greek words for spectus and exploro). The apologists of innovations justified what appeared to be a new medical technique by linking it with earlier procedures, and by validating its historical continuity, thus making it more acceptable to a profession which venerated its long and respected tradition. References to a Hippocratic or Galenic passage or to one cited by their contemporaries and subsequent commentators were employed to link new medical instruments or techniques with traditional medical practices.

Listening to sounds within the chest and abdomen was reported in ancient medical literature and referred to at the time of R. T. H. Laennec. Among the earliest references is the Ebers Papyrus (1500 B.C.), which mentions within the body audible signs of disease.[1] A millenium later, Soranus of Ephesus distinguished some uterine diseases by the sound produced when the hand was pressed on the abdomen.[2] Aretaeus of Cappadonia characterized the abdominal sounds produced by dropsy as drumlike, and therefore, they were called tympanic—of or like a drum or drumhead. Caelius Aurelianus (A.D. 200) listened to the chest by placing his ear in direct contact with it to diagnose bronchitis.[3] William Harvey, when concentrating on the structure and function of the heart, presented a description of cardiac sounds. In his lecture of 1616 he compared the heart's function to "two clacks of a water-bellows to rayse water." In describing the organ's motion he noted the sounds "with each movement of the heart, when there is

delivery of a quantity of blood from the veins or the arteries, a pulse takes place and can be heard within the chest."[4] With few exceptions, it remained until the eighteenth and nineteenth centuries for the internally generated sounds to be associated with specific structural or organic changes, and consequently for these sounds to be used as diagnostic signs of specific diseases.

Laennec's countryman Pierre-JeanGeorges Cabanis provided historical justification for the stethoscope when he attributed to Hippocrates the plan to search for philosophical and practical instruments to improve medicine. Cabanis claimed: "If the disciples of Hippocrates had understood his lesson well, they might have laid the foundation of that analytical philosophy by the aid of which the human mind will be henceforth enabled to create to itself, as it were daily, some new and improved instruments of advancement."[5] Cabanis viewed, as a good example of the Hippocratic desire for medical progress, Laennec's invention of the stethoscope or, as Laennec called it, a baton. William Stokes, early English proponent of the stethoscope, found the Hippocratic thrust for new medical knowledge well illustrated in not only Laennec's discovery of the stethoscope, but also the program for the advancement of physical diagnosis he constructed for it.[6] William Addison, who used the microscope to inspect lung tissues,[7] awarded Laennec the premier position in medicine for introducing methods of physical diagnosis. He wrote: "were I to affirm that Laennec contributed more towards the advancement of medical art than any other single individual, either of ancient or of modern times, I should probably be advancing a proposition which, in the estimation of many, is neither extravagant nor unjust."[8]

Laennec claimed full credit for the invention of the

stethoscope. He was originally inspired to use a paper cylinder to listen to the heart of a young female patient after noticing that a log scratched at one end with a pin sounded clear to someone listening at the other end. Laennec was wary of ancient theories and could not see any precedent for use of his auscultatory technique in medical diagnosis. Instead he claimed: "It is easy to prove that all preconceptions and all the popular errors in medicine owe their origin to the general acceptance of the theoretical opinions expressed by physicians of the past."[9]

Laennec's invention appeared to stand preeminent among nineteenth-century physical diagnostic instruments because the stethoscope made use of the faculty of hearing, a sense of novel application in medical diagnosis. More importantly, Laennec discussed and identified a spectrum of sounds associated with diseases and interpreted them for physicians who would apply the stethoscope. He introduced a new terminology, including the words stethoscope, rales, fremitus, cracked-pot sound, metallic tinkling, aegophony, bronchophony, cavernous breathing, puerile breathing, veiled puff, and bruit.[10] Laennec's teacher Jean-Nicolas Corvisart, who used Auenbrugger's diagnostic technique of percussion of the chest, set a precedent for Laennec in correlating clinical histories with postmortem observations related to heart diseases.

In 1761 Leopold Auenbrugger proposed the use of percussion or the process of tapping the chest wall with a finger or an implement to note the sounds emitted. His suggestion inspired one contemporary physician to conclude that Auenbrugger had been anticipated by Hippocrates who, in fact, had discussed a different procedure that entailed shaking a patient by the shoulders (succussion) and listening for the sounds evoked in the chest.[11]

The method of applying the ear directly to the chest, or immediate auscultation, also was employed by Hippocrates, who found this procedure useful to distinguish between the accumulation of water and pus within the chest. Water bubbled like simmering vinegar. Distinguishing between internal fluids based on their sounds remained a viable method for millenia. Ambroise Paré reiterated in the sixteenth century, "If there is matter or other humors in the thorax, one can hear a noise like that of a half-filled gurgling bottle."[12] The presence and accumulation of secretions within the chest were also studied by tieing a string around the chest to note its increase or decrease in size.[13] However, the major internal sounds described by early physicans were those generated by the beating of the heart. Simple auscultatory

methods growing out of the ingenuity of Hippocrates and others were brought to bear on the sounds from the internal organs to understand and recognize disease.

These direct methods of physical examination of the chest requiring no special devices continued to be applied during the intervening centuries. Evidence appears in paintings. For instance, friezes and other pictorial representations from the Middle Ages depict physicians examining patients by placing their ears to the individual's chest.[14] These procedures were to evolve into sophisticated methods with mechanical devices that enable physicians to tune in the sounds of the human body.

By the end of the seventeenth century, the diagnostic potential of auscultation had become explicit among a group of English experimentalists. Robert Hooke applied his talent for physiologic experimentation to ferret out the consequences of listening to the sounds emitted by the internal organs. After listening to the beating heart, Hooke speculated, "who knows, I say, but that it may be possible to discover the Motion of the Internal Parts of Bodies . . . by the sound they make; that one may discover the Works performed in the several offices and shops of a Man's Body, and thereby discover what Instrument or Engine is out of order."[15] John Forbes, who first translated Laennec's text into English, was aware of Hooke's curiosity about the body sounds and the potential Hooke thought they offered for diagnosing internal diseases.[16] Generations of physicians before Forbes were also aware of Hooke's special interest in body sounds and referred to Hooke's passage repeatedly, prior to Laennec's publication announcing the discovery of the stethoscope.

Laennec transformed these suggestive ideas into a program of describing the different sounds produced in the chest cavity by the circulation of air, movement of the lung tissues, accumulation of fluids, reverberation of the voice, and beating of the heart and large blood vessels. Auscultation, as one of six methods including observation of the movements of the chest, percussion, mensuration, succussion, and abdominal probing, was recommended to clarify the condition of the torso and uncover disease throughout the nineteenth century.

THE DIAGNOSTIC SIGNIFICANCE OF THE STETHOSCOPE:

The stethoscope remained the symbol of the physician for more than a century because it enabled practitioners to hear the symptoms of a variety of common and persistent internal diseases, especially those attacking the respiratory and circulatory systems in the chest and abdomen. The refinement of diagnosis initiated by the stethoscope led to recognition of earlier stages of disease previously of little or no concern to most physicians. John Forbes[17] reflected, in his own assessment of disease, the shift in the delineation of disease facilitated with the introduction of the stethoscope. The transformation of Forbes' thoughts on the relationship between diagnosis and pathology occurred in the course of studying Laennec's treatise. Forbes learned rapidly what some of his contemporaries were never able to understand.[18] Richard Quain, who presented the Harveian Lecture in 1885, commented on the suspicion and distrust of the stethoscope by those who were already practicing medicine when it was introduced. Quain wrote: "The stethoscope, introduced by Laennec in 1819, was used by but a few at the commencement of the second quarter of this century; and I well remember how an eminent physician to St. George's Hospital, whom I met in consultation little more than thirty years ago, characterized it as a dangerous instrument."[19] Forbes and William Stokes of Dublin were the main disseminators of Laennec's views on the stethoscope to English-speaking physicians,[20] although another English translation was edited by Theophilus Herbert in 1846.

As did other early nineteenth-century practitioners, Forbes relied on the pathologic evidence discovered in autopsy to designate and confirm the disease process. To correct what he at first assumed to be Laennec's misunderstanding, and to evaluate the function of pathologic signs in the delineation of disease, Forbes rearranged the chapters of Laennec's book *On the Diseases of the Chest*. Forbes' objective was "to improve the pathology at the expense of the diagnosis."[21] Claiming that Laennec had written the treatise so that the pathologic part was subservient to the system of diagnosis, Forbes restored it to what he "humbly conceived it ought always to have been, two independent treatises,—the one on Pathology, the other on Diagnosis,—mutually adapted to each other, *yet, each complete of itself and not necessarily connected with the other.*"[22] (Italics mine.)

Before he published the translation of Laennec's text, Forbes discovered the unequaled clinical value of Laennec's diagnostic system. Forbes explained: "Almost all other diagnostic signs are furnished by symptoms which, for the most part, have only a remote connexion with the morbid lesion, and are, indeed, frequently present in other and very different diseases. M. Laennec's diagnostics, on the contrary, are the immediate and almost physical result of the

individual derangement of parts; and if they shall be proved by the experience of others to be as certain and invariable as he affirms, there can be no question of his having conferred on Medicine, by their discovery, one of the greatest benefits with which it has ever been enriched."[23]

Not until Forbes had completed his translation did he become as impressed as Laennec was with the importance of the internal "diagnostic measure," discovered with the aid of the stethoscope and other physical methods such as immediate auscultation and percussion. Forbes admitted that he had abridged some of the "diagnostic details" and promised to include all the "valuable diagnostic material if a second edition were to appear."[24] His immediate corrections were presented in an appendix in the form of cases he had omitted entirely, as well as fuller information on some of those he had included in abbreviated form. Forbes fulfilled his promise when he published in 1824 an English version of *Original Cases with Dissection and Observations illustrating the Use of the Stethoscope and Percussion in the Diagnosis of Diseases of the Chest*, with cases originally described by Auenbrugger, Jean-Nicolas Corvisart, and Laennec.[25]

The medical community accepted Laennec's invention in stages. Those who used the stethoscope shortly after its invention include English, German, Russian, and American physicians, some of whom brought wooden models back from Paris. Among these physicians were C. J. B. Williams (1805-1889) and Alexander Hannay (1787-1848). A summary of the early literature on the use of the stethoscope reveals both caution and eagerness to adopt the instrument, coupled with an awareness of the major pitfalls in learning to apply it successfully.

In Britain, John Forbes complained in the *British Medical Journal* about the lack of interest in auscultation. Three years after his translation of Laennec appeared, some accounts of the use of the stethoscope emerged. Apparently, "the new light was too strong for older eyes."[26] George Rosen found an account of the stethoscope in the *London Times* of 19 December 1824, in which the instrument was reported to have been "invented a few months ago."[27] Dr. Peter Mere Latham's case notes of 1824, compiled at the St. Bartholomew's hospital, show that he used the stethoscope.[28] James Hope (1801-1841) concentrated all his efforts to get the stethoscope accepted as a diagnostic tool through his writings and public demonstrations.[29]

In America, the first mention of Laennec's auscultatory method appeared in 1820 in the *Journal of*

Foreign Medical Science and Literature when Laennec's forthcoming publication was announced. In 1821, the same journal published a review of Laennec's book taken from the *Quarterly Journal of Foreign Medicine and Surgery*. Forbes' translation was republished in Philadelphia in 1823. Among the earliest American physicians to discuss the stethoscope was Luther Vose Bell, who practiced at the New York City Dispensary. Publishing in 1824, he recognized the difficulties of learning to use the instrument without being instructed in a hospital, in which the student could listen to a variety of heart and lung sounds and correlate them with postmortem observations.[30] Auscultation and percussion were discussed in lectures given at the Jefferson Medical College in Philadelphia in 1827.[31]

James Jackson, Jr., reported using the stethoscope in the 1820s at the Massachusetts General Hospital in Boston. Henry I. Bowditch taught auscultation in the same city upon returning from studies with Pierre Louis in Paris.[32] In general, auscultation was promoted in Philadelphia and Boston, in the two major centers of clinical instruction in the United States. Austin Flint, who graduated from the Harvard Medical School and studied clinical medicine at the Massachusetts General Hospital under James Jackson, became the most influential teacher of auscultation in the century. He was called the "American Laennec" by Samuel Gross. In 1886, William Osler summed up the contributions Flint made to American stethoscopy: "Not one of you who takes a stethoscope into his hand but is a debtor to Dr. Flint for simplifying much that was complicated in the auscultation of heart and lungs."[33] Flint's contribution was a text, published in 1856 that stressed auscultation and percussion in healthy individuals. Previously, all texts had emphasized the abnormal sounds detected with the stethoscope.

If use of the stethoscope was occurring cautiously, by 1830 the literature on auscultation was ample. A reviewer in 1831 of *A Treatise on Auscultation, illustrated by Cases and Dissections*, written by Robert Spittal, House Surgeon of the Edinburgh Royal Infirmary, claimed "so much has lately been written on auscultation, that it would be difficult to produce much new matter on this subject, and accordingly, the treatise before us is chiefly a compilation from other works."[34]

Throughout the rest of the century, the story of Laennec's discovery of the stethoscope appeared frequently, sometimes with slight embellishments. In the "Foreign Correspondence" section of an issue in the third volume of *JAMA* (1884), it was deemed newsworthy to relate the story of Laennec's invention of the stethoscope as an episode linked to his observation of children amusing themselves by holding a cylindric piece of wood to their ears to increase the sound of a pin being scratched across the other end. The next day, at the hospital, Laennec tightly rolled up paper into a cylinder with a small central opening and applied it over the heart of an obese young female patient. The paper stethoscope was used until Laennec replaced it with a solid wood model, which he considered to be the best conductor of sounds. Laennec's account of his discovery does not mention how he first observed the sound-intensifying properties of a solid substance, nor does he state his awareness of the physical principles of acoustics, except that he "happened to recollect a simple and well known fact in acoustics and fancied at the same time that it might be turned to some use on the present occasion."[35]

Many physicians continued to rely on pathologic evidence as the final arbitrator of a diagnosis, believing that the actual inspection of an organ after death provided the only definite confirmation or negation of the original diagnosis. Previously, intuition and experience gained through observation of similar cases, as well as of a few external signs, provided the basis for diagnosis. Listening to amplified, overlapping, and unmusical body sounds gave clues to disease formerly only discovered through vivisection, the study of diseased experimental animals, and deduced from inspection of diseased organs in an autopsy.

Laennec himself extended the emphasis in the second edition of his book on the diseases of the chest studied with the stethoscope to include pathologic evidence. In the first edition (1819), he analyzed signs elicited by percussion and auscultation. In the second version (1823), he described each disease in detail, including diagnosis, pathology, and treatment in a book Fielding H. Garrison has called "the most important treatise on diseases of the thoracic organs that was ever written."[36] Laennec's more thorough analysis of diseases, from their remote signs to the observations made in autopsy, added essential information that postmortem inspection alone could not supply. The most perplexing disease phenomena were expected to be elucidated with the stethoscope. James Clark, whose inspection of Paris hospitals led to Forbes' translation of Laennec's book, singled out fevers for intensive investigation: "as a knowledge of fever stands in the same relation to physics as that of inflammation does to surgery . . . what disease comes under the care of the physician in which fever is not liable to occur at one period or another during its progress, and even to become the prominent feature?"[37] The thermometer and stethoscope jointly were to be applied to unravel the mysterious elements of fever.

Laennec's stethoscope ushered in an age of new and varying diagnostic criteria. The stethoscope forced the physician to concentrate on distinguishing sounds. In the process of learning the value of each sound for what it indicated about the structure and function of an organ, the medical practitioner began to set standards and establish criteria for the diagnosis of disease, which were not always directly related to the pathologist's criteria. The diagnostic concept of disease evolved gradually.

Theories of diseases are integral to the interpretation of the physical signs expressed by these diseases. A few examples of those who tied theory and disease signs together show what aspects of disease were emphasized in the nineteenth century and what signs the stethoscope was expected to reveal. Laennec's conclusions for auscultation were originally based on the pathologic theories and descriptions of Gaspard Laurent Bayle and Pierre Louis, who assumed that the most common fatal disease, pulmonary phthisis or tuberculosis, was a single disease transmitted by inheritance. These views were accepted during the first half of the century and overlapped with the period during which there evolved a more complex description of tuberculosis as a disease having three forms (catarrhal, fibroid, tubercular) or combinations of these, together with the conviction that vitiated air and food, toxic substances, and infected material caused the disease. Inheritance was believed to be less important than unsanitary conditions or the constitution of the person's tissues exposed to the unsanitary environment. Andrew Clark of England and Alfred Loomis of the United States taught this new conception, which led E. D. Hudson in 1885, who was a professor of general medicine and diseases of the chest in New York, to recommended a thorough examination of the chest before making a diagnosis of the disease. "An exact diagnosis should include, *in extenso*, an exact knowledge of the condition of each portion of the respiratory apparatus, including the air passages, vesicles, interstitial tissue, and pleura."[38] Therefore, physical examination of the chest had "to admit new facts and new interpretations of the old acoustic laws, in the light of a broader and changing pathological view."[39]

Hudson reviewed the methods of examination that represented "the opinions and convictions which I have reached, first as a faithful student and observer

of our several authorities on the subject and, concurrently, by independent observation in private practice during the past eighteen years, and in my clinics during the past twelve years at the Women's Medical College, the New York Polyclinic, and in my wards in Bellevue Hospital."[40] Hudson explained the physical signs in detail but emphasized the role of the physician, who was advised to depend on inspection for the information he needed to make a diagnosis in most diseases.[41]

Medical texts stressing the use of the stethoscope as an instrument to provide diagnostic signs were beginning to appear in the late 1820s. Karl Gustavus Schmalz was among the earliest German authors to write a text on diagnosis, depending, in part, on the use of the stethoscope. He coupled his criticism of nosology, which implied that diseases are separate entities, with an emphasis on evaluating diagnostic signs of all types. From his conception it followed that treatment was to aim for removing a "peccant entity," rather than restoring the healthy action of the organs, which had suffered no physical change except in their performance.

John D. Goodman of the Rutgers Medical College in New York commented in 1828 in his review of the third edition of Schmalz's book that "a part of his introduction is occupied with an excellent and perspicuous account of auscultation and percussion as a means of distinguishing diseases of the chest, and bears a very decided testimony in favour of their usefulness, now no longer doubted, except by those who are too indolent to derive advantage from their ears."[42] Goodman challenged physicians to produce a treatise on diagnostics founded on a proper study and application of the principles of general anatomy and physiology for which the stethoscope would provide original information. One text by J. Lisfranc in French translated into English by Alcock in 1827, asserted "that the stethoscope ranks among the most valuable acquisitions to our science, and that the extent of its usefulness is, as yet, far from being ascertained. It is true, a complete practical acquaintance with mediate auscultations is to be attained only after numerous trials, long experience, and persevering employment and study of the stethoscope."[43] Among the growing list of diagnoses made possible with the stethoscope were confirmation of pregnancy, recognition of dropsies and internal aneurisms, and verification of doubtful fractures and stone in the bladder.

With the introduction of physical diagnosis and increasing refinement of equipment for the purpose came a greater sophistication in teaching the scientific principles of physics and physiology. In learning the signs of disease that could be detected without the use of physical aids, memorization was essential. To inspect a patient and recognize signs similar to those of a previously examined patient, or to those described in a textbook was a large part of the method of medical diagnosis based on experience, sometimes described as intuitive, especially if the signs were more subtle. To apply an instrument and recognize the information it revealed with an appropriate interpretation entailed a different process and required an ingenuity based on the principles of science and technology. Charles Scudamore described aspects of the process in 1826: "A skillful use of the instrument requires much practice. It is not, as some may imagine, a simple matter of hearing a delicate sound. *Tact* is necessary, but this will be acquired by perseverance."[44] Scudamore's own awkwardness and disappointing experiences had made him acutely aware of the difficulty in learning to use the instrument and the principles upon which it functioned.

By the beginning of the twentieth century, memorization of the characteristics of diseases was challenged in a number of medical texts. In 1905, Egbert Le Fevre's textbook on physical diagnosis was singled out for introducing a new era in diagnostic procedures and laying the basis for relying on reason rather than memorization to make a diagnosis.[45] The reviewer of Le Fevre's text urged that the quadrad diagnostic pattern, beginning with inspection, palpation, percussion, and ending with auscultation, be replaced by auscultation used by itself. This was the strongest recommendation for stethoscopic examination, coming almost one hundred years after the announcement of the instrument.

METHODS TO DETERMINE HEART SOUNDS:

The stethoscope offered advantages over other methods for the study of the functions of all four chambers of the heart. Laennec pointed out that the stethoscope provided information about the functions of all the heart's chambers, whereas feeling the pulse only provided information about the function of the left ventricle.[46] Laennec wrote: "The mere state of the pulse then is far from indicating the state of the circulation in general; it does not even certainly indicate its condition in the whole heart, as it merely corresponds with the construction of the left ventricle, which may be regular at the time when that of the auricles and right ventricle is irregular."[47]

The stethoscope inspired physicians to search for the causes of the various sounds produced by the

motions of the heart chambers and the blood flowing through them. The British Scientific Association organized a committee, which reported to the Bristol meeting in 1836 on their experiments to determine the nature of heart sounds. The committee declared: "That the first sound of the heart, as heard in the chest, is generally complex in its nature, consisting of one constant or essential sound, and one perceptible only under certain circumstances. This constant element of the first sound may be considered as intrinsic, appearing to depend on the sudden transition of the ventricles from a state of flaccidity in diastole, to one of extreme tension in systole; while the extrinsic or subsidiary sound, which in a variety of circumstances contributes largely to the first sound, arises from the impulse of the heart against the parietes, chiefly of the thorax."[48]

Arthur Leared, who undertook extensive investigations of the same phenomena in 1852, described the sources of the sounds observed in the circulatory system as (1) the circulatory apparatus and (2) the circulating fluid in which are included (a) current sounds and (b) concussion sounds.[49] Typical of these experiments is one Leared set up to simulate the sound "bruit de soufflet." He described his apparatus:

To the neck of an India rubber bottle, a tube of the same material, two feet long, was adapted. With an aperture in the side of the bottle, a brass box, provided with a valve opening inwards, was connected; the other extremity of the box being attached to another, . . . caoutchouc tube. . . . The free extremities of both tubes having been placed in a large vessel containing water; the end of the longer one was fixed horizontally with the surface, equidistant between it and the bottom of the vessel, and at a distance from its sides. . . . On alternately strongly compressing and relaxing the bottle, an active circulation ensued, at first attended by loud gurgling, but speedily on the expulsion of air assuming a steady and uniform progression. . . .

A stethoscope was now partly introduced beneath the water in the reservoir, and the bell-part approached to the extremity of the longer tube, care having been taken that there should be no contact, and that the current should not impinge on the instrument. There was heard through it, when the ear was applied, a perfect rhythmical *bruit de soufflet*, loudest near the mouth of the tube, and decreasing in intensity as the stethoscope was moved from this position.[50]

Austin Flint, who played a central role in America in the teaching of cardiac diagnosis, also encouraged experimental model building for diagnostic purposes. He claimed that to find

explanations of cardiac murmurs . . . it is not necessary to be profoundly conversant with the science of acoustics. Comparisons on a large and a small scale are at hand. The ocean, if not lashed into fury, is silent, except when its waves are broken by the shore or by rocks. A brook, with its bottom and borders smooth, flows silently, but it is murmuring when the current is interrupted. Coming nearer, in respect of magnitude, to the heart and blood vessels, murmurs may be produced by forcing fluids into rubber tubes and bags of varying size. Valvular-like sounds are produced by forcible tension of pieces of linen or muslin held below the surface of a liquid. Musical notes may be caused by a stream of liquid acting upon a vibrating body in a closed cavity. It is perhaps not impossible by ingenious contrivances to represent artificially all the vibration in intensity, pitch and quality of the cardiac murmurs, together with the normal heart sounds and their abnormal modifications.[51]

Other devices for imitating the sounds of the heart, as well as other organs, were developed throughout the century both to investigate the causes of unusual sounds and to demonstrate the details of normal sounds to students learning to diagnose chest diseases with the aid of the stethoscope. Mechanical models were constructed to duplicate the physical conditions that produced the chest sounds. Among the earliest models were those used to carry out experiments, completed in 1830. The experimenter, Robert Spittal of Edinburgh, agitated and then listened to the sounds of thirteen different fluids. He found that sounds produced by the fluids of a consistency and viscosity most like those fluids present in the chest when an individual suffered from pneumonia were similar to those sounds detected with the stethoscope when this disease was present.[52]

Sounds created by the motions of the heart and described in such terms as triple rhythm, opening snap, rumble of mitral stenosis, harsh systolic murmur of the aorta, and blowing soft diastolic murmur of the aorta or pulmonary insufficiency had all been identified before the end of the nineteenth century.[53] These terms did not always reflect the common meanings ascribed to them. For instance, Cabot explained that "the presence of any of several types of lesions in or near the valves of the heart gives rise to eddies in the blood current and thereby to the abnormal sounds to which we give the name murmurs. No one of the various blowing, whistling, rolling, rumbling or piping noises to which the term refers, sounds anything like a 'murmur' in the ordinary sense of the word."[54] D. C. Hawley of Vermont had noted in 1892: "Murmurs are not modifications of the normal heart sounds, but are new sounds, which are added to, or take the place of the normal sounds, on account of mechanical defects in the action of the

heart."[55] Clinically significant sounds would only be changed after new techniques and more information proved that some of these early audible traces of disease were incomplete or inconclusive.

The procedures and tests evolved for eliciting additional information from the heart and chest sounds began with those of Leopold Auenbrugger, Joseph Skoda, and Adolf Weil and extended to many other inventors who revealed an increasing sophistication in the techniques and refined descriptions of the various chest sounds. Techniques varied from the simple—positioning the stethoscope on the chest—to the complex—masking specific sounds with electrical filters so that some sounds could be heard in artificial isolation. For instance, to locate the exact areas on which to place the stethoscope for pinpointing a chest sound, researchers designed the cardiometer and other instruments. Similar in construction to an aesthesiometer, the cardiometer consisted of two pointers hinged together, which were to be placed at specified locations on the chest and the distance between them measured and read from the instrument (see figure 5.1).[56]

For standardizing the loudness of the heart tones to enable a physician to differentiate the normal tones from the erratic ones in 1899, Albert Abrams of San Francisco proposed to apply the physical principle "that the intensity of sound varies inversely as the square of the distance from the sounding body, hence the distance to which a heart sound may be heard depends upon its intensity."[57] Abrams placed a series of vulcanized rubber rods between the stethoscope and the chest. These rods varied in length between six and twenty-six centimeters. Then, over the areas where the heart tones were heard with maximum intensity, he placed a rod of medium length and gradually increased the length of the rod until the heart tones were no longer audible. He constructed a table containing the sizes of the rods applied and the loudness of the sounds heard at the location of each heart valve. Every physician was encouraged to construct his own table to use with his stethoscope and the conditions under which he applied it. This method, which Abrams termed *stethophonometry* was an attempt to introduce standardization into heart tone designations.[58] Later, Abrams devised an electrical device to help distinguish muscular and valve-induced heart tones, which is discussed below.

Howard A. Kelly worked out a system of mapping chest sounds by applying an aniline dye directly to the chest. He found that the markings remained clear from one to several weeks. For the diagnostician, for the medical student, and even for the patient anxious

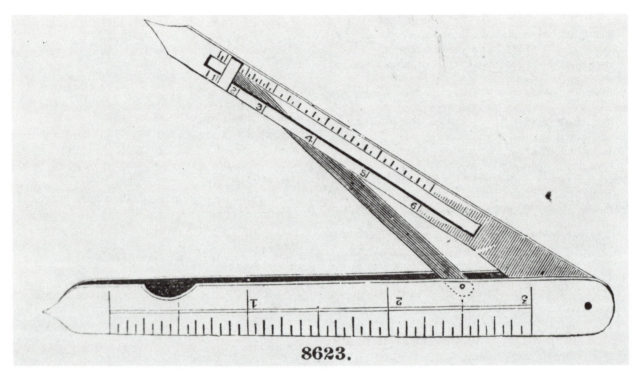

Figure 5.1. Cardiometer 1893 from A. S. Aloe Catalogue, p. 625.

to see progress in the cure of his or her disease, marking the chest was useful.[59]

An ingenious application of the stethoscope was the technique of "intrathoracic auscultation" suggested by Benjamin Ward Richardson. By placing a stethoscope at the open end of an esophageal tube introduced into the stomach, sounds from the stomach, heart, and blood vessels were heard more distinctly. Richardson explained:

I withdrew the tube until the opening on the left side came in contact with that portion of the oesophagus that lies in immediate proximity with the heart. By previous auscultation of the heart over the thoracic wall I had failed to detect clearly the two cardiac sounds owing to the feebleness of the cardiac action, but now both sounds were as distinct as they would have been from a normal heart. They were not, however, the same precisely as the sounds we hear through the thoracic wall. . . . At the same time, they were loud and were singularly distinct.[60]

Procedures combining stethoscopy and percussion became standard modes of examination. The practice of striking (percussion) the chest and listening with the stethoscope for the changes in sounds produced by lung tissue, while the patient held his breath, was standardized in the United States by James M. DaCosta of Philadelphia. He called the technique "respiratory percussion" to describe the changes in pitch and resonance of the sounds determined by percussing and placing the stethoscope over different portions of the chest and listening for echoes during inspiration and expiration. He outlined the location and type of sounds to be expected in some common diseases—bronchitis, pulmonary emphysema, pneumonia, pleurisy—and equated the presence and severity of disease with sounds produced through "respiratory percussion."[61]

STETHOSCOPE CONSTRUCTION:

Until the twentieth century, changes in the design and the materials out of which the stethoscope was constructed were only occasionally based on the principles of acoustics as demonstrated in the laboratory. Some unusual-looking stethoscopes, as well as some less than satisfactory sound-conducting instruments, were produced. The stethoscope does not selectively conduct sounds but, when properly constructed, conveys sounds free of distortion. A simple test of quality applied to all stethoscopes in the nineteenth century was to fix the bell of the instrument on a ticking watch and note if these sounds were conveyed clearly to the ear. Charles Dennison proposed an even more exacting test by suggesting that the watch be placed on a table, covered with the palm of the hand and the bell of the instrument applied to the back of the hand. "The clearness with which the working of the machinery is heard is the criterion of perfection in the instrument."[62] This test seemed suitable, but it was inconclusive. It was difficult to construct an apparatus that magnified equally all the tones produced within the body. Instruments introduced in the early twentieth century appeared to make diagnosis more artificial, since emphasis was placed on magnifying the sound picked up by the instrument, rather than distinguishing between sounds.[63] The human ear is sensitive to sound vibrations between twenty and twenty thousand cycles per second. Tests reveal that the sounds generated within the heart, chest, and abdomen range from 20 to 1,000 cps, which is, therefore, the sound variability of most value in a stethoscope. However, sound vibrations produced within the chest and abdomen lie in an inefficient portion of the human hearing spectrum. Therefore, designing a stethoscope to increase its efficiency in frequency, intensity, loudness, and masking, as well as the variation and duration of sound stimuli and quality of sound, was a prerequisite. Four principles for constructing a stethoscope to provide the maximum performance for each of these sound characteristics discovered early in the twentieth century were elaborated by J. B. Dawson of Australia in 1964:

First, the loudness of the derived sounds varies inversely with the volume of the medium [air] through which con-

duction takes place. The volume of the space between the 'business end' of the instrument and the ear drum must consequently be as small as is practically convenient. Secondly, the transference of sound energy depends upon the elasticity, viscosity and density of the medium through which it is travelling. . . . Thirdly, the stethoscope must be capable of transferring all the sounds from the surface of the emaciated or obese, normal or barrel-chested, male or female, young or old, so that the quality, intensity and frequency are familiar to the observer. . . . Fourthly, the stethoscope as a system for transferring energy vibration across interfaces separating different media can be stimulated to determine the effect of changes in sound frequency, intensity and background noise.[64]

An essential part of the stethoscope whose design combined all these physical criteria was the chest-piece. A chest-piece combining a high-frequency responding diaphragm and a low-frequency responding bell made from materials that were durable, rigid, and poor heat conductors constituted the basic unit.[65] Sound is collected in proportion to the area of the chest-piece, but for the purposes of concentrating on a small area and a specific sound, the chest-piece was usually limited to two inches or less in diameter.[66] Robert C. M. Bowles of Boston patented several binaural instruments in the late nineteenth and early twentieth centuries before he satisfactorily solved the problem of selectively focusing on sounds. In 1902, he received the first patent for a double chest-piece consisting of a bell and a diaphragm, which could be alternately switched into position (see figure 5.2).[67] Howard B. Sprague, a student of Paul

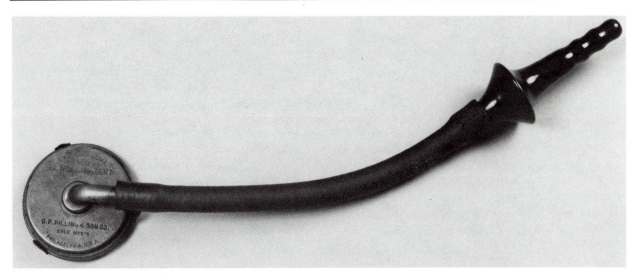

Figure 5.2. Bowles patent chest piece on monaural flexible tube with ebony ear piece. *NMAH No. 11499, SI Photo No. 78-5067.*

Dudley White in Boston, improved this dual chest-piece four years later by arranging the chest-piece so that the examiner could either use the open bell or diaphragm by switching a valve.[68] This model, known as the Sprague-Bowles chest-piece, remained the standard chest-piece throughout the first half of the twentieth century.

To interfere minimally with the transmission of sound, the instrument's tubing had to contain the least possible volume of air. Therefore, the ideal tube is short and single with a small rigid bore that is internally smooth. For instance, an instrument with a tube 3 inches long transmits sound eight times louder than one with a tube 26 inches long.[69] The latest model that best approaches these criteria was designed by David Littman in 1961 and was produced commercially by the Cardiosonics Medical Instrument Co. of Belmont, Massachusetts. This aesthetically appealing stethoscope weighs 109 grams, is 22 inches (55 cm) long, and contains an open bell and diaphragm chest-piece placed back to back. The remainder of the instrument consists of plastic tubing molded into a single rigid piece, which is threaded with earpieces also made of plastic (see figure 5.3).[70]

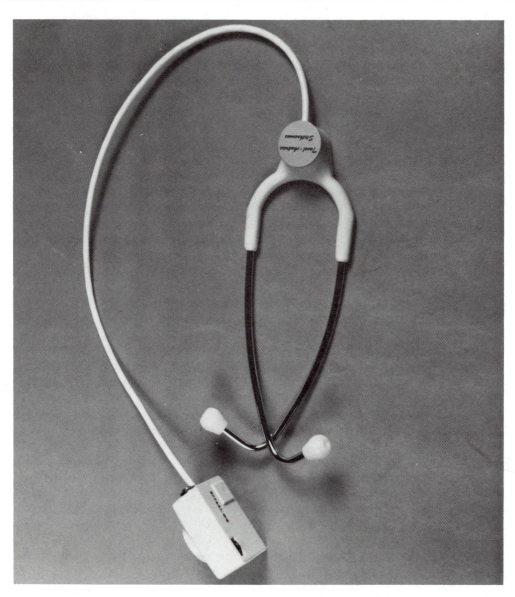

Figure 5.3. Modern Binaural stethoscope. *NMAH No. 322621.04, SI Photo No. 78-5076.*

VARIETIES OF STETHOSCOPES:

MONAURAL:

It was undoubtedly known to a number of individuals in a number of contexts that a solid extended piece of wood, metal, or other material would conduct and increase the faint sounds to which it was exposed by direct contact. Leonardo da Vinci realized the sound-conducting properties of an oar dipped in the water and held to the ear. "If you cause your ship to stop, and place one end of an oar in the water and the other end to your ear, you will hear ships at a great distance from you. You can also do the same by placing the end to the ground, and you will then hear anyone passing at a distance from you."[71]

The sounds heard through the stethoscope depended on the construction of the instrument used, the method employed in using it, the ear listening with it, and the brain interpreting the sounds. While diagnosis of disease was always an individual and uncertain, if an unpredictable, process, the addition of an instrument to provide data presented a variable that appeared to offer precision, but equally could confuse and complicate the signs presented by the diseased patient. The limitations of each type of instrument and the information it revealed were among the facts physicians had to assimilate as physical diagnosis when the stethoscope was incorporated into the diagnostic process.

The stethoscope has always provided some of the most difficult data for physicians to interpret. Physicians have had to develop an acute sense of hearing, one of the senses least used in diagnosis, and learn to fractionate their hearing so that some sounds were excluded and slight changes noted in others. Variations in instruments testify to the many attempts to make the stethoscope more useful in distinguishing between sounds and less difficult to apply in a variety of circumstances.

Laennec briefly discussed the principles of sound transmission that explained why the stethoscope was important for listening to internal chest sounds. Investigators since the seventeenth century who had studied sound transmission had concluded that sound traveled through solids at a greater velocity than through liquids or gases.[72] Laennec adopted the form of the instrument that he empirically proved best served the purposes of diagnosis. The instrument's ability to conduct sound, he opined, "is perhaps contrary to the law of physics."[73] It was not. Laennec's original design for a stethoscope, consisting of a firm cylinder made of a quire of paper rolled up (28.8 cm long, 3.6 cm in diameter, and 3.6 cm deep at one end) and pasted together, was soon changed to a model made of wood (see figures 5.4 and 5.5).[74] Laennec described the wooden instrument:

It consists simply of a cylinder of wood, perforated in its centre longitudinally, by a bore 3 lines in diameter, and formed so as to come apart in the middle, for the benefit of being more easily carried. One extremity of the cylinder is hollowed out into the form of a funnel to the depth of an inch and a half, which cavity can be obliterated at pleasure by a piece of wood so constructed as to fit it exactly, with the exception of the central bore which is continued through it, so as to render the instrument in all cases, a pervious tube. . . . This instrument I commonly designate simply the *Cylinder* (baton) sometimes the *Stethoscope*.[75]

Charles Haden, using a lathe, modified the tube by dividing it into two halves joined by a screw formed from the edges of the split cylinder.[76] This type of cylinder was used until Pierre Piorry in 1828 designed a lighter tube by hollowing out the ends of the tube. This thinner, hourglass-shaped, and eventually, shorter tube was capped with flat, ivory ear and chest-pieces. Piorry's model was made even more slender and elegant by other designers and became very popular, although it was less effective in transmitting clear sounds while simultaneously magnifying their intensity.[77] The single cylinder or monaural stethoscope continued to be used and manufactured throughout the nineteenth and into the first half of the twentieth century.

The single-tube stethoscope was constructed out of a variety of woods. Laennec had made stethoscopes out of glass and metal but found them less effective.[78] The last model made by Laennec was made of walnut wood, which he turned on a lathe that he had learned to use.[79] Laennec preferred a medium dense wood like India cane and even paper to denser substances. Others, like the Parisian Marc Hector Landouzy, who in 1843 compared stethoscopes made of wood, metal, and glass, concluded that the lighter and more elastic types of wood, such as fir, logwood, and boxwood, produced the best instruments.[80] For Landouzy, the best stethoscopes were made of solid, unadorned light wood.

One of Laennec's more unusual models was made out of goldbeater's skin inflated with air, which was a conspicuous failure.[81] Laennec had planned to make stethoscopes to sell, but his deteriorating health did not permit him to carry out this plan. The diagram of his stethoscope that appeared at the end of his text was complete enough for a woodturner to follow in constructing the instrument.

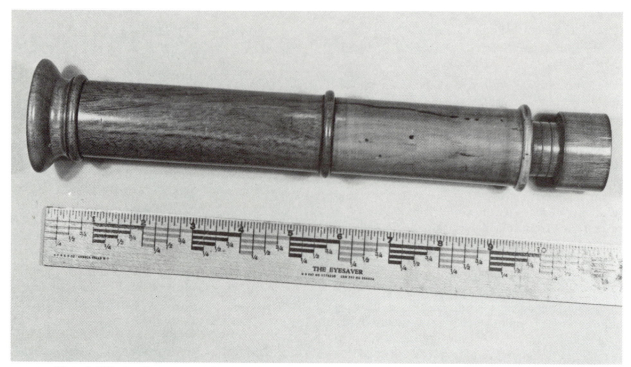

Figure 5.4 Nineteenth-century wood monaural stethoscope made by Collin of Paris and stamped to indicate the maker. Owned by Dr. W.R. Chitwood of Wytheville, Virginia.

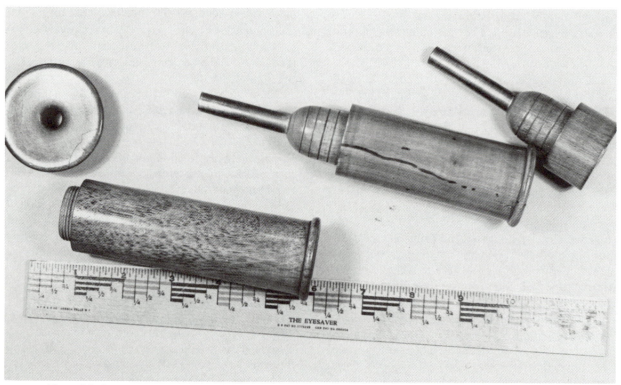

Figure 5.5. Same monaural stethoscope disassembled. The long dark streak in the middle piece is not a crack in the wood and may be a stain due to the varnish.

Other sizes and shapes of stethoscope tubes, made of papier-mâché, aluminum, chrome-plated metal, and other alloys, combined with ebony, ivory, and vulcanite (hard rubber) chest- and earpieces, were constructed as these materials were obtainable. Pine and cedar woods were especially good materials because they did not conduct heat rapidly, and therefore, did not feel cold when touched to the skin, nor did they break easily when dropped.[82] The lightness of these woods and the small number of imperfections (knots) they contained made them easier to fashion into small tubes. Most polished wood models measured from six to nine inches in length and contained one hollowed end either flared like a trumpet or straightened to apply to the chest and one flat rimmed end to place against the ear (see figure 5.6).

The small wooden stethoscope met the specifications placed by physicians on these instruments: light, small, and easily carried.

C. J. B. Williams and others who studied the acoustical principles of stethoscopy after attending the clinical lectures of Laennec concluded that several forms of the instrument were required for the primary uses to which the instrument was put by the diagnostician. For conveying the sounds originating in the denser parts of the chest, such as from the heart, a light, rigid, and solid wood cylinder was best; for those sounds produced in less compact areas, the same instrument perforated longitudinally with a thin air column served better.[83] So that the diffused sounds of respiration could be concentrated, the cylinder was scooped out at the end placed on the body, as originally suggested by Laennec.[84]

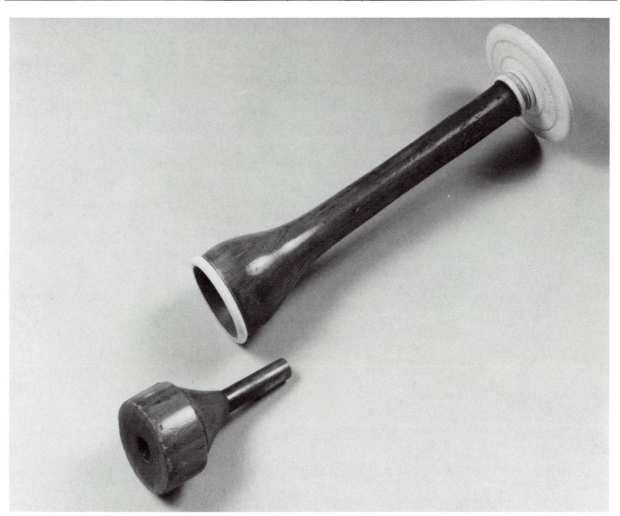

Figure 5.6. Monaural stethoscope with ivory ear pieces and wooden insert for bell. Gift of the Maryland Medical and Chirurgical Faculty. NMAH No. 302606.20, SI Photo No. 78-5066.

Among the more than thirty types of monaural stethoscopes that attempted to meet the different requirements of physicians, not all of which were conducive to accurate auscultation, were those designed by Barclay, D. M. Cammann, Adolphe Piorry (trumpet-shaped), C. J. B. Williams, Alfred Loomis, William Stokes, William Ferguson, Burrows, Hawksley, John Elliotson, A. S. Walsh, Clark, Arnold, Dobell, Richard Quain, Boeker, J. M. DaCosta, Ludwig Traube (hard rubber), Pinnard (aluminum), Freudenthal (hard rubber with soft rubber bell),

Heinrich Quincke of Kiel,[85] and Oertel (combination monaural and binaural with graduated monaural tube), which were sold by American manufacturers and importers, including George Tiemann,[86] Charles Truax and Greene,[87] and Kny-Scheerer.[88] (See figures 5.7, 5.8, 5.9, and 5.10). The cedar wood stethoscope with a bell chest-piece resembling an egg cup in size and shape was a popular model sold in both full and shortened versions. However, a shorter bell with a longer and thinner tube was a more satisfactory stethoscope. The thinnest tubes were made of metal.

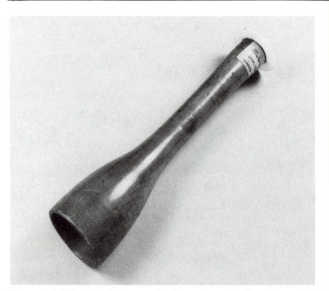

Figure 5.7. Wood stethoscope with ivory tip and hollowed-out bell. Gift of Maryland Medical and Chirurgical Faculty. NMAH No. 302606.1, SI Photo No. 78-5064.

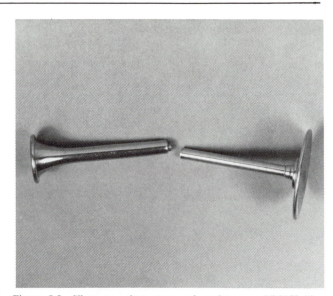

Figure 5.8. Silver two-piece monaural stethoscope. NMAH No. 322774.01, SI Photo No. 78-5062.

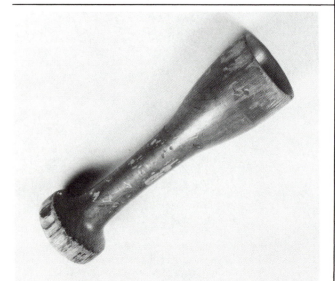

Figure 5.9. Wood monaural stethoscope. Gift of Maryland Medical and Chirurgical Faculty. NMAH No. 302606.2, SI Photo No. 78-5063.

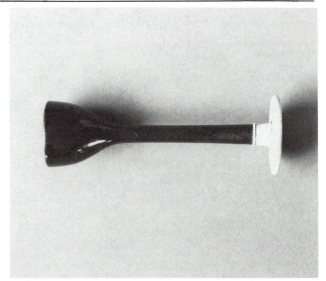

Figure 5.10. Wood monaural stethoscope with ivory earpiece. NMAH No. 302606.01, SI Photo No. 36399.

Williams provided explicit instructions to stethoscope makers. He cautioned that all stethoscopes should have at least one inch or two of a perfectly cylindrical tube to concentrate the vibrations. Those that were wholly conical or bell-shaped revealed confusing sounds not unlike those heard in a hollow sea shell when held up to the ear.[89] Williams used an abridged version of Laennec's instrument that was four inches long, to which he added a trumpet-shaped end, which confined the air column and gave less discomfort to the patient.[90] The English maker who most succeeded in meeting Williams' exacting standards was Grumbridge of London. For constructing the body of the instrument, Williams preferred mahogany or walnut wood, and for keeping the instrument sterile, ebonite.[91]

The use of metals permitted the manufacture of a one-piece monaural stethoscope of variable length. One aluminum model telescoped from seven inches fully extended to an intermediate position of five inches, and in its least extension, to three inches. These positions were locked into place by a bayonet catch. Another telescoping model was adjustable to varying lengths. The outer tube carried the earpiece and the inner one terminated in the chest-piece.[92] The mounts were made of celluloid colored to resemble coral, amber, or tortoise shell.[93] These forms of the monaural stethoscope have not been saved, possibly because the materials have not lasted over the past one hundred years, and certainly, because they were not as commonly used as were the plain wooden types.

Arnold produced a long flexible rubber tube called a conversation tube, which was used to communicate with a deaf individual. Hard rubber mounts were placed on each end. A single tube two to three feet long, containing an ear peg at one end and a removable chest-piece at the other end, served two purposes: as a conversation channel and as a stethoscope.[94] The end placed on the chest or given to the person speaking was usually an elongated cone and the other end was shaped to be inserted into the ear. In the seventeenth century, the New England Puritans required young people who were courting to speak to each other across a table. To make these meetings more private, they used a device with a cup at each end to alternately speak and listen to each other, foreshadowing the speaking tubes produced in abundance in the nineteenth century.[95] The adjustable conversation tube offered the maximum convenience to conversationalists and deaf people, as well as to the examining physician (see figures 5.11 and 5.12).

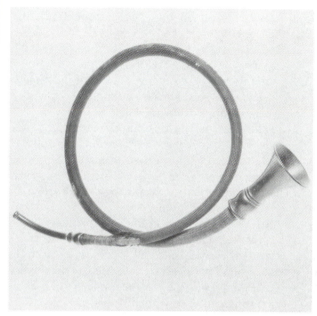

Figure 5.11. Conversation tube and hearing aid. *SI Photo No. 71-3-16.*

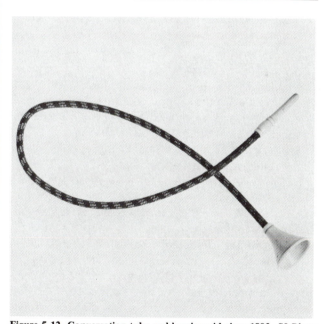

Figure 5.12. Conversation tube and hearing aid circa 1893. *SI Photo No. 71-3-15.*

The instrument with a flexible shaft could be rolled up and carried in the pocket. However, this and other tubes did not conduct all sounds equally well. The diagnostician seeking to hear and interpret the details of sounds produced by the respiratory and circulatory systems was advised to use the more traditional stethoscope.

Modifications to monaural stethoscopes made them more useful, and therefore, more attractive to the practitioner. To encourage the use of the monaural instrument and provide maximum portability, designers combined other related and unrelated instruments with it, such as the thermometer, nasal speculum, anal speculum, female catheter, ophthalometer, reflector, and *porte-caustique*.[96] The most fashionable were combination stethoscopes that included a percussor or pleximeter, which came assembled with the instrument and could be used with the stethoscope or detached for use separately. Piorry saw an advantage in making his new pleximeter a part of the stethoscope to call his new method to the attention of all physicians.[97] Jules de Dervieu, assistant to Piorry, was among the earliest to combine Laennec's stethoscope with Piorry's pleximeter. De Dervieu inserted an ivory plaque at the end of the stethoscope, which was moved by a *ressor venait* (a spring). Piorry found this ingenious double instrument inferior to the simple plessimeter.[98] Many English and American physicians preferred to use their index fingers instead of the ivory plessimeter to percuss their patients. It was possible to convert a wooden hollow tube stethoscope into a solid conducting tube by the addition of a solid substance such as an India-rubber bag filled with water (hydrophone), which was inserted into the bell end of the tube. This arrangement changed the acoustic properties of the tube and usually intensified the sound.[99]

Typically, the stethoscope was constructed with either an earpiece or a bell, which was screwed into the stem. When either end was removed, it was possible to find a thermometer or other instruments stored in the stethoscope stem. One combination stethoscope, a somatoscope, was designed by V. Huter of Marburg in 1877, which combined a percussion hammer, pleximeter, and stethoscope.[100] Solger produced a combined stethoscope and percussion hammer by 1872, as did Felix von Niemeyer in 1868.[101] An unusual combination of a stethoscope, plessimeter, thermometer, syringe, and assorted pills were stored in a walking stick, owned by a Viennese physician, Edlen von Gunz-Zwelthof in 1870 and presently preserved in Vienna.[102] A walking staff,

containing drugs and instruments, had been exhibited in 1851 at the London Exhibition.[103]

Temporary substitutes for the physician who had forgotten his monaural stethoscope, suggested by those who found these items useful in an emergency, included a wineglass and a clinical thermometer case six inches long by half an inch in diameter. V. Poulain recommended that a thermometer can be used as a stethoscope by placing its rounded end into the ear.[104] These unusual devices were also recommended to those wishing to avoid having to carry an additional instrument.

BINAURAL OR BIAURAL:

Debate over the quality of sound carried through a solid cylinder or through a partially opened single tube led to the realization that, although an air column would carry a smaller variety of sounds, some of these were of foremost value to the physician. One difficulty in using the solid wood type of stethoscope was that the tube vibrated in response to the surface of the chest wall where it rested, thus the physician had to separate the sounds produced on the exterior of the chest from those that were produced within the chest. The superiority of an air column in conducting some internal body sounds of greater interest to the clinician motivated physicians and manufacturers to design stethoscopes that could be placed in one or both ears simultaneously. When both tubes were combined into one instrument, the stethoscope became known as a binaural stethoscope.

A few prototypical binaural stethoscopes were constructed before 1850. The son of C. J. B. Williams, C. Theodore Williams, described an unwieldy precursor constructed in 1829.[105] It consisted of a trumpet-shaped chest-piece of mahogany screwed into a connection into which were attached two bent lead pipes without earpieces. This may have been the instrument designed by Nicholas P. Comins, a medical student in Edinburgh, who produced a "flexible stethoscope" in 1829 because, as he explained, "it can be used in the highest ranks of society without offending fastidious delicacy" (see figure 5.13).[106] While it was essentially a bent tube, it was complex. It consisted of two tubes seven inches in length and five-eighths of an inch in diameter. The diameter of the aperture was an inch and a half. Earlier, C. J. B. Williams of London had used an instrument with flat earpieces and two metal tubes attached to the bell of a stethoscope. The sounds the instrument conveyed were exaggerated and its inflexibility made it awkward to apply. Another one was

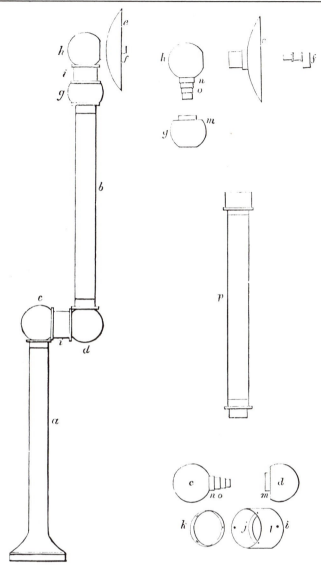

Figure 5.13. 1829 Illustration. From *London Medical Gazette*, vol 4, of Comins stethsocope.

Comins description follows:

These pieces are united by a perforated joint (C,D), three inches in length, at right angles to their extremities: and the two pieces of which the joint consists, being united like the joint of a flute, permit the limbs of the cylinder to form any angle. The upper end of the instrument is provided with an ear-piece, (E), sufficiently large and concave to envelop the ear. Its central portion (F) being angular and moveable, admits the extremity of the cylinder as nearly as convenient to the meatus auditorius externus. The ear-piece can, by means of a moveable joint, (G, H), be placed laterally with respect to the extremity of the tube. The moveable joints, (C, D, G, H), were they formed of brass, could, by a simple contrivance, be rendered in any position air-tight. But as this, and perhaps every substance that would deviate from the homogenousness of the cylinder, would injure the sound, external securities are necessary. The following has been devised: each joint is covered by a metallic ferrule (iii) 5/8ths of an inch in length, and 6/6ths of an inch in diameter, except at one extremity, (J), where it is reflected inwards, at right angles, and where the diameter decreases about 3/16ths of an inch. Within the ferrule, and in contact with the reflected extremity, is placed a small flat ring, (K), which is secured through an aperture in the ferrule, (L), at three points, to one side of the joint (M). The other end of the ferrule is screwed also at three points to the other side of the joint, (N). The ferrule, and the enclosed ring are by this contrivance permitted each to move freely with respect to the other; while with respect to the joint, they preclude the possibility of its opening, or of its not being air-tight. Should friction, however, eventually cause it to become too free, the screws can be withdrawn from the pieces, (D, G), and by means of silk coiled in the depressions, (O, O) the joint can again be rendered air-right (N. P. Comins, *New Stethoscope*, p. 420.

designed by Marc-Hector Landouzy of Paris in 1841. It contained a number of gum-elastic tubes, which enabled ten students to listen to the chest sounds simultaneously.[107] The instrument required at least two people to apply it. Teaching stethoscopes were abandoned until special multi-ended stethoscopes were designed at the end of the century. Dr. Golding-Bird at Guy's Hospital in London used a stethoscope with flexible tubes in 1843, which he found convenient since he had arthritis and preferred to sit in a chair while examining patients.[108]

The early 1850s was a rich period for the development of the binaural stethoscope. The first acceptable binaural model was composed of gutta-percha. It was designed by Dr. Arthur Leared of Dublin and displayed in London at the International Exhibition of 1851.[109] Its two tubes were fitted with flat earpieces and a single chest-piece. The elasticity of the tubes made the instrument easier to apply and to hold in place within the ears. This model was not produced commercially. In 1851, Marsh of Cincinnati received a patent for a double stethoscope. The chest-piece was constructed of a membrane stretched over a disk and connected to two gum-elastic tubes leading to the ears. The earpieces were unsatisfactory and the sounds conveyed were muffled.[110] The leading designer of a binaural stethoscope in the nineteenth century was George Cammann of New York. Cammann was familiar with the Landouzy and Marsh stethoscopes. Since he did not approve of patenting a medical instrument as Marsh had done, he designed a binaural stethoscope that could be available without patent restrictions (see figures 5.14, 5.15 and 5.16). Cammann's superior stethoscope became the most widely respected binaural stethoscope of the century and is the most easily recognized nineteenth-century binaural stethoscope today. In a report published in 1855, he claimed to have perfected his instrument in 1852.[111] Among Cammann's improvements were the substitution of ivory or ebony knobs for insertion into the ear and the use of a spring to keep them in place and thus free the examiner's hands. A segment of each tube was made of flexible material—wire coiled between layers of soft rubber and coated externally with silk or cotton—for greater maneuverability of the instrument. The original Cammann stethoscope resembled a squashed monaural instrument attached to elongated tubes of varying construction. It consisted of

a wooden cylinder, resembling a dumpy little uniaural stethoscope. (A) One end of the cylinder expands into a cup (B), which is applied to the chest for collecting sound, while

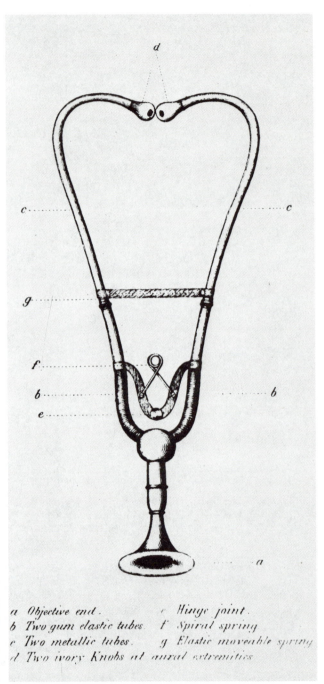

a Objective end.   e Hinge joint.
b Two gum elastic tubes. f Spiral spring
c Two metallic tubes.   g Elastic moveable spring
d Two ivory Knobs at aural extremities

Figure 5.14. Illustration of binaural stethoscope with parts labeled. *SI Photo No. 43567-E.*

to its other extremity are attached two tubes (C, G). These tubes communicate with the hollow cylinder, are about 10 inches in length, and consist of 3 inches of flexible (D), and about 7 inches of metallic tubing (E). The former is joined to the wooden cylinder, while to the free ends of the latter the small ivory knobs (F) are attached. The two metallic tubes are connected by a jointed bar (G).[112]

Furthermore "all joints were either screw or slip lathe turned to exact fit."[113] Added to its qualities of lightness, durability, and good sound conduction was ease in handling, facilitated by the attachment of a chest-piece encircled with soft rubber—the suggestion of Dr. Snelling—to make it more secure on the uneven surface of the body.[114] Cammann's stethoscope was criticized by Austin Flint in 1856 because the instrument made it difficult to compare the pitch of sounds. Flint eventually endorsed the stethoscope.

Dennison's stethoscope resembled the Cammann type except that it was larger and contained a removable chest-piece with a number of interchangeable bells and an adjustable screw mechanism for regulating the tension of the earpieces.[115] A model designed by Harvey Hilliard in 1875 and also claimed by Ferris and Co. for Dr. Spencer of Clinton, England[116] adjusted the earpiece tension by a low hinge attached to each earpiece, which encircled the back of the head or could be placed under the chin.[117] In imitation of the conversation tube, the diameter of Dennison's conducting column of air tapered through the length of the tube up to the earpieces. Making the inner surfaces of all these parts smooth was essential to high fidelity sound conduction. Tiemann and Co. of New York was the most successful in concealing the wire coil at its attachments at either end of the tube[118] and produced the model publicly acknowledged by Dennison as the best: "All the joints, bells, tubes and arms are constructed on the principle of a slightly conical tube, each portion fitting evenly and tightly into the other, and the fastenings of the flexible portion to the gutta-percha are so perfect that there is no interruption in the transmission of sounds from the chest to the ear."[119] Although more cumbersome in appearance than the Cammann stethoscope, Dennison's model was comfortable and extremely efficient.[120]

Numerous changes and improvements in the construction of binaural stethoscopes were announced in medical journals.[121] Later in the century, inventors attempted to incorporate the principles of acoustical theory. Materials permitting the construction of flexible, sound-channeling tubes were essential to the creation of a useful binaural stethoscope. In the second half of the nineteenth century, rubber strength-

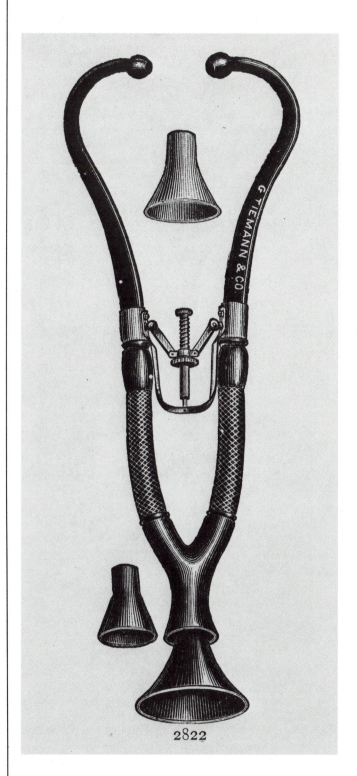

Figure 5.15. Illustration of Cammann-type stethoscope, circa 1889 from Tiemann's catalogue. *SI Photo No. 79-5035.*

INSTRUMENTS FOR PHYSICAL DIAGNOSIS.

FIG.
*2813 Arnold's Stethoscope..$ 1 00
 2814 Boeker's   " 1 00
 2815 Martin's Combined Stethoscope........................... 3 75
*2816 Cedar Stethoscope... 40
 2816-A "   "   with rubber ring........................ 85
*2817 Ebony   " 1 00
 2817-A "   and Ivory Stethoscope............................... 1 50
 2818   "   Stethoscope, with rubber ring.................... 1 25
*2819   "   "   with Pleximeter and Hammer............ 2 50
*2820 Hawksley's New Stethoscope............................... 1 00
*2821 University Stethoscope, Improved........................ 2 25
*2821A   "   " 2 25

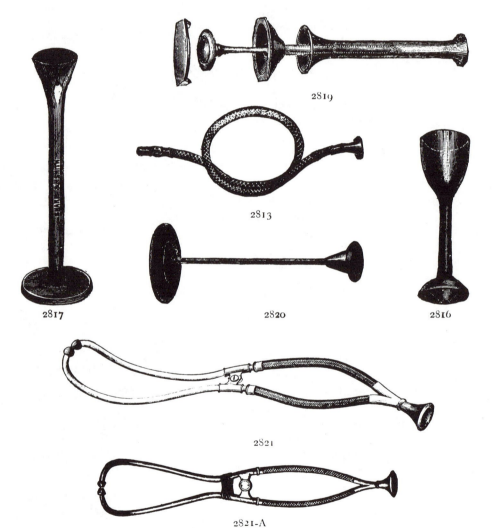

Instruments designated by a * are illustrated.

Figure 5.16. 1889 Illustrations. From Sharp and Smith Catalogue, Chicago, includes Arnold's conversation tube. *SI Photo No. 79-5029.*

ened with coiled wire, encased in a silk or fabric cover, was used in the manufacture of the most successful flexible single and double stethoscopes.

Not all designers of binaural stethoscopes were successful. T. C. Blackwell of Edinburgh persuaded Mr. Lewis of Allen and Hanburys to make what turned out to be a clumsy-looking model. The appearance was marred by having the sectional area of the larger tube equal the sectional area of the two smaller tubes. The Y-shape of the binaural instrument was retained, but the narrowing of the tube beyond the joint was eliminated. This was accomplished by placing the worm of the chest-piece on the outside, which made the tube more bulky at that point. A knife edge was placed at all joints to prevent the constriction that occurs beyond the attachment of a rubber tube to a rigid tube.[122] The basic shape of the binaural stethoscope remained throughout the period, although some of the claims for particular modifications indicated that the changes were intended to have a major impact on the auscultatory procedure. A review of some of the more interesting improved binaural stethoscopes reflects some of the conceptual and mechanical problems recognized by nineteenth- and early twentieth-century stethoscope designers.

The most unique invention among binaural stethoscopes was the differential stethoscope. Introduced by Scott Alison in 1859 to the Royal Institution of Great Britain, it was based on Cammann's stethoscope in size and materials, but contained one essential difference: it consisted of two stethoscopes joined together for convenience but terminating in separate chest-pieces, thus enabling both ears to function independently as they normally do. George Carrick described it in 1873:

Of these two acoustically separate instruments, one transmits sounds from one point of the chest to one ear, and the other from another part of the chest to the other ear, the auscultator being thus enabled to listen to two parts of the chest at the same time. . . . the differential stethoscope plainly demonstrates the interesting law in acoustics, that if, of two sounds, of like quality but varying in intensity, one sound is conveyed to one ear, the other to the other ear, only the major or louder is heard. . . . When the two sounds are the same in degree and in quality, then we hear them equally well with both ears. The value of this acoustic law, in its application to medical practice, must be obvious to every physician. In auscultating the lungs, he is frequently called upon to compare the intensity of two sounds, and to decide which is the louder; and yet how difficult, almost impossible in some cases, it is to do so correctly with any stethoscope but the differential one.[123]

Alison was in communication with John Tyndall concerning the acoustical principles upon which the instrument was constructed.[124] "The great advantage of the differential stethoscope . . .," claimed Carrick, "over all others is, that by allowing us virtually to place each ear on a different part of the chest at the same time, it enables us to differentiate sound easily, i.e., to recognize the stronger from the weaker."[125] This procedure was a major departure from all previous methods of applying the stethoscope and demanded that the physician possess excellent hearing in both ears. Several decades earlier, Andrew Clark already had pointed out to Samuel Wilks that if two earpieces are employed in a stethoscope, "the sound is heard at the spot where it is produced."[126] Using both ears to recognize the source of an internal body sound was explained as being in conformity with the most efficient functioning of the human ear.

Harvey Hilliard and Spencer proposed a binaural stethoscope that could be used as a simple binaural or a differential stethoscope, depending on whether one or two chest-pieces were attached to the tubes. Another method of changing the standard binaural stethoscope into a differential form was to add a crosspiece to the distal ends, which in turn, would connect two or more elastic tubes of convenient length. The tubes could be applied over the chest or lifted when it was desirable to stop a particular sound. Hilliard explained that it differed "from that of the ordinary differential stethoscope in that the sounds are brought to the two ears simultaneously, and the whole of the auditory power is, therefore, at work on the same subject, which, as I have said, is analyzed by a process of exclusion to the very great advantage and ease of the listener in forming his judgment."[127] William Ewart called this instrument a "comparing stethoscope." One model to Ewart's design was made by Matthews in 1886. Ewart claimed that he was forestalled in 1881 by Constantin Paul, who exhibited a type of comparing stethoscope before the Académie de Médecine in Paris.[128]

Two more differential stethoscopes containing built-in mechanisms for measuring the differences in loudness between several sounds were constructed in the early twentieth century. Max Joseph Oertel designed a special chest-piece, which contained a metal tube for changing sound perception into visual perception. It was explained that

in this tube there is a slit which can be opened, and . . . read on a scale. A second tube slides over the one with a slit, and can make the slit of any length up to four centimeters. To the end of this tube a Y tube is fitted which is attached to the tubes of a binaural stethoscope. The arrangement provides a stethoscope with a window, [whose] area . . . can be varied . . . and measured accurately. The method of using it is to make the width of the slit one millimeter, and then slide the outer tube towards the graduated end until the slit is covered . . . The chest piece is then applied over the apex of the heart and the slit uncovered until the first sound cannot be heard. On shortening the slit the sound is heard again; the length of the slit when the first sound is just lost is noted. The slit is once more covered by the sliding tube, and then the chest piece is transferred to the aortic site and the slit uncovered again until the second is just lost. The length of the slit is noted again. . . . If the heart is beating vigorously, and making very loud sounds, the slit must be opened to two or more millimeters.[129]

Heinrich Bock designed a differential stethoscope that also converted sound into visual stimuli. The stethoscope consisted

of a conical chest piece attached to a circular box which is divided into two compartments by a thick metal diaphragm, which is pierced by a small hole. Into this hole a cone of metal can be inserted. When the hole is closed, air-borne sounds are stopped. . . . The pointer should be set at 100 when the hole is closed. [To use] the instrument open the aperture by one complete revolution of the screw, place the chest piece over the apex of the heart, and turn the screw until the first sound is no longer heard. The position is noted; the average position is 80. The pointer is turned back again to about 10, the stethoscope is applied to the aortic site, and then the pointer turned until the second sound is lost. This occurs on the average at about 60.[130]

The Bock stethoscope proved to be more useful because it could be applied in a comparatively noisy environment, whereas the Oertel model required an absolutely quiet room, although it could be used to compare very vigorous heart sounds.[131] Bock stated that "the first mitral sound is a comparative sound and indicates whether the left ventricle is enlarged or insufficient in its musculature; at the same time it indicates the strength of its contraction. The strength of the heart muscle may be deduced from the first aortic sound as well as from the relations of the sounds to each other."[132]

The ability of the differential stethoscope to localize sound was first evaluated in 1936 according to physiologic and physical principles. Lateralization and comparison of sounds were studied in special experiments undertaken by William J. Kerr. Kerr applied the principle that "lateralization of sounds depends chiefly on differences of phase or timing of the sounds perceived and differences in intensity of the sounds in the paired organs of hearing."[133] He constructed a stethoscope "consisting of two similar chest pieces connected by rubber tubing through 4 'Y' shaped pieces with a headset of the ordinary binaural stethoscope."[134] His final model contained crossed and direct tubes made of rigid metal tubing connected to rubber tubing of equal length, which ended in the chest-pieces. Rubber tubing was also placed between the earpieces and the metal tubes. While not of value to anyone with defective hearing in one ear, the Kerr "symballophone" was important to detect and localize slight clinical differences and to time events accurately.

In the early twentieth century, double stethoscopes were introduced by Muralt (1910), Froeschels, Nicolai (stereostethoscope), and in 1935 by Hawthorne.[135]

Binaural stethoscopes were not combined with other instruments as commonly as the monaural types had been. By the twentieth century when the binaural stethoscope was popular, portability was less of a problem. Physicians could carry a greater assortment of instruments, as well as heavier ones, in their carriages and automobiles. They also placed greater emphasis on the quality and function of their instruments, goals which were less attainable in a multi-purpose gadget. Furthermore, it was convenient to hook the binaural instrument around the neck and carry it at all times, especially after it became a symbol of superior medical practice. For those who preferred to fold up their stethoscopes, Salt and Son of Birmingham introduced in 1881, a Cammann-type model with sliding tubes, which extended and locked into position and could be collapsed, making the stethoscope compact and easy to carry.[136] Nevertheless, a few ideas for adding special attachments to the binaural stethoscope were implemented. For instance, F. W. Koehler of Louisville, Kentucky, with an aim similar to that of Piorry, attached a plessimeter to the margins of the bell. When a physician wanted to obtain a percussion sound, a bulb forced air on a rod placed on top of the pleximeter, which then fell and created the sound that was conveyed directly to the examiner's ears through the stethoscope.[137]

Laennec introduced the stethoscope as the instrument par excellence for detecting and categorizing the sounds within the chest, which could be linked to normal and abnormal structures and functions. Within the nineteenth century, the instrument had been applied to every cavity and organ in the body. By the end of the century, obstetrics provided the basis for the most significant new application of the instrument. Many sounds could be heard in almost any disease of the chest. These were not easily sorted out; however, the fetal heart was a clear indication of pregnancy. One American observer explained: "An auscultatory sign means not a certain disease, but a certain condition of the lungs, a condition which may be produced by a great variety of diseases. Whereas, auscultation of the foetal heart means always, absolutely, beyond dispute the existence of gestation and the life of the foetus."[138] Among the plethora of instruments produced for diagnosticians of all specialties, many stethoscopes poorly served the purpose of isolating and carrying the body sounds to the ears of the physician. For those who realized that the *auditus eruditus* was not merely "question of mechanics but of the perceptive faculties of the intellect,"[139] the variety of instruments was inconsequential. Physicians continued to listen to body sounds and learned to ascribe meaning to them, while paying less attention to the structure and function of the stethoscope. Ignorance of the mechanical details that made the stethoscope a good conductor of sound, coupled with the interest in the weight and portability of the instrument, encouraged manufacturers and designers to emphasize its lightness and small size, while minimizing the effect of these externally imposed constraints on its performance as an accurate sound conveyor. The physician's concern with the ease in transporting the stethoscope made it difficult to design a proper instrument in a period when the materials available for its construction were limited or not readily available and often expensive. Inventors were critical of manufacturers who did not follow their plans exactly or who used improper materials in the construction of stethoscopes. Charles Dennison, designer of a popular stethoscope, could, therefore, claim that only one manufacturer, George Tiemann & Co. of New York, had produced a creditable model of his binaural stethoscope by 1892.[140]

ELECTRIC STETHOSCOPE:

An effective incentive to a new exploration and interpretation of chest sounds was the invention of the electric-powered stethoscope. Electricity transmits sound waves about twenty thousand times faster than air; therefore, there is no overlapping of sound waves and they are heard more distinctly. An electric stethoscope is able to magnify sounds not heard with the mechanical instrument.

A simple early electric stethoscope, known as the "heartphone," was invented by Gottschalk in the late nineteenth century and consisted of a transmitter,

receiver, battery, and a regulating controller. By arranging the casing of the transmitter, a physician could examine different-sized surfaces. The sound was conducted through soft rubber tubes enclosed in metal and was regulated by a controller, placed on the cord between the transmitter and receiver.[141] Albert Abrams of San Francisco in 1899 discovered, with another instrument of his invention, that blood pressure measurement with a tonometer was unreliable when the individual being tested was afflicted with arteriosclerosis. While conceding the additional difficulty in learning to apply the electric instrument, Abrams emphasized the fact that "the trained ear can never replace a carefully gauged instrument for determining and registering the intensity of respiratory or cardiac sounds."[142] His controller consisted of twelve resistance units with a thumb slide, providing a range of adjustment to suit the individual and permitting the examiner to mask the louder sounds when desirable.

To select and interpret heart and lung sounds for the purpose of monitoring medication, Abrams improved the instrument he had introduced in 1899. The original purpose of electric stethoscopes was to increase the intensity and permit the selection of individual sounds for closer analysis. By 1902, Abrams had developed a stethophonometer, which he attached to a stethoscope for the purpose of regulating and recording on a scale the intensity of the chest sounds. By increasing the resistance to the sound in measured stages, reflected in the scale of the stethophonometer, Abrams concluded "that the intensity of the heart tones is no accurate gauge of cardiac strength."[143] The important distinction between sounds made with the instrument was "the muscular and valvular elements of the heart sound," which were almost impossible to distinguish with the conventional stethoscope at that time.[144] As increased resistance was interposed with the stethophonometer, the muscle-induced sound of the heart was gradually eliminated, thereby allowing the physician to listen to the flapping sounds of the heart valves.[145]

INSTRUCTIONAL STETHOSCOPES:

Teachers required a stethoscope that would allow a number of students to listen to the heart sounds of a patient simultaneously. One of the first multiple-ended stethoscopes was designed by Landouzy in 1841 to permit ten students to be linked to the patient at one time. Constructed of an iron alloy, it was 120 cm in length and contained flexible arms. It proved useful in a period when the stethoscope was first being taught to medical students on a regular basis. Landouzy called his instrument the polystethopolyscope or polyscope.[146] In the early twentieth century, Aitchison Robertson in England connected a binaural stethoscope to one sound collector enabling 10 to 12 auscultators to listen to one patient simultaneously.[147] By the beginning of the twentieth century, the multiple stethoscope had been improved only slightly, so that devices to simulate heart sounds were also being constructed.

In 1900 Charles W. Larned of Johns Hopkins introduced techniques "to produce outside the body, tones which when conveyed to the ear would represent with a reasonable degree of exactness, at least in force and rhythm the sounds heard through the stethoscope placed upon the patient's chest."[148] He described four methods, which included using the forearm and stethoscope as the conductors for the sounds generated by tapping or percussing with the index or middle fingers. Larned outlined the procedures for producing specific heart sounds, including mitral and aortic valve insufficiency, mitral stenosis, and normal heart sounds. The distinguished cardiologist and teacher, Richard Cabot of Boston, in 1904 taught his students to distinguish the heart sounds with a mechanism composed of levers, drums, and an organ bellows connected to a megaphone.[149]

The use of artificially induced sounds was replaced by the electric receiver and multiply linked stethoscope, which was hooked up to a patient and the sound distributed through a series of receivers located in a lecture room, clinic, or linked to a loud speaker. Able to supply one thousand or more receivers with sounds of the intensity heard with the stethoscope, the electromagnetic device was incorporated into a portable unit. This teaching device was initially used in 1923 by Cabot and C. J. Gamble at the Massachusetts General Hospital.[150]

Phonograph records of heart sounds were made with the stethophone and a special electric recorder, which extended the teaching function of these electric instruments (see figure 5.17). By the method of phonocardiography, in which all vibrations of the chest are recorded[151] on film, auscultation on a broader scope becomes feasible. Sound vibrations could be slowed down by the recording film and correlated with electrocardiographic events. However, since the vibrations of sounds made by the lungs and those made by the heart overlap in their frequencies, the trained ear has an advantage over the phonocardiograph in distinguishing the sounds of these two

organs, in that the ear can select those sounds on which to concentrate (see figure 5.18).[152]

CONCLUSION:

S. Weir Mitchell summed up the reliability of the stethoscope in medical practice a half century after its introduction. "Every physician who deserves the name," he claimed, "now uses the stethoscope but, as yet, few men of the mass of physicians have trained themselves to learn to use the many other means which, in later years, have come to our aid."[153] Mitchell urged adoption of all types of medical equipment and techniques, a theme which had prompted the earliest followers of Laennec. Victor Collin, who had studied at the Neckar Hospital in Paris with Laennec, adhered to the view that "a single type of examination [using one type of instrument or test] is rarely sufficient; and that it is only in calling to our aid two or more of them and comparing the symptoms that they provide"[154] that a correct diagnosis can be made, provided that all instruments be avoided when not particularly necessary.

Nineteenth-century physicians applied instruments with discretion and distinguished between those models that gave poor results and those forms that deserved wider application. The physician's desire for improved performance expressed itself in continual attempts to redesign and modify even basic instruments. Laennec provided a stimulus for this cautious attitude toward medical instruments when he complained about early microscopic data. "If the causes of severe disease are sought for in mere microscopical alterations of structure, it is impossible to avoid running into consequences the most absurd and, if ever cultivated in this spirit, pathological anatomy, as well as that of the body in a sound state, will soon fall from the rank which it holds among the physical sciences and become a mere tissue of hypotheses founded on optical illusions and fanciful speculations, without any real benefit to medicine."[155] Both the data generated by the stethoscope and the observations gathered with the microscope were unclear, unorganized, and difficult to understand until they had been studied, interpreted, and verified by many physicians.

Laennec's invention stood preeminent among nineteenth-century physical diagnostic instruments because the stethoscope made use of the faculty of hearing, a sense of novel application in medical diagnosis, but mainly because Laennec provided an interpretation of the sounds associated with diseases and their diagnostic significance for the physician to learn

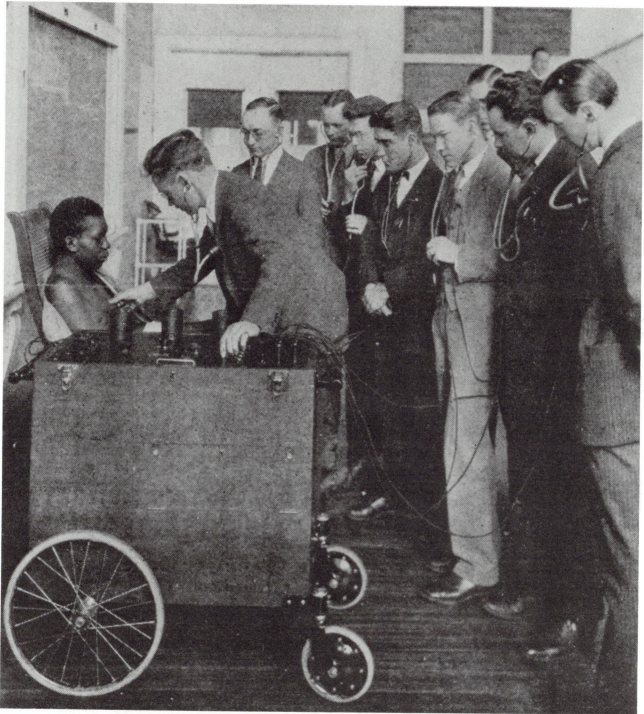

Figure 5.17. Multiple electrical stethoscope used to instruct a small group from C. J. Gamble "Multiple Electrical *Stethoscope and Electrical Filters as Aids to Diagnosis," JAMA* 83 (1924), p. 1230. *SI Photo No. 80.13929.*

as he applied the stethoscope. The public demand for the stethoscope forced physicians who were unable to use the instrument to at least carry one and apply it. Professor Trousseau told his student, C. Theodore Williams, that he knew a deaf physician who always used a stethoscope. "Il ausculte toujours et il entend jamais."[156]

The endorsement of diagnostic instruments was often qualified with the demand that instruments be chosen with care and avoided unless believed to be essential—a decision which was not easily made in the period of their introduction. By the end of the nineteenth century, the physician puzzled over the many models of monaural and binaural stethoscopes. (See figures 5.19, 5.20, and 5.21). It was generally agreed that a binaural stethoscope composed of an inner tube of smooth metal covered with a rubber outer layer connected to a diaphragm-shaped chest-piece responded best to the higher frequencies of the chest sounds and a bell-shaped chest-piece picked up

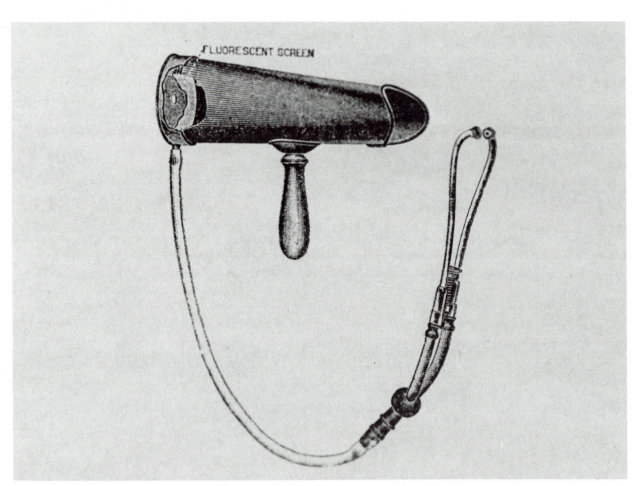

Figure 5.18. The See-Hear, a combined fluoroscope and stethoscope which enabled the operator to see the movements of the heart while listening to its sounds. *SI Photo.*

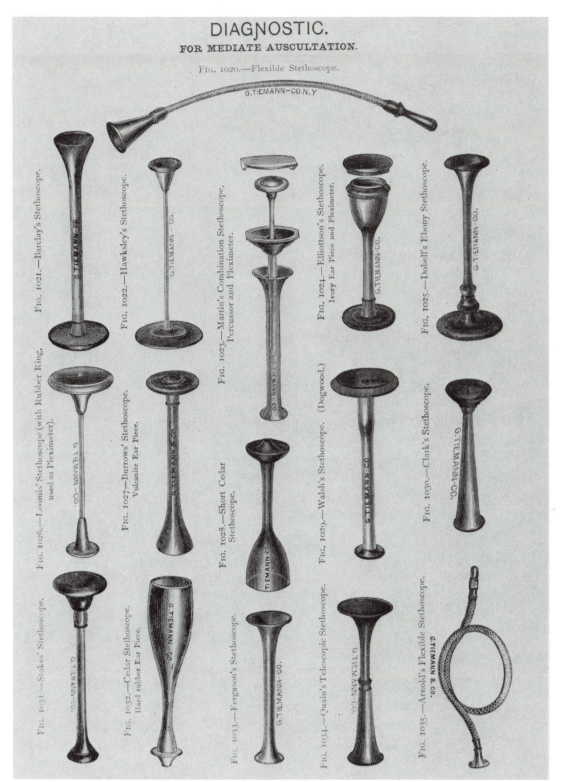

Figure 5.19 Assortment of 1889 monaural stethoscopes. From George Tiemann and Co.'s *Surgical Instrument Catalogue*, 1889, p. 5. *SI Photo No. 80-13427.*

DIAGNOSTIC.

FOR MEDIATE AUSCULTATION.

Many other modifications of Cammann's Binaural Stethoscope have been suggested, of which that of Mr. Irvin Palmer deserves special notice. This instrument is adapted for use as calipers and the elastic band of Cammann's is replaced by a circular box spring at the hinge. Attached to the joint is a dial plate, which registers the divergence of the two metal arms—thus at once enabling diametric and other measurements to be accurately and readily made without the addition of a separate instrument. It will recommend itself to the profession for the facility with which it permits anatomical measurements to be registered: as, for example, in estimating the relative expanding power of the two sides of the chest, in lung disease, &c.

London Medical Record, May 15, 1881.

FIG. 1044.—Ware's Stethoscope.

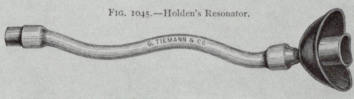

FIG. 1045.—Holden's Resonator.

FOR MEDIATE PERCUSSION.

FIG. 1047.—Hoffmann's Pleximeter.

FIG. 1046.—Flint's Pleximeter.

FIG. 1048.—Glass Pleximeter.

FIG. 1049.—Ivory Pleximeter.

FIG. 1050.—Flint's Percussor.

FIG. 1051.—Gerne's Pleximeter.

FIG. 1052.—Percussor with Whalebone Stem.

FIG. 1053.—Winterich's Percussion Hammer.

FIG. 1054.—Speir's Echoscope (to intensify sounds produced by percussion).

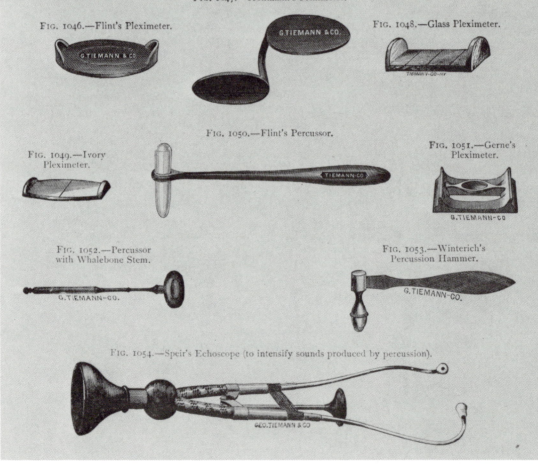

Figure 5.20. Diagnostic equipment for mediate auscultation from George Tiemann and Co.'s *Surgical Instrument Catalogue*, 1889, p. 7. *SI Photo No. 80-13425.*

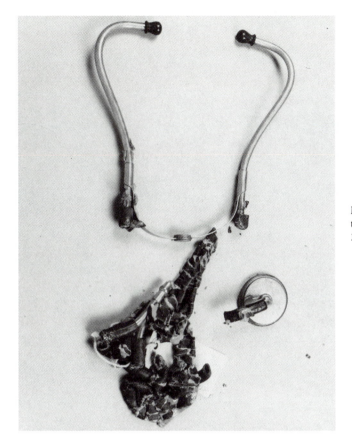

Figure 5.21. Binaural Stethoscope, deteriorated to show how rubber tubing may crack after drying out. *NMAH No. M 7824, SI Photo No. 78-5069.*

the lower frequencies with greater clarity. These two chest-pieces combined in a single unit when attached to two flexible tubes in a binaural stethoscope, became the most reputable instrument by the twentieth century.

A prime user of the stethoscope was to become the experimentalist.[157] Physiologists employed the stethoscope and other diagnostic equipment to measure and understand the various animal systems that they were exploring. Measurement of the intermediate phases and ultimate changes in bodily functions assisted diagnosticians and experimentalists in their quest for precision in an age that came to regard precision as highly desirable. Sound-locating instruments used to define the stages of disease and to distinguish between closely related maladies, which made the diagnostic process more precise, included, by the twentieth century, the electric stethoscope with filters to select specific sounds for study, and the cardiometer for accurately positioning the stethoscope on the chest. Physiologic and pathologic studies esca-

lated in the nineteenth century because of the availability of special instruments to measure finer details, with the result that the borderline between physiology and pathology became refined into increasingly complex components.

The location of the heart and other internal organs was determined by percussing the chest and marking the echo. Thousands of examinations were compiled to give an estimate of the normal positions of all organs and the sounds they made. Sound-recording and sound-locating instruments were applied extensively to formulate tables of measurements, which indicated the boundaries between abnormal and normal sounds. Now that the most widely used early diagnostic instruments have been discussed, a host of specialized and unique instruments that assisted in determining other borderlines between health and disease in other parts of the body is taken up in the next chapters, which center on issues that assess the impact of instruments on physiology and pathology.

6

CONCEPTS OF THE PULSE AND INSTRUMENTS

INTRODUCTION:

Among the most basic physiologic phenomena for which instruments were developed is the pulse. Nineteenth-century physicians, who were aware of "valuable contributions of the past, none the less real because based on wrong theory,"[1] helped to preserve useful older methods of physical examination and to encourage improvements in these techniques through the use of instruments. Feeling the throb of an artery near the surface of the body is perhaps the most fundamental of these techniques. All that was required was the fingers and a sense of rhythm. After being overshadowed by other diagnostic criteria in the early to mid-nineteenth century, the pulse took on a new importance when instruments were developed to measure and record its intricate characteristics as well as the rate of its motion. The history of pulse observation and interpretation in Western societies in the last half of the nineteenth century reveals the introduction of an array of special instruments to measure and record the pattern of the blood flow in the heart and blood vessels. Previously, the pulse had been interpreted and designated by a variety of terms applied to describe its characteristics, including rhythm, frequency, amplitude, and regularity. In tracing some of these early descriptions, we set the stage for understanding the complexity and clarity introduced through the use of instruments designed to measure, record, and interpret the pulse. Before special pulse instruments were introduced in the latter half of the nineteenth century, the physician had neglected this phenomenon in favor of giving increasing attention to other physiologic events that became more accessible through the application of instruments.

In 1867, Eduoard Seguin claimed that "the pulse as the external expression of circulation has always been the beacon of physicians."[2] In tracing the medical profession's attitudes toward the pulse and the instruments devised for observing and measuring it, it appears that the fundamental phenomenon of the arterial pulse had to be magnified and "rephrased" to regain a major role as an effective element in diagnosis and treatment in the nineteenth century among physicians in Western societies. Seguin argued for the use of instruments to reassess the pulse when he explained that "the pulse may finally remain what it primarily was, if we improve the means of perceiving and reading it as we have the other clinical signs."[3] Francis Adams, who translated some of Galen's statements on the pulse in 1834 and published them a decade later, pointed out that a lack of care in using the pulse as a diagnostic sign had overtaken contemporary physicians: "It is to be borne in mind that the ancients performed the operation of feeling the pulse more methodically than is now generally done, which may in part account for our having lost sight of some of the nicer shades of distinction which they recognized."[4] Throughout the nineteenth century, a lack of appreciation of some of the basic characteristics of the pulse—rhythm, strength, volume, and frequency—would remain the basis for encouraging physicians to use special instruments devised to record the pulse, especially as it could be detected in the wrist or radial artery and the neck or carotid artery, or in a combination of these vessels and the heart itself. Pulse data had already been gathered centuries earlier, some of it with simple tools and timers.

For millenia the pulse had been regarded as a basic sign of life, as well as an indicator of disease. The term for the study of the pulse, *sphygmology*, is derived from the Greek word *sphygmos*, which means to beat or pulse. The study of sphygmology was broadened by Hippocrates to include all movements of the pulse, not just its violent forms, which originally attracted the attention of physicians.[5] Sphygmology and urology (the study of the color and consistency of the urine) are among the oldest of the diagnostic signs developed in all cultures, including the Egyptian, Greek, Arabic, Indian, Chinese, and Western nations.[6] In the East, physicians accepted the range of pulses as the foundation for elaborate and definitive diagnosis and prognosis but never developed devices to assist them in measuring and describing the pulse. The distinctions Eastern physicians noticed among different types of pulses were as detailed as those that evolved from applying a variety of mechanical pulse recorders many centuries later. In over one hundred Ayurvedian treatises, six hundred types of pulses are enumerated. The unique attributes of the pulse noted in different parts of the body remain among the most important theoretical components of Chinese and Indian medical practice.

The sensitivity of Western physicians in applying fingers to pulsating arteries close to the skin diminished as devices were interposed between the physician and the patient's pulse. One of the earliest attempts to amplify the pulse through an intermediary device was made by the Polish physician, Joseph Struthius, who in the sixteenth century suggested putting a leaf on an artery or vein to make its pulsations easily visible.[7] This simple arrangement would be extended and multiplied to include complex devices to record and print data. There is reason to believe that the increased use of instruments led to an estrangement between the patient and the physician, culminating in the mechanization of medical practice related to cardiology by the twentieth century. The development of methods to study the pulse in the East and the West provides an illuminating case study, contrasting medicine that has ignored mechanical aids and medicine that depends on their assistence.

Ilza Veith, who translated the oldest Chinese text related to sphygmology, the *Nei Ching* (circa 250 B.C.), claims that sphygmology was "the chief means of diagnosis employed in the *Nei Ching*."[8] The basis of this practice was the belief that each organ of the body has a proper pulse, which prevailed at different times of the year. The relationship between the pulse, organs, and months of the year led to the creation of an official pulse-calendar. Taking at least half an hour to feel the pulse to make a diagnosis and a prognosis, the Chinese physician brought the method to a fine art. Pulses were represented graphically as they appeared to their Chinese observers by symbols or hieroglyphs representing such natural events as the jump of a frog, the movement of the tail of a fish, or a drop of rain falling on a roof.[9]

Notation of pulses based on simile and analogy was repeated in other cultures and would expand to include musical notes, shorthand symbols, and special terms. Indian pulse descriptions were linked to the motions of serpents, swans, and peacocks. These descriptions were carried over into the Galenic Corpus in designations such as pulsus formicans (ant-like or scarcely perceptible pulse) and pulses dorcadisans (leaping like a goat).[10] Picturesque descriptions did not satisfactorily characterize the pulse for Western commentators of the eighteenth and nineteenth centuries including the physician Sir John Floyer, the inventor of the pulse watch in the early eighteenth century. He criticized those who described the pulse as being similar to "a flying Ribband or Feather or to the motion of cock's wings."[11] Later, the pulse and the heart sounds were described in terms of the sounds and noises familiar to physicians in other cultures and ultimately were based on the sounds and graphic patterns obtained with the aid of pulse magnifying and interpreting instruments. Precision and objectivity were the goals of those who changed the pulse nomenclature.

The Chinese have defined disease as a dynamic chain reaction affecting the whole organism. The Chinese belief that all diseases have an impact on the entire organism is directly linked to their understanding of the pulse. The pulse reveals to the Oriental physician the earliest signs of disease and quickly indicates the effectiveness of any treatment that may be applied. The radial artery of the right wrist in the male and the left wrist of the female was examined for compressibility, frequency, regularity, size, and the impression that it made upon the fingers.[12]

After the flurry of activity in analyzing the pulse with the aid of mechanical instruments and devices, the twentieth-century physician employed the pulse as a diagnostic aid but as only one of a series of disease markers. Thus, the pulse once more became less significant than it had been in the past to the medical practitioner. The differences between the Eastern and Western physicians' views of the pulse as they remain up to the present have been summed up by Amber and Babey-Brooke:

To the Western physician the pulse in its relation to health and disease is relatively unimportant. The average doctor uses the pulse as one of a series of diagnostic aids to the diseases of the heart and circulation, and often a minor one at that—just another in a series of laboratory tests to be fitted into the jigsaw puzzle of health. But to the Ayurvedic, Unani and Chinese doctor of yesterday and today, the pulse was and is a subject of primary importance; and all other diagnostic techniques are ancillary to the pulse readings.[13]

ANCIENT PRACTICES:

To discover the earliest sources of the Western physician's attitudes toward the pulse, it is necessary to turn to two of the oldest medical documents, the Ebers and Smith Papyri, in which appear references to the pulse.[14] Praxagoras (340-320 B.C.) was the earliest to distinguish between the arteries and veins and to formulate a science of the pulse by confining his observations to pulsating arteries.[15] Herophilus was the first to recognize the pulse as a clinical sign useful in diagnosis and prognosis. His description of the different classes of pulses and their qualities and variations were central to the later teaching of Archigenes, Rufus, and Galen.[16]

A knowledge of music was important to interpret the pulse, according to Herophilus. In singling out four of its qualities, size, frequency, force, and rhythm, he emphasized the rhythm. By rhythm, he meant the relative duration of the diastole (arterial expansion) and systole (pause) of each pulse beat.[17] To delineate these components of a pulse beat, Herophilus employed the metrical scheme invented by Aristoxenus, a philosopher and musician at the beginning of the third century B.C., who proposed the concept of "feet" to include a pattern of long and short syllables. Variations in the discerned normal pattern were taken to be signs of disease.[18] Herophilus timed the pulse by the clepsydra or water clock, but little is known of the conclusions he drew from this procedure.[19]

Hippocrates differentiated the pulse into a sphygmos and a palmos.[20] The sphygmos corresponded to the perceptible movements of the arteries and the palmos or palpitation corresponded to arterial motion, which was later denied by Galen. Initially, the sphygmos or violent movements was associated only with disease, but after the descriptions provided by Herophilus, the sphygmos began to be recognized as part of the normal sequence of pulsation.[21] Markellinos before Galen discusses the types of pulse associated with specific diseases. One pulse he mentioned was the "gazelling" pulse, which is dicrotic or giving two beats during a single motion of the diastole. The first beat is softer, followed by a stronger pulse just like the gazelle, which takes a small step before taking a sudden big jump. Rufus, another pre-Galenic

expositor, described the pulse associated with a double beat found in healthy people after violent exercise and in those individuals with rising temperatures.[22] The dicrotic pulse remains a useful sign for the pulse altered by disease.

Commentators and translators of Galen's pulse treatises, in attempting to simplify his explanations, introduced confusing descriptions of the pulses. These transformations are in part responsible for the misunderstanding and eventual rejection of the pulse descriptions devised by Galen.[23] Galen defined the pulse as an expansion and contraction of the arteries taking place in two motions designated by the terms *diastole* and *systole*. By the diastole he meant "as it were, an unfolding and expansion of the artery, the cold air enters, ventilating and resuscitating the animal vapour, and hence the formation of the vital spirits; and by the systole, which is, as it were, a falling down and contraction of the circumference of the artery towards the centre, the evacuation of the fuliginous superfluities is effected."[24] Galen distinguished between two separate and independent movements by the terms diastole and systole which terms are used in the reverse sense today.[25]

Harvey in *On the Motion of the Heart and Blood in Animals* distinguished the diastole and systole in the modern sense. He found that

inasmuch as it is generally believed that when the heart strikes the breast and the pulse is felt without, the heart is dilated in its ventricles and is filled with blood; but the contrary of this is the fact, and the heart, when it contracts, is emptied. Whence the motion which is generally regarded as the diastole of the heart, is in truth its systole. And in like manner the intrinsic motion of the heart is not the diastole but the systole; neither is it in the diastole that the heart grows firm and tense, but in the systole, for then only, when tense, is it moved and made vigorous.[26]

Galen confronted the difficulty of distinguishing the characteristics of the pulse. Responding to the body's varying physiologic needs, the pulse varied in its size, speed, and frequency. These three attributes of the pulse were related so that "the size of the pulse is measured by the quantity of dilation and contraction, the speed by the time taken by each of the two movements of the single beat, and the frequency by the time interval between successive beats, which is determined largely by the length of the intervals between the time of quiescence and their variations. . . . there are twenty-seven varieties of each of the two movements in each single beat."[27] When the variations in other than the spatial qualities are considered, there are five different classes, including its size, strength or force, speed of each single movement of diastole or systole and speed of a series of pulses, and finally, hardness or softness, which depends on the coats of the arteries.[28] Knowing the normal intervals and the proportions between them, in addition to recognizing their alteration by disease, was essential in discerning the intricacies of the pulse. Only through experience could the physician learn to recognize these subtle distinctions.[29]

One method devised to assist the physician in learning the components of the pulse was introduced by Joseph Struthius in 1555. Struthius represented the pulse graphically for the first time in Western literature in his *Ars sphygmica, seu pulsum doctrina supre 1200 annos perdita et desiderata omnibus tamen Medicinam . . .*, which depicted the pulse in symbols. The use of symbols probably occurred earlier, although no record of any earlier symbols exists. Herophilus in ancient Greece called attention to the similarity between the arterial pulsation and musical cadences. The Chinese had represented the pulse by drawing circular figures with radiating lines to distinguish the different pulses, although their intention was not to represent the tactile pulse in the manner of Struthius. Robert Flood in 1630 and Struthius described the pulse by a series of musical notes. A twentieth-century historian of sphygmology has constructed graphs of the pulse described by Struthius. These are the *pulsus dicrotus* and the *pulsus caprazans*, which derived their names from the ancient Greeks (see figure 6.1).[30]

Difficulty in determining certain aspects of the pulse would remain into the nineteenth century, even after a series of instruments were invented to magnify and transform the component parts of the pulse from a tactile to a visual observation. Instruments would refine recognition of the qualities of the pulse and introduce new opportunities for error. Certainly, the demands made upon the observer were as sophisticated as those required by Galen's system and were best learned through experience and practice. Contradictory results obtained by investigators or by the same investigator at different times were also part of the harvest of applying machines to observe and record the pulse.

PULSE TIMERS:

Among the earliest instruments to be used in connection with the pulse were those that registered the frequency of the beats by measuring the weight of the water flowing into a container while the number of pulsations were counted. The weight of the water was proportional to the number of beats per unit of time. The clepsydra or water clock was the instrument used by Herophilus for this purpose.[31]

Nicolaus Krebs, better known as Cusanus, introduced a novelty into the tradition of Herophilus when he used the water clock to compare the pulse of a healthy young man and that of a weak man in 1476 in *The Experiments on Statics*, one of a collection of four papers or "Idiota libri quatuor."[32] The water clock was the least expensive and most reliable time measurer in use and would remain so until the eighteenth century. Cusanus recommended that the pulses of individuals be counted up to one hundred beats and the amount of water that flowed through the clock for each person be weighed.

From the weight of water therefore, the differences of the pulses would be arrived at, in the young, old, healthy, infirm, and so a truer knowledge of the disease; since there necessarily turns out to be one weight in one infirmity, another in another. Wherefore a more accurate judgement might be arrived at by such a difference resulting from an experiment of the pulses, and by the weight of the urine, than by touching of a vein and the color of urine at the time.[33]

It was the physician's task to discover the weight of the water that flowed through the clock while one hundred pulses were counted in a healthy boy or young man, as well as in other individuals suffering from different diseases, so that he could use these observations as standards in diagnosing illnesses.[34] Up to the seventeenth century, clepsydras existed in several forms, but all were produced for communal use. They were large and placed in a permanent public location.[35] Portable table clepysdras were introduced in the seventeenth century when the mechanical clock achieved its greatest advances. The earliest record of a portable clepsydra is a description by Fulgenzio Micanzio, provided in a letter to Galileo in 1630.[36] Athanasius Kirchner of Rome provided the earliest published description of the table clepsydra in 1646 and added more detail in his publication of 1654.[37] Kirchner recognized the value of timing the pulse. Since clepysdras had to be turned over to drain the water back, they were designed to measure periods of at least half an hour or more. This fact may account for the then-current practice of measuring the pulse for 30 minutes at a time.

Among the earliest instances of a pendulum being used to compare the frequency of the pulse was the swinging chandelier in the Pisa Duoma, which Galileo

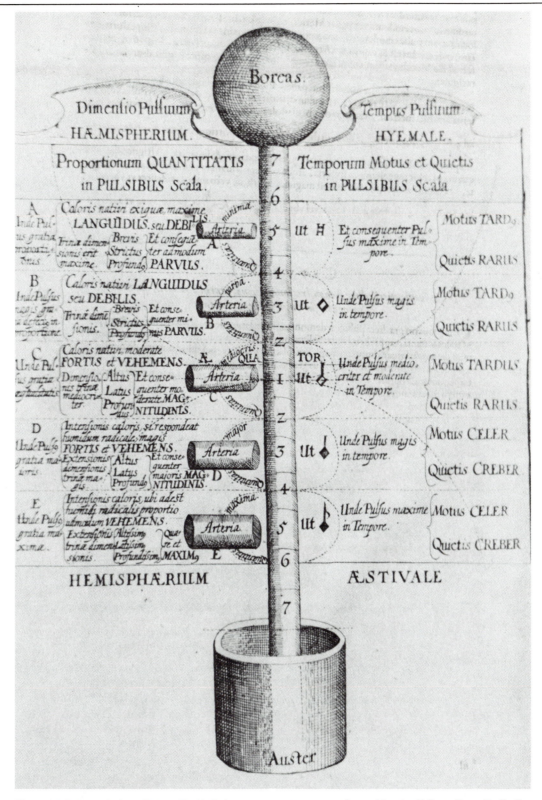

Figure 6.1 Pulse scale from Robert Fludd, Pulsus seu nova et arcana pulsuum historia, E Sacro Fonte Radicaliter Extracta, nec non medicorum ethnicorum dictis et authoritate comprobatu. Frankfurt: W. Hofmanni, 1630. The scale shows the equivalencies between the proportional quantity of pulse and the speed of the pulse. Photo by the author from text in *Collection of Maryland Medical and Chirurgical Faculty Library*.

timed by comparing it to his own pulse in 1582. He counted his pulse to be eighty beats per minute. The pendulum clock was the first scientific instrument devised by Galileo. Its first practical application was as a small pendulum used to time the pulse, which was called a pulsilogium. Galileo observed the isochronism of the pendulum or the fact that an unobstructed pendulum will make equal motions from side to side about a center point of suspension in equal amounts of time.[38] The only description of Galileo's discovery is provided by Vincentio Viviana in his letter of 20 August 1669 to Prince Leopold de Medici.[39] Santorio Santorio, who may have met Galileo at Padua, since their careers at the university overlapped, devised a pulsilogium to use on patients with fevers. His descriptions appear in his 1625 publication.[40] Perhaps also familiar with the work of Struthius, Santorio described the pulsilogium, which could be regulated so that its rate of motion from side to side could be changed until it coincided with that of the pulse. Behind the pendulum, whose length was variable, was placed a scale marked with appropriate diagnostic inscriptions, which therefore, provided a measure of the pulse's rate, of value to the physician. The pulse was described in the diagnostic terms assigned to the length of the pendulum with which its beat coincided or the amount of shortening or elongating necessary from one observation to the next. A pulse of x number of inches could be differentiated from one of y number of inches by this pulsilogium.

Several of Santorio's pulsilogia were illustrated. One, called a cotyla, had a bowl shape at the bottom and a dial divided into twelve equal parts.[41] A second one possessed a dial divided into twenty-four parts or "the number of divisions of public clocks of the time."[42] Santorio planned to explain these clocks in De medicis instrumentis, which was never published.[43]

Marin Mersenne of Paris explained the function of the instrument:

if the doctors wish to note whether the pulse of their patients is going faster or more slowly the second, third, fourth or fifth day, etc. than the first and by how much it is going too fast, the string fixed by one end will show it to them, for if the pulse beats the first day, or the first hour more slowly, etc., the string must be shortened to show the faster speed, and according to the shortening one gives it, he will recognize by how much the pulse is going faster.[44]

The various types of pulsilogia which depended on the accuracy of the swing of a pendulum over short periods of time were used primarily to indicate the acceleration or de-acceleration of the pulse without indicating a specific number of beats per unit of time. Even by the time Harvey was seeking quantitative confirmation of the circulation theory, he did not find it essential to count accurately the number of pulses per unit of time, nor to compare the different pulse rates among various animals. In chapter nine of De motu cordis, Harvey's count of the pulse during half an hour varied between one thousand and four thousand beats.[45] These variations may be ascribed in part to individual variation and the possible inaccuracy of the clock he used. In one passage of the First Discourse, written in 1649 to answer Jean Riolan's questions about the circulation of the blood, Harvey quoted Riolan's proposed rate for the human pulse of two thousand beats per hour without contesting this figure.[46] Harvey's own effort to demonstrate that blood was not continuously created, which bore witness to the fact that the same blood circulated repeatedly, was also based on his observations that if phlebotomy was performed for half an hour, the body would be almost drained of its blood.[47] To demonstrate the force, frequency, volume, and rhythm of the pulse, Harvey suggested that a piece of intestine be filled with water and closed at both ends. When a tap was given to one end, the movement at the other end was immediately noticed, just as the thrust of the blood from the heart into the arteries was noted in feeling the pulse.[48] Similar mechanical experiments would be carried out in the last quarter of the nineteenth century to understand the motion of the pulse and to appreciate the information given by the sphygmograph invented to record graphically the motion of the arteries and the heart.

JOHN FLOYER AND THE PULSE-WATCH:

John Floyer was the first physician to write several volumes (1707, 1710) on the pulse and to explain a timer that he called a pulse-watch. By counting the number of pulses occurring within one minute, he created a demand for watches capable of registering the passage of time in seconds. Physicians who adopted his technique were the prime users of such watches over the following fifty years.[49] Floyer devised an entire system of medicine (prognostic, diagnostic, and therapeutic) on the basis of the pulse rate. The foundations of his system lie in the iatro-mechanistic theories of the period, which he understood, but did not embrace wholeheartedly. To Floyer it seemed unessential that a successful practitioner understand iatro-mechanism. Floyer's stated goal was to fulfill the medical program envisioned by

William Harvey, which remained uncompleted.[50] The second part of his program led to a reexamination and interpretation of many diseases previously classified by the ancient Greeks. Floyer explained all diseases in terms of the function of the circulatory organs and their expression by the rate of the pulse.[51] Floyer's plans were optimal for the early eighteenth century. There is no need for the apology Floyer's most recent biographer makes in his assessment of Floyer's contributions. Gary Townsend claims that: "Floyer's great problem was his inability to place pulse numeration in its proper perspective. Having little else but the pulse to rely on and lacking a proper knowledge of pathology, he was apt to deduce too much from his observations on one subject."[52] The fact is that the diagnostic technique Floyer concentrated on was the most outstanding one to be brought to the attention of physicians at the time, since they had learned to understand the circulation but had not been taught how to apply it in their practices. Floyer's pulse theories provided a system for accomplishing this goal. As Thomas Willis, the English iatrochemist-mechanist two generations earlier, and others did, Floyer attempted to carry out Harvey's own intentions to make the discovery of the circulation useful in medical practice.

As incomplete and over-simplified as it seems in retrospect, Floyer's interpretation of pulse counting as a practical application of the circulation theory was an anticipated consequence of the discovery of the circulation. Floyer defined the pulse as "that sensible motion which is given to the Artery by the Blood, which the Heart injects into it or . . . is the motion of the Heart and Arteries, and the Original of all the Animal Motions."[53] Floyer summarized Harvey's position:

Dr. Harvey gave the first credit, if not the first rise to the opinion about the circulation of the Blood, which was expected to bring in great and general Innovations into the whole Practice of Physick, but it had no such effect. I'm satisfied that Dr. Harvey did design a Tract about the Pulse, as he intimates, which if he had done, he would have pursu'd his scheme, and drawn it into Practice. I hope what I have done will excite the young Physicians to improve this subject, which will be very useful, by improving the Notion of many Diseases, and will reduce them to a Circulation too slow or too fast, and we shall discover hereby the true and real effects of all Specifics, as they either stop or accelerate the Pulse.[54]

Diseases of the blood were those emphasized in Floyer's description of the circulation running "too fast or too slow."

The pulse provided an early bridge between older and newer medical concepts and indicated aspects of internal diseases not evident to the senses in other ways. Floyer reintroduced the Chinese terms for different pulses and simplified some of their distinctions. He emphasized the obvious characteristics of the pulse because he believed that the more intrinsic pulses would not be apparent to many physicians, and therefore, would not be useful in medical practice.[55] In taking this position, Floyer recognized a major problem that was to reoccur in other methods of physical diagnosis—the difficulty in defining the qualities and quantities of the organs and their functions in terms that could be learned and understood by the majority of physicians without unusual effort and that could be simplified and applied to most patients.

Another reason Chinese pulse lore impressed Floyer was its reputed foundation in the blood's circulation, although Floyer recognized that the Chinese did not know the route of the circulation as Harvey had revealed it. Understanding that the blood circulated, combined with monitoring the pulse, Floyer was satisfied that the Chinese were superior to the Greeks in developing diagnosis on the basis of the pulse and refraining from therapeutic practices like bleeding, cupping, and giving clysters. Floyer blamed the confused ideas about Chinese pulse doctrines on those who translated them into Latin.[56]

The most compelling association Floyer found between the Chinese doctrine of the pulse and his own observations was their measurement of the pulse. The Chinese recorded the pulse at a rate of forty-five to fifty beats per minute or about twenty to thirty beats per minute less than Floyer had observed it to be. Floyer constructed a table of the pulse rate and related it to the latitude in which the individual lived when his pulse was recorded and found that the pulse decreased with decreasing latitude, which supported the lower rate for the pulse discovered by the Chinese.[57]

The Chinese had not developed a special timer for the pulse, but Floyer found such a timer essential. Encouraged by Santorio's publications, Floyer used a standard watch with a single hand like a pendulum clock to time the pulse. Lacking facility in using this type of watch for the short time span during which the pulse was counted, Floyer had a craftsman produce a pulse-watch that registered sixty seconds.[58]

The publication of his first volume on the pulse-watch induced an anonymous benefactor to send Floyer a watch, which Floyer illustrated in his second volume (see figure 6.2). Floyer claimed that unlike his own pulse-watch, which was four to five seconds slower than his minute glass, the one sent to him was only one second slower.[59]

One of the most illustrious critics of timing the pulse for diagnostic purposes was R. T. H. Laennec.[60] Unlike ancient commentators on the pulse, Laennec understated the difficulties in learning to understand the circulatory and respiratory sounds through application of the stethoscope. His estimation of the time needed to master the stethoscope—a few weeks or at most a few months—was not adequate for many practitioners. The problems of teaching students how and when to apply the stethoscope continued over the next century as new models and special teaching techniques were designed. The sounds produced within the chest were mystifying and subject to misinterpretation just like the force, rhythm, and other aspects of the pulse.

Critical assessment of existing diagnostic modes characterizes the introduction of new methods, including methods employing instruments. In the rush of enthusiasm to introduce the instrument, the value of former methods is diminished when unbiased assessment would have shown that some of the older techniques retain a usefulness that may even be enhanced when combined with new equipment. The stethoscope, when used to magnify the sound of the pulse, provided some of the most generally useful diagnostic data—the force of the blood pressure—in a technique worked out by the Russian physician N. L. Korotkoff in 1905.[61] Discovered while preparing his thesis for the doctorate in medicine, Korotkoff's technique (described in chapter seven, below) became the foremost method of recording the blood pressure, employed universally by physicians up to the present.[62]

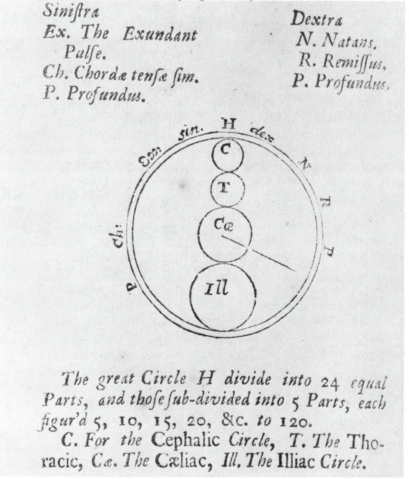

Figure 6.2. 1710 Illustration from John Floyer's *The Pulse Watch,* **vol. ii p. 328. From the** *National Library of Medicine, Bethesda, Maryland No. 78-117.*

Nineteenth-Century Pulse Technology:

Timing the pulse was only one way to quantify it. The ancient terms charactrizing the pulse's strength, speed, and patterns of beats defined qualities of the pulse that would be made explicit and numerical in the nineteenth century through the application of instruments, which could amplify, trace, and select specific patterns of the pulse and produce permanent records of them. The pulse was described according to the components of its frequency, strength, rhythm, volume, and the shape of the curve it produced when permitted to trace a path on paper through the use of amplifying instruments.

By 1867, the value of quantifying the pulse for diagnostic accuracy appeared important, especially when compared to taking the temperature with the thermometer. Seguin claimed that: "The pulse, as the external expression of circulation, has always been the beacon of physicians, and though pathologically temperature, as expressed by the thermometer; bids fair to take the lead in diagnosis, the *pulse* may finally remain what it primarily was, if we improve the means of perceiving and reading it, as we have the other clinical signs."[63] The fingers not only lacked training in feeling the pulse, but also, unaided, were not adequate to determine all of the pulse's components. Austin Flint agreed with Seguin: "It is evident that few of the characters of a pulsation, occupying as it does but a seventieth part of a minute, can be ascertained by the sense of touch alone."[64]

Learning the characteristic of the pulse more precisely was crucial to understanding the exact distinction between a normal and abnormal pulse. The goal of obtaining fine distinctions among the pulses was reinforced by the fact that the body temperature could be determined to within one or two degrees with the use of the thermometer. As we show in chapter seven, finding the standards for normal and abnormal pulses was important to all physicians in their daily contact with patients. The relation between the normal and abnormal pulse was described by Eduaord Seguin in 1867:

Whilst physiological temperature, once established for our race, holds good as the standard of health for everybody, physiological circulation presents such changes above and below its mean reckoning that, when we are called to a new patient, we never know, and can only suspect, what—if any—was the deviation of the healthy pulse from the would-be average. In this trying and frequent occurrence, we know very well what the pathological pulse is; but how can we form a judgment upon the distance which separates this pulse from the healthy one? Since to establish our proportion we miss the most important term, the normal pulse.[65]

Stephen Hales in the eighteenth century first measured the arterial force by opening an artery and inserting a tube to conduct the blood driven by the force of the heart. While this led to measurement of blood pressure, it also contributed to the recording of the pulse. A series of experiments employing tubes of various types were undertaken in the nineteenth century by Fick, von Reichert, Du Bois-Reymond, Ludwig, Vierordt, and others. The most important of these instruments was devised by Carl Vierordt and Carl Ludwig in 1828 and 1847, respectively. Vierordt was the earliest to construct a sphygmograph to record graphically arterial movements, which were communicated to a lever. The tracings registered as simple vertical strokes. Ludwig recorded in his Marburg laboratory the arterial pressure from a dog's artery. Using Poiseuille's bent tube and mercurial column, he put a float on top of the mercury from which a stem arose and to which a needle was attached. This device, called a kymograph, traced the movements communicated to it by the fluctuation of the mercurial column onto a strip of soot-blackened paper stretched across a revolving drum. Hoff and Geddes, who studied the development of physiologic recording instruments, described Ludwig's kymograph as a new tool, which gave a basis for quantitative analysis of physiologic functions and a means of communication free from barriers of language.[66] The laboratories of Marey at the College de France, Starling in London, Bowditch in Boston, and others applied the kymograph to numerous problems of research related to bodily systems including the pulse and the circulation.

The sphygmometer was among the first pulse amplifiers that could be applied without opening an artery, and therefore, was of potential use to the diagnostician. Invented by Jules Hérisson and constructed by the engineer Paul Gernier in 1834, it provided a measurement of the volume, strength, and frequency of the pulse but did not provide a permanent record of these measurements.[67] The sphygmometer consisted of a straight glass tube, filled with mercury and covered at the other end with an elastic membrane. The mercury moved vertically in response to the movements of the artery. L. Waldenburg's pulse-clock, which resembled a clock barometer and registered the movements of the artery on a dial, was another instrument for transforming the pulse into a visual phenomenon.[68]

The first clinically useful pulse recorder was introduced by Étienne Marey in 1860 and improved over the next several decades (see figure 6.3).[69] While the instrument no longer recorded the actual volume, strength, or rhythm of the pulse, it presented a permenent record of the waves of the curve transmitted to a stylus by the motion of circulating fluid. Marey's sphygmograph consisted of a long spring furnished with a pelotte or button to be fastened over the radial artery. The spring's motions were communicated to a lever approximately six inches long, furnished with a stylus or pen that traced the movements on a strip of smoked paper or glass, which was moved by a clock mechanism underneath the pen. The Marey sphygmograph was difficult to apply because it extended up the arm longitudinally. Modified by Burdon San-

derson and F. A. Mahomed, it became the model most used in England until 1882, when the homeopathic physician Robert E. Dudgeon designed a compact and sensitive instrument that could be applied to the wrist without a support (see figures 6.4 and 6.5).[70] Dudgeon's sphygmograph measured two and a half by two inches and weighed four ounces. A hand-wound clockwork pulled a piece of smoked paper six inches long by an inch in height through the instrument in ten seconds. The smoked paper record was varnished with gum damar in bezodine to preserve its tracing.

The instrument consisted of a series of levers, the shorter arm pressed over the artery and the longer arm carrying the recording apparatus. The size and shape of the tracing was determined by the lengths of

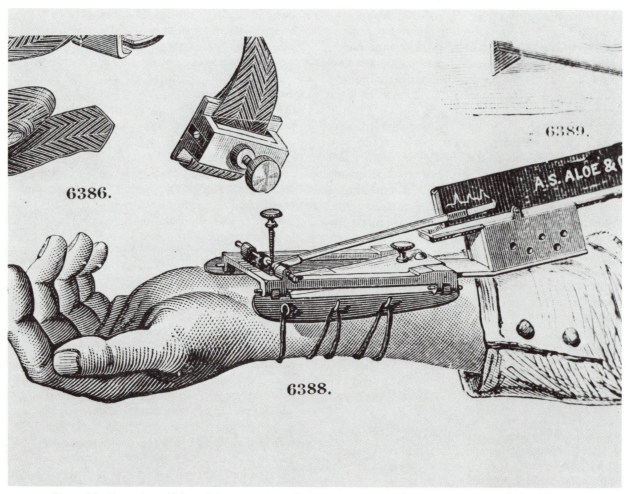

Figure 6.3. Illustration of Marey Sphygmograph applied to wrist circa 1893, from A. S. Aloe Catalogue, p. 351. *SI Photo No. 78-10551.*

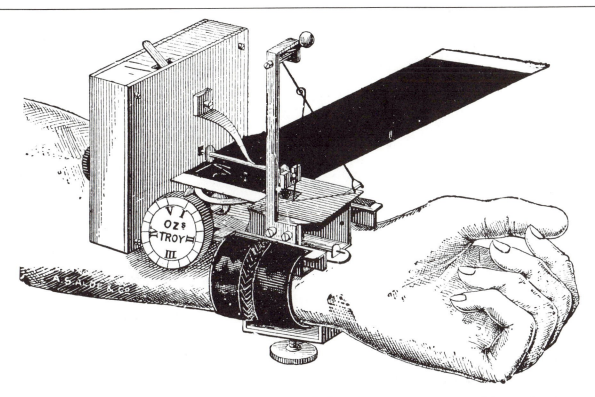

Figure 6.4. Illustration of Dudgeon's sphygmograph circa 1893, in place on the wrist showing dial to regulate the pressure of the lever applied to the pulsating artery. From A. S. Aloe Catalogue circa 1893. *SI Photo No. 78-10551.*

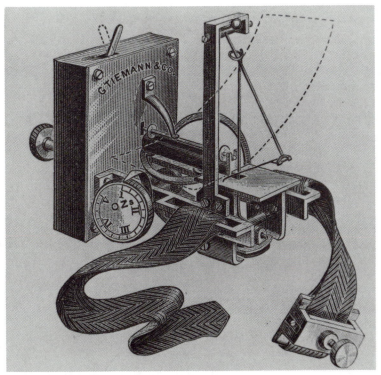

Figure 6.5. 1889 Illustration of Dudgeon sphgmograph from George Tiemann Co. Catalogue, 1889. *SI Photo No. 80-13424.*

the lever arms, the vessel size, variations in arterial tension, and the degree of pressure exerted on the artery. As a pressure control, a dial graduated in ounces or grams was fixed to the lever and could be set for the tension required to keep the lever on the artery and not obliterate the pulse (see figure 6.6). B. W. Richardson proposed a more manageable tension regulator by fixing the sphygmograph with a pressure gauge that projected as a weighing bar varying from one to six ounces. The weight could be moved along the bar as in a metronome.[71]

To make the recording easier to read and to compare each record with other tracings, Richardson added a row of sharp points to the roller bar, which moved the smoked paper along. The points cut a series of lines equidistant from each other along the entire length of the paper. With these guide lines as a background, the traces made by the ascending, or ventricular, and the descending, or auricular, pulse could be described accurately.[72]

The pulse in the veins was also measured by special instruments. One device called a hemarunascope was designed by Octavius A. White of New York in 1877 and was manufactured by F. G. Otto and Sons of New York. The instrument, which had similarities with Poiseuille's hemodynameter,[73] consisted of a glass tube of small caliber, open at both ends and bent symmetrically in half. This bend created a sufficient column of air to use as a highly sensitive and elastic spring. One end was expanded into a bell shape to be placed over the vein while excluding air during observation. The shaft of the tube was graduated in centimeters to facilitate quick estimation of the features noted. Filled with a drop of filtered aniline in an unbroken column, the "instrument [was] made to rest firmly and steadily upon the trunk of a superficial vein of sufficient dimensions, the peculiar movement of the stream of blood beneath the bowl of the instrument setting the sensitive fluid column within the tube into sympathetic motion, clearly demonstrating that the blood within the vein receives the shock and experiences augmentaion of contents nearly isochronous with the arterial throb."[74] Among the prospective uses for this sensitive manometer were extending physiologic research, detecting deviations from a healthy standard of the circulation, and indicating when to prescribe various drugs.

JAMES MACKENZIE AND PREVENTIVE MEDICINE:

By the turn of the century, physicians who were skilled in using the pulse-related instruments to explain physiology and pathology of circulatory disease

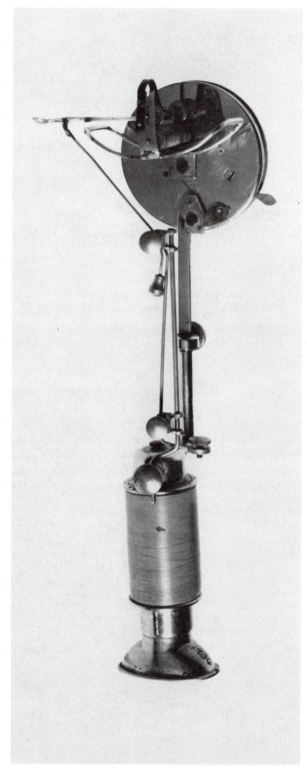

Figure 6.6. Pond's sphygmograph. *NMAH No. M 1603, SI Photo No. 72-756.*

realized that there had been an over-emphasis on cure and treatment and a relative neglect of counseling to prevent diseases of the circulatory system. Such counseling, they believed, could also be furthered by the use of these instruments. These experts claimed that diagnostic hardware revealed the presence of disease only after it had made inroads into the normal structures and functions of the body. James Mackenzie, English clinician and cardiologist, and the American, William S. Thayer, are among those who published these views in the hope of establishing prevention as the foremost concern of medical practitioners. Mackenzie focused on diseases of the heart and circulatory system and brought his views to the United States and Canada on several visits.

Physicians recognized some of the loss of diagnostic skill they suffered by employing instruments to register the pulse. The increasing use of instruments led to a call for programs to sharpen the senses of physicians who would be expected to function without these delicate instruments when the number of patients precluded the use of such instruments and the remote location made it difficult to obtain and service instruments regularly. Combining information received with the sphygmograph and that obtained directly through the fingers was encouraged.[75]

James Mackenzie made early diagnosis, based on observation of the pulse, a key element in his preventive medicine program. Mackenzie invented a successful pulse recorder and understood the pulse and its implications for health and disease better than most of his contemporaries. Intensive use of the polygraph to record and study the pulse led Mackenzie to conclusions similar to those of Oriental physicians who had studied the pulse without the aid of any instruments. Mackenzie appears not to have been aware of Chinese pulse doctrines.

Mackenzie, whose name is most often associated with the polygraph, indicated in 1909 that he never wanted his name to be linked with the polygraph in a conversation with J. W. Linnell, his resident medical officer at Mount Vernon Hospital in London. The polygraph, in Mackenzie's opinion, was a research tool, not designed to be of use to the general practitioner, who was expected to understand the significance of the heart sounds and changes in rhythm without applying the polygraph to all of his patients.[76]

Mackenzie considered his own successful studies with the sphygmograph and polygraph a preliminary stage in medical research. The polygraph provided a diagrammatic representation of the variations of the simultaneous pulsing cycle in the arteries, veins, and heart. The instrument became a symbol for twentieth-century American and European heart specialists, thus realizing Mackenzie's worst fears for its impact on medical practice.

Mackenzie continually stressed his own preference for medical practice over medical research. By close observation of the patient, he believed, the earliest signs and symptoms of heart disease could be noted. Mackenzie discovered that the heart muscle compensated for loss of function and first revealed its weakness through other organs when placed under strain. The earliest signs of disease of the heart were expressed in the functional limitation in other body parts that depended on proper circulation of the oxygen-bearing blood, which the heart was no longer able to supply in sufficient amounts.[77] As a result of his clinical experiences, he believed that instruments applied to the heart were of little use in diagnosis of disease in its earliest stages, whereas observation of the patient's behavior provided the evidence to understand developing heart failure. He explained:

for a time being under the delusion that instruments were the most scientific method, I spent much time in recording the rate of the heart, and studying the changes in the character of the pulse by graphic records and blood pressure instruments. These did not help. Then it occurred to me to ask of the individual, healthy and ailing, 'Why have you to stop?' and they all replied, 'Because of a feeling of distress.' This gave a new turn to my inquiry, and I then investigated this sensation of distress.[78]

One of these studies concentrated on women who had died of heart failure in the course of giving birth after appearing to be healthy during their pregnancies. Mackenzie studied the circulation of pregnant women with the intention of preventing some of these deaths.

Mackenzie collected records of irregular heart action with the Dudgeon sphygmograph and differentiated several forms of irregularity. By comparing the pulse in the heart and in the jugular vein, he traced the progression of an abnormal circulation. The venous pulse, itself a pathologic sign, provided information about two chambers of the heart—the right auricle and ventricle; the arterial pulse reflected the condition of the left ventricle. Mackenzie described his method in 1892: "After much labour I hit upon a plan almost ridiculous in its simplicity. This method consists in placing a hollow lead cone or funnel (called a 'receiver') over any pulsating part where the surface of the skin permits the cavity of the funnel to be hermetically closed. The base of the receiver I have mostly used has a diameter of one inch and a half."[79] When Mackenzie reduced the funnel to a small round box, he realized that he had reinvented Marey's tambour, which he had observed as a student. Then he continued:

This receiver is connected by means of an india rubber ink tube to a Marey's tambour and lever, the latter of which can be made to write on the smoked paper of a Dudgeon's sphygmograph or revolving cylinder. The advantage of this method is enhanced by the fact that several such receivers can be used to take tracings, at one and the same time, of heartbeat, and of arterial, or venous pulse. In this manner the time of the occurrence of the various incidents in a cardiac revolution can be discerned with certainty even in a pulsation at some distance from the heart.[80]

The function of the instrument led to the name "clinical polygraph." Mackenzie stated, "Inasmuch as the whole arrangement can be used for taking, at the same time and on the same recording surface, tracings of the radial pulse, with tracings of the apex beat, carotid, venous or liver pulse, or the respiratory movements, and as its size is such as to permit its being carried about with the greatest facility, and readily employed in general practice, I will refer to it as the 'clinical polygraph.' "[81] Krohne and Seseman of London made the first clinical polygraph for Mackenzie.

Other changes in the pulse-recording instrument made it easier to carry and able to record a tracing over an extended period. Improvements to the instrument culminated in the ink polygraph, perfected in 1906 by a Lancashire watchmaker, Sebastian Shaw of Padiham. Mackenzie used the polygraph to make recordings lasting up to one and a half hours. The American cardiologist, Paul Dudley White, testified to the popularity of the polygraph. White had studied cardiac arrhythmia and the jugular pulse with the instrument in 1912. Yet, on his first visit to the United States in 1906, Mackenzie failed to find a local manufacturer to supply the polygraph to American users. He tried to enlist the interest of W. T. Porter of the Harvard Medical School, who owned an instrument-making business, but was unsuccessful.[82]

In his first book published in 1902, *The Study of the Pulse, Arterial, Venous and Hepatic and of the Movements of the Heart*, Mackenzie related his observations and the conclusions to which they led. Allbutt, who reviewed the text for the *British Medical Journal* on 26 July 1902 commented that "so far as we are aware, this collection of three hundred and thirty-five tracings, nearly all of them perfectly taken by the author and as carefully reproduced, is unrivalled."[83] Allbutt praised Mackenzie for proving that medical research can be done by a busy physician. He explained: "We often hear that in the bustle of general practice scientific work is impossible; if Dr. Mackenzie had done no more than dispel this error he would have done good service."[84]

Although recorders were crucial to Mackenzie's study of the heart and pulse, he denounced their use by the general practitioner. He claimed: "For routine practice no instrument is necessary, and as soon as I found out the knowledge it could convey, I set about discovering means by which the information could be obtained by the unaided senses."[85] Instruments to diagnose and explain the course of disease represented a preliminary stage in the development of medicine. For Mackenzie, "the employment of mechanical devices as a rule represents a stage in the evolution of medicine, a necessary stage no doubt, in most cases, but still a stage, and a crude and elementary one."[86]

Improving instruments did not provide the means for better medical practice. Mackenzie felt that efforts over the last years of the nineteenth century and early twentieth century were misdirected in improving the stethoscope, the thermometer, and other instruments. Sir Thomas Lewis, who advanced Mackenzie's attitude toward the study of heart diseases, encouraged his students to take a more leisurely and intelligent interest in phenomena encountered in everyday practice, rather than to rely overly on laboratory research. A similar spirit of caution had occurred to surgeons in the nineteenth century when concepts including "rational surgery," "conservative surgery," and "preservative surgery" were announced with the intention of eliminating and reducing surgical procedures.

Medical instruments provided an opportunity for advances in understanding aspects of disease but also extra opportunities for error to which Mackenzie called attention. "While it may be claimed," he said, "that we may have one hundred new methods for investigating disease in the living, each of which adds to the sum of our knowledge, it must also be recognized that we have one hundred more ways for going astray."[87] Mackenzie insisted that certain criteria be applied before introducing instruments into practice. The inventor must demonstrate the bearing which the new facts an instrument uncovered would have upon knowledge of the disease condition it revealed. Furthermore, this information must provide a guide to treatment. Then, the inventor, after recognizing the value of his device in clinical medicine, must find a means to function without it in routine practice. While this advice seemed to verge on the absurd, which Mackenzie acknowledged, he could not understand how any physician could practice medicine with all the devices available in the early twentieth century. He singled out the Johns Hopkins Medical School for exposing students to too many instruments. Some of the instruments included: Roentgen ray apparatus, bacteriologic apparatus, various endoscopes, the sphygmograph, uretal catheters, equipment to test the senses, and calorimeters. Even though ranked as the most respected medical school in the United States, Johns Hopkins was not providing a desirable curriculum, Mackenzie reasoned, with so much emphasis on instruments and laboratory techniques. In his report on his second trip to the United States in 1918 as a guest of the American Medical Association, he remarked of Johns Hopkins physicians, "I never was more surprised to find such a stupid outlook as they possessed . . . so far as my own work is concerned, they had not even realized the elementary principles necessary to guide them in understanding the meaning of the symptoms which their numerous methods revealed."[88]

Mackenzie's criticism of the way in which instruments were used by physicians extended to all medical instruments. He wrote in his book on *Heart Disease and Pregnancy*, a summary of his intensive research on the heart, published during the last years of his life in 1921:

The coming of the stethoscope was the beginning of a method in clinical research which has greatly hampered the practice of medicine, in that the introduction of mechanical methods has led to a confusion as to the kind of knowledge which these methods are capable of affording. This criticism applies not only to the stethoscope and its various modifications, but to all other instruments which have since been employed in the examination of the patient. I need only mention the sphygmograph, polygraph, electrocardiograph, and blood pressure instruments.[89]

German, American, and French physicians accepted Mackenzie's views earlier and more wholeheartedly than did his countrymen. William Sydney Thayer of Baltimore explained in 1914:

And much of the information which these procedures give us can now be obtained by the simplest clinical observation. Nowhere is this more striking than in the study of cardiac irregularities. . . . The newer anatomical and physiological studies, the introduction and perfection of polygraphic and electrocardiographic methods has given us a very considerable amount of information which is not only of diagnostic but of great prognostic and therapeutic value. We are able to recognize with considerable accuracy, irregularities due to respiration, extra systoles of various sorts. . . . But comparing the results of these studies with that which is to be observed at the bedside, it becomes clear that most of

these conditions may be recognized with a considerable degree of accuracy, by the simpler methods of inspection, auscultation and percussion. By combining auscultation with the palpitation of the carotid pulse and the observation of the venous undulations of the neck it is usually possible to detect extra systolic irregularities and even with some degree of accuracy to separate different kinds.[90]

Having been alerted to important aspects of disease through instruments, the astute clinician learned to function without instruments in his daily practice.

Mackenzie discovered after following the lives of one thousand patients that the diseases which brought people to the physician's office were not the ones which caused their deaths.[91] He realized that physicians could recognize the third and fourth stages of disease using pathologic and clinical methods and instruments that were in vogue, but that they had not developed the concepts and methods essential to uncovering the first and second stages of disease, which accounted for this discrepancy in apparent and fatal illnesses.[92] The early stages of disease were the most difficult to detect because they were only detected by subjective methods. In addition, instruments and tests designed to study one organ did not provide information about changes in the functions of other organs. Therefore, the specialist who concentrated on diagnosing and treating one organ was at a disadvantage, which was underscored by the selection of recruits for World War I. Many physical diagnostic and laboratory tests proved incapable of detecting future disease and the body's ability to withstand the stress of war.[93]

Progress in medicine was not to be gauged by the tests for disease set up in the laboratory and hospital, in addition to the mechanical devices used to perform them. Rather, these artificial aids demonstrated the unnecessary complexity constantly intruding into medical practice "and as the employment of instruments is supposed to give a scientific accuracy to the observations it is imagined that in this way medicine is becoming more scientific."[94] However, far from enhancing the scientific nature of medicine, complexity and specialization were "darkening the understanding in a cloud of detail."[95] For Mackenzie, simplification was the test of real progress in medicine and its development as a science, which was not fostered by medical technology.

CONCLUSION:

Early descriptions of the pulse emphasized its rhythm, which was described by patterns of motion such as a leaping gazelle or a thundering elephant. By the seventeenth century, when the circulation of the blood was demonstrated, the rate, as well as the rhythm, of the pulse began to be of importance, especially for distinguishing between a normal and abnormal circulation. Counting the pulse for periods of one minute was facilitated in the early eighteenth century by the design of a pulse watch the physician could carry. Understanding the periodicity of the circulation and the function of the heart muscles provided justification for counting the pulse for one or two minutes and extrapolating this information for longer periods.

The nineteenth century witnessed a major reevaluation of the pulse among Western physicians. The introduction of instruments and devices enabled a

visual form of analysis to be added to observation based on the feel of the pulse. The implications of the circulation as indicated by changes in the pulse took on new significance when the pulse could be visualized, as well as timed, and compared to other sounds. Recording instruments, especially the sphygmograph, polygraph, and kymograph, enabled physicians to stop the motion of the pulse for intensive study and comparison with other observations and measurements of the cardiovascular system (see figure 6.7).

The sphygmograph made knowledge of the circulation useful to the physician in the sense that he could study the heart and vascular motions controlling blood and discover the changes that resulted in a disease requiring treatment (see figure 6.8). The

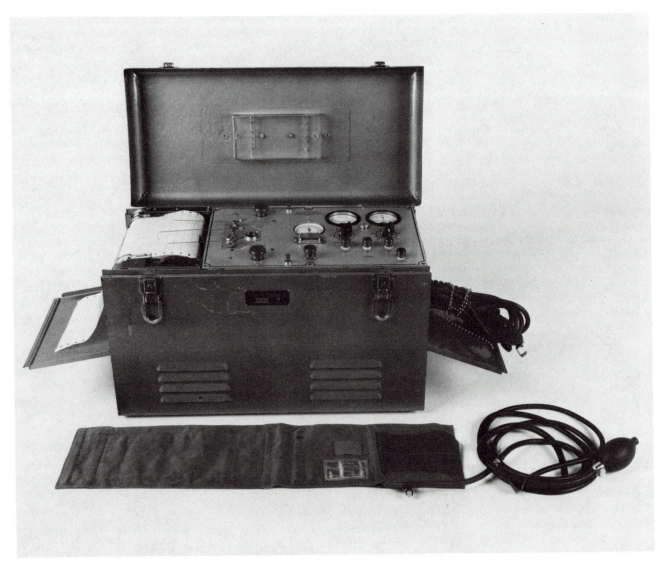

Figure 6.7. Keeler polygraph circa 1950. *NMAH No. 321, 642.02, SI Photo No. 76-6043.*

effect of the treatment applied (usually some type of drug) could then be studied through the tracings provided by the sphygmograph.

The next stage in refining the analysis of the vascular system grew out of recording the electrical pulses generated by the heart muscle as it contracted and expanded in pumping the blood. George Burch and N. P. Pasquale have provided a short but incisive account of the development of the electrocardiograph from the first cumbersome unit assembled by Weller in England to the many portable units manufactured by the largest American supplier, the Cambridge Instrument Company.[96] (See figures 6.9, 6.10, 6.11, 6.12, 6.13, 6.14, and 6.15).

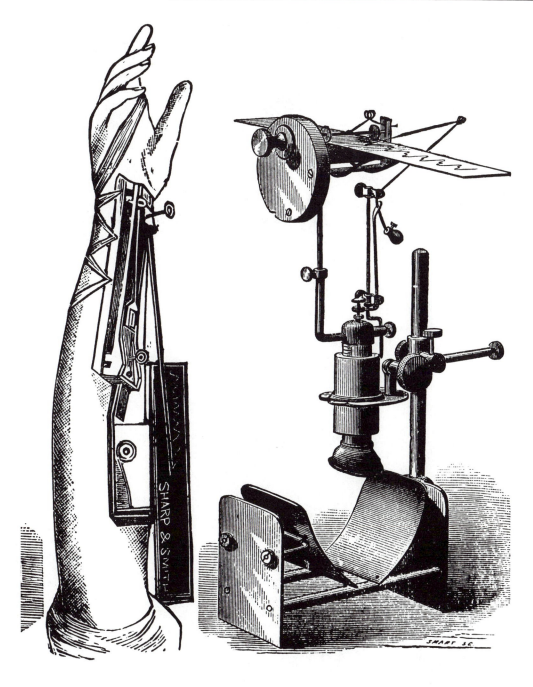

Figure 6.8. Marey and Pond sphygmographs, illustrated in 1889 in Sharp and Smith Catalogue, *SI Photo No. 79-5031.*

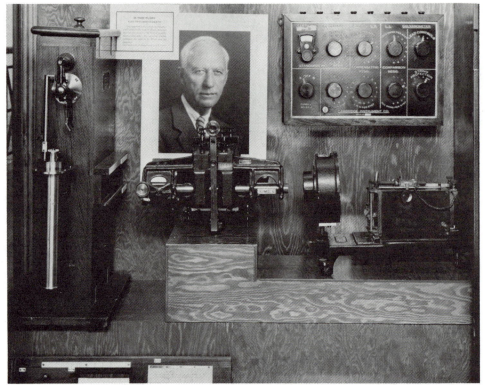

Figure 6.9. Display of Frank Wilson's electrocardiographic equipment in the National Museum of American History, Smithsonian Institution. *SI Photo No. 43361-C.*

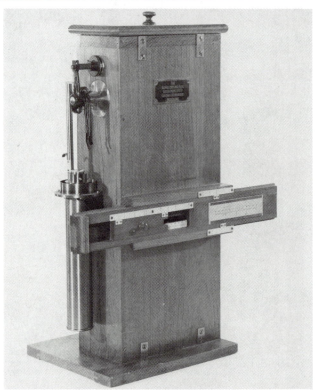

Figure 6.10. Original electrocardiograph of Frank N. Wilson. Cambridge Camera purchased in 1920s. *NMAH No. M-6775, SI Photo No. 651069.*

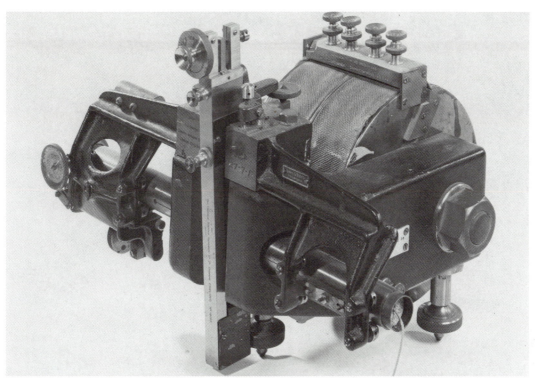

Figure 6.11. Galvanometer of Frank Wilson's electrocardiographic machine according to the design of Mr. Duddell. Purchased in 1914. *NMAH No. M-6773, SI Photo No. 651069-C.*

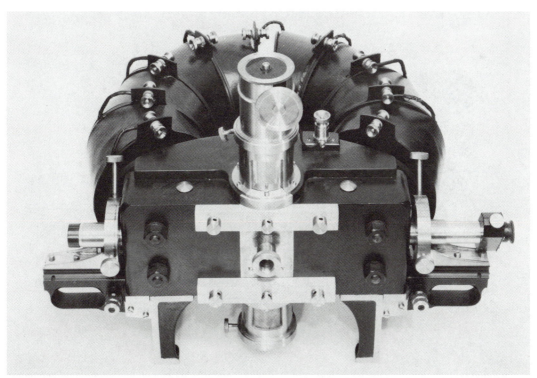

Figure 6.12. The original American string galvanometer designed by Horatio B. Williams and made by Charles Hindle for Alfred E. Cohn of Rockefeller Institute Hospital. *NMAH No. M-6777, SI Photo No. 43361-D.*

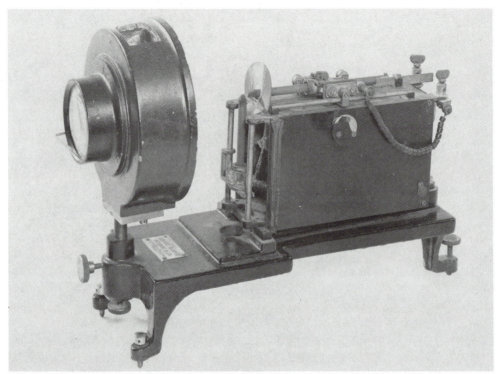

Figure 6.13. Carbon arc lamp which furnished the necessary light for photographing the magnified movements of the quartz string. *NMAH No. M-6776, SI Photo No. 651069-A.*

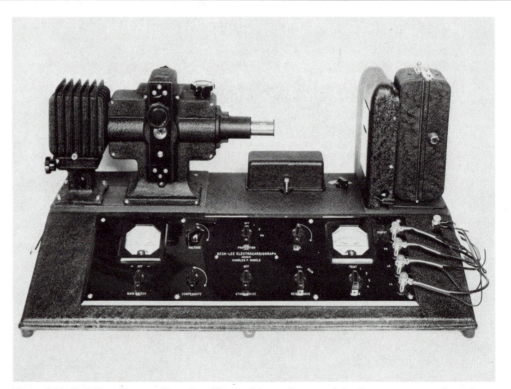

Figure 6.14. Beck-Lee electrocardiograph, office model contains one of the first permanent string galvanometers. *NMAH No. M-6772, SI Photo No. 43361-B.*

The development of the thermometer, stethoscope, and cardiovascular instrumentation, along with the increasing knowledge of body functions that preceded or accompanied these instruments, led to significant changes in medical diagnosis, fundamental biological concepts, and the societies in which the technology was applied. Some of these changes have been alluded to; they are discussed in greater detail in the following chapters.

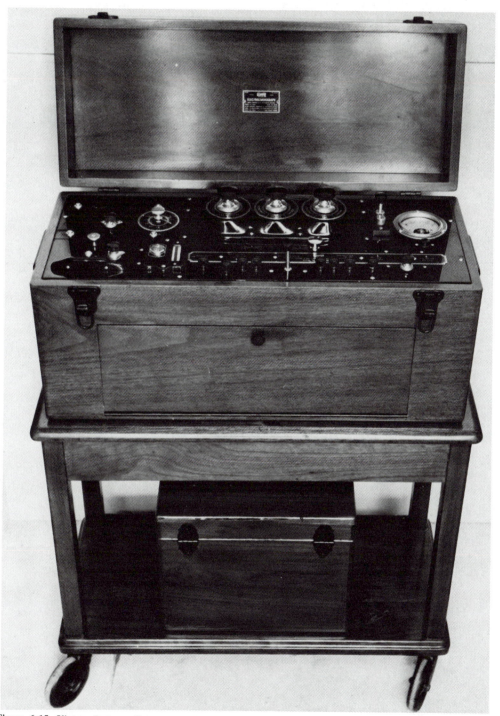

Figure 6.15. Victor electrocardiograph in the 1930s. Manufactured by General Electric with rolling stand, battery case and amplifier unit (in upper case). *NMAH No. M 6803, SI Photo No. 43361-A.*

PART III

EXPLORING THE IMPACT OF MEDICAL TECHNOLOGY

7

DIAGNOSIS AND INSTRUMENTS

INTRODUCTION:

Traditionally, technological developments were closely associated with the discoveries and reconceptualizations that became known as scientific medicine. Exploring a number of examples suggests some of the kinds of·interrelationships that developed between formal scientific medicine and specific technological innovations.

Instruments introduced and developed in the nineteenth century provided new methods for measuring and recording the structures of organs and their functions within the body. Instruments provided measurements by which calculations leading to specific and objective criteria were possible for distinguishing between normal and abnormal structures and their functions. Physiologists primarily determined the instrumentally derived methods and techniques for studying the physical relationships within the normal organism, and pathologists extended these methods to the abnormal being. Physiology and pathology underwent a dramatic evolution as contributing sciences to medical practice when instruments and the institutions to which they gave rise were established. It is the goal of this chapter to suggest why the study of physiology and pathology was changed by the introduction of technology and, in turn, had an impact on medical practice and, in some instances, to indicate how this change occurred.

The major expectations for applying the data collected from physiologic and pathologic research to medical practice included clarification and amplification of the knowledge of diseases, a greater capacity to distinguish diseases from each other, earlier identification of the signs of disease, and wider application of established and newly discovered therapeutic measures. All these desiderata were furthered by the new methods of diagnosis; some of which had their roots in tests worked out by physiologists and were made possible with the aid of instruments, chemicals, devices, and other aids.

Diagnosis, prognosis, and therapy had been cornerstones of medical practice for millenia. Diagnosis was reevaluated in the seventeenth century when new terms began to be applied to the functions and changes produced by diseases, which were revealed through animal experimentation and those observations that had been previously overlooked or misunderstood. Instruments made it possible to study the physiology of animals and to obtain more information from these experiments. Subsequently, diagnosis began to play a larger role in the physician's approach to the patient in the sense of requiring more time and giving more satisfaction to the physician, who could uncover and respond to specific physical events within the diseased body. Differing philosophical viewpoints and new discoveries related to the cure, alleviation, and prevention of diseases spawned debate over the nature and scope of medical diagnosis when undertaken with the aid of technology. The nineteenth-century physician reassessed diagnosis in terms of instruments and the medical records to which these tools contributed.

The physical manipulation required by diagnosis with instruments led to special programs to train individuals in their use. Intensive laboratory work associated with experimental physiology provided practice in applying instruments to animals for those who would later use instruments on their human patients. Using laboratory animals to familiarize diagnosticians with living organisms and to test and sharpen their manual dexterity became accepted to the point that twentieth-century critics could argue that there existed a surfeit of laboratory courses in the pre-medical and medical school curricula.

Medical and laboratory instruments made it possible not only to diagnose, cure, and alleviate disease, but eventually, to prevent disease, thus bringing to reality a health goal only dimly realized up to this period. Sharpening the senses of touch, hearing, and vision with the aid of instruments revealed signs of disease previously unknown or unvalued and, in some instances, at an earlier stage in the disease cycle. Campaigns to prevent certain diseases, therefore, were initiated and maintained by physicians, as well as by public health authorities. Medical practice with instruments and the technical skills to apply them contributed to the emphasis placed on accurate diagnosis and effective treatment while offering greater opportunities to halt disease in its earliest stages. Anemia, detected by counting red blood cells and corrected by diet, and lung diseases detected by measuring the vital capacity of the lungs and arrested with rest, diet, and drug treatment, were among the serious diseases readily detected and confirmed with instruments in the last quarter of the century.[1]

A host of diagnostic facts obtained with instruments emerged from the discoveries in experimental physiology and pathologic anatomy made in nineteenth-century European laboratories and hospitals. These basic sciences were introduced into American medical schools by physicians who had studied in Germany, France, and England.

PHYSIOLOGY AND INSTRUMENTS:

Observation of physiologic systems in living organisms became feasible with instruments that could monitor and record changes over a limited time period and in response to varying conditions of control and stress. The linkage between organs was demonstrated by the simultaneous recording of their behavior with instruments sensitive to the unique functions of each organ. For instance, as described in chapter six, the motions of the heart, blood vessels, and blood during the course of a single pulsation could be transcribed into a series of lines traced out by a sensitive lever attached to the body, so that it would respond to muscular movements produced by the organs of circulation. Among the most successful instruments applied to study the simultaneous motions of the blood, blood vessels, and heart chambers were the sphygmograph, polygraph, and kymograph. In the course of discovering the complex and interdependent relationship between these and other organs, the study of anatomy became more distinct from the study of their functions or physiology. Charles Robin in 1878 summed up the distinction between physiology and anatomy established by experimentalists. He explained that "a system is a

complexity from the anatomical point of view, it is a functional unit from the physiological point of view."[2] Finding suitable techniques for posing and finding answers to functional or physiologic questions was an evolving process, which the historian Joseph Schiller has analyzed as consisting of four stages based on the disciplines that contributed to the shaping of physiology. Before physiology became a distinct study, Schiller claims, "scientists [had to become] conscious of the fact that chemistry and physics could offer procedures and not a methodology, that anatomy provided the ground for experimentation and not the explanation of phenomena, that medicine could raise problems and not offer solutions, and that physiological laws were unlike the laws of any other science but nevertheless not metaphysical."[3]

Instruments made it possible for physiologists, physicists, and chemists to communicate with each other and to obtain information in a form appropriate to the particular uses of each specialist. For example, the thermometer used by the physician registered temperature on a standardized scale limited to the extremes that the human body could tolerate. The physician's function was to apply the generalities derived from experimental studies to specific patients.

Laboratory and diagnostic instruments were vehicles for establishing physiologic laws. These instruments included those to measure and record the beats of the heart, the capacity of the lungs, the flexions of the muscles, the electric patterns of the brain, the fluctuations of the temperature, and other functions. The laws were formulated in terms of the collected data and expressed in the language based on the function of the instrument. The form in which the data were received was determined by the mechanical boundaries of the equipment used in each instance. For instance, the sphygmograph registered the pulse produced by the heart beat as a series of vertical peaks and depressions traced on paper by a lever responding to the swelling and emptying of an artery located near the surface of the body. The tactile and auditory expression of the pulse was transformed into a visual observation which became permanent when recorded on specially prepared inked or waxed paper. So that physiology and anatomy could be related, correspondences were made between an anatomic structure and its function by formulating the data into a pattern so that the structure and its functional ability could be determined on a comparative scale. The scale was described within the physical terms appropriate to the instrument, such as millimeters of mercury for blood pressure, degrees of temperature on the Fahrenheit or Centigrade scales, centimeters of contraction or expansion of a muscle, and the shape of the wave pattern traced by the pulse on a piece of paper ruled with a time and pressure axis. Within the end points of each instrument's scale, the measurement was relative. To make the physiologic scale meaningful to the physician, it was necessary to record many individuals, although this was not always possible. One example of a standard derived from a very small sample of individuals is the standard developed for hemoglobin content in the red blood cells. The history of hemoglobinometry shows that the method of estimating hemoglobin concentration by reference to a standard of diluted blood was based on actual studies of fewer than fifty individuals. The method was introduced by W. R. Gowers in 1878 and modified by J. Haldane in 1901 when he tested thirty-eight men and women in Belfast to arrive at the normal standard of the capacity of the blood to carry oxygen, and thus, its hemoglobin concentration. This standard was accepted for the next thirty years.[4] As the number of individuals tested and measured increased, the data provided by instruments became more precise and statistically relevant, since the information could be compared for a wider group of people and the idiosyncracies associated with small proportions of the population tested could be made obvious.

The experimental procedures crucial to physiology and the conclusions to which these led were discussed primarily in the nineteenth-century scientific and medical journal literature. Descriptions of laboratory apparatus, new techniques, and modifications of equipment and medical treatment were almost exclusively introduced through medical, physiological, biological, and chemical journals, all of which included articles related to physiology.

Journals evolved so that those solely concerned with only one area of interest to medical specialists multiplied and replaced the general texts and journals. It was predicted in 1889 that "in the twentieth century the science of medicine will be studied in these journals. The general journal [of medicine] is of the past; the special journal is of the future. [In fact] on the growth and development of special journals many of the great problems of medical science will depend."[5] The first physiologic journal emphasizing experimentation and apparatus was François Magendie's *Journal de physiologie expérimentale* (1821-1831). The growth in the study of physiology is quickly summarized by noting that, at the time of the first International Physiological Congress in Basel in 1889, seven hundred publications were presented and

by the time of the fiftieth anniversary meeting of the congress in Boston, twenty thousand publications were contributed.[6] The rapid increase in the early twentieth-century physiologic literature is also indicated by the sixfold rise in the published papers between 1900 and 1926 in the *Zentralblatt fuer Physiologie*.[7] By 1926, 20 percent of the papers were contributed by Americans. The growing impact of physiology and its attendant technology on medicine is displayed in this periodical literature.

Searching the periodical literature to locate and explain all the types of instruments used in physiologic and other studies related to medicine would be a useful, although difficult, task. Dietmar Rapp[8] has demonstrated how this type of study might be done. He selected ten significant physiologic texts published or translated into German between 1784 and 1911. From these, he listed all the techniques and equipment used to study physiology in this period. These texts, written by leading German, French, Italian, and Swiss physiologists, appeared approximately a decade apart, and therefore, provide a sense of the development of physiologic research techniques and equipment throughout the nineteenth century. Rapp organized the instruments discussed in each text into three groups, namely, operating equipment (vivisection), equipment derived from physics and chemistry, and special equipment devised for exploring physiologic processes directly. Within the last category, he divided the equipment into nine areas corresponding to the special studies of the blood, heart (circulation and lymph), lungs, digestion, nutrition, metabolism, muscular movement, peripheral and central nervous systems, sense organs, and speech. The earliest text selected was published by the Italian Leopold M. A. Caldani (1725-1813) and was entitled *Physiologie des menschlichen Koerpers*, which appeared in Prague in 1784. Rapp listed from Caldani's text five pieces of apparatus used in surgical operations, six pieces derived from physics and chemistry, and four pieces applied directly to physiologic studies of the circulation, respiration, and muscular movement. In each instance, Rapp noted the pages in the text on which an instrument was discussed and briefly summarized the way in which the equipment was employed. The other texts chosen for similar analysis included those by Johann H. F. Autenrieth (1801-1802), Francois Magendie (1826), Johannes Mueller (1835-1840), Gustav Gabriel Valentin (1847), Carl Ludwig (1858-1861), Ludimar Hermann (1870), Leonhard Landois (1881), and Luigi Luciani (1904-1911). The use of specialized physiologic equipment grew from the original four pieces described by Caldani to 280 pieces discussed in the four-volume text of Luciani, which was published in Jena. Magendie utilized thirty pieces of equipment for his physiologic experiments related to the blood, heart, lungs, digestion, metabolism, muscle motion, the venous system, and sensory organs. These included thermometers, galvanic batteries to coagulate serum, a microscope to observe the circulation, a bellows to measure lung capacity, a calorimeter, a gasometer, and electrical stimulators to excite the nervous system. The authors of these texts were not the only designers of the described equipment. Some of the apparatus was widely known to experimentalists and bore the names of their inventors, such as Poiseuille's instrument for measuring the volume of blood expelled by the heart in one beat, Volta's batteries, Santorius' instrument for measuring metabolism, Spallanzani's tubes for extracting stomach fluids, and Young's optometer.

The secondary literature related to European physiology frequently discusses the internal history of physiology from a theoretical viewpoint, which is illustrated by famous experiments. The laboratory environment centering around instruments and apparatus is barely mentioned. It would be useful to know the structure of the leading laboratories supervised by Hermann Helmholtz, Johannes Mueller, and Justus Liebig among the German centers, those of François Magendie and Claude Bernard among the French, and that of Michael Foster in England. Liebig spent a decade beginning in 1824 in designing and building up his chemical laboratory in Giessen, in order to undertake analyses of tissues and organic compounds.[9] He was a pioneer in developing and equipping laboratories from which a multitude of physiologic studies would flow. The German laboratory became the pinnacle of a well-stocked environment for the cultivation of advanced physiologic experiments. Bernard's studies, on the other hand, provide examples of novel interpretations and solutions to problems posed by a lack of sufficient instruments and equipment.

A number of Bernard's published lectures reflect his use of instruments that are illustrated in the published text. In his *Leçons de Physiologie Opératoire*, which appeared in 1879, a year after his death, a variety of cutting instruments, syringes, and cannulas are displayed, especially in the ninth lesson devoted to instruments of general use in vivisection. Bernard insisted that physiologic laboratories must work with phenomena at three levels: vivisection, physio-chemical analysis, and anatomico-histologic study,[10] but both Magendie and Bernard favored vivisectional experimentation, in contrast to the emphasis placed on chemical and physical analysis by their German

colleagues. Bernard encouraged his students to study the inner or internal environment of the animal, but such studies required other types of instruments. He insisted that "to analyze the phenomena of life, we must necessarily penetrate into living organisms with the help of the methods of vivisection."[11] Bernard recognized that the tools available to French investigators for sophisticated vivisection experiments and other studies were primitive and difficult to obtain. He even lacked adequate microscopes and microtomes to study the details of bodily tissues. To overcome the limitations of his vivisectional and observational tools, Bernard turned to poisonous compounds, which could be used to probe bodily tissues in ways not directly observable, but which altered the function of these tissues, and therefore, supplied information not unlike that provided through the use of an instrument such as the microscope. He regarded himself as being the first to understand "poisons as the veritable reagents of life, extremely delicate instruments which dissect vital units" by their ability "to alter histological units."[12]

Bernard's methodological and conceptual rationale for vivisection as an essential component of physiology gave the greatest impetus to those studies and provided a climate of acceptance that would extend into the twentieth century. Bernard viewed a number of medical treatments as forms of physiologic experimentation and extended this view to include vivisection as long as it was performed for the welfare of the patient. The harshness of these methods forced physiologists to evaluate the practical consequences of their results and to concede that only a few of their discoveries were of direct value to medicine. The eradication of one type of skin disease and the insertion of a ligature to treat an aneurysm were among the few examples brought forth by 1875. Therefore, it was difficult to justify the role of physiology in medicine, especially of the more unpleasant techniques like vivisection. Instruments helped to mitigate and circumvent some of the unpleasant aspects of research on the animal and human body and to make these experiments more acceptable to society.

Michael Foster's physiologic course at University College London became the model for teaching physiology to English physicians and surgeons, especially after the Royal College of Surgeons in 1870 required that all college candidates be instructed in laboratory physiology. English physiologists into the 1870s had earned their living as medical practitioners because the institutional support for experimental physiology, which existed in Germany and France since the early nineteenth century, was not available in England. Gerald Geison has analyzed the social, reli-

gious, and scientific factors contributing to the delayed emergence of physiology as a profession in
England, as well as Foster's special experimental concerns.[13]

Americans who brought back the techniques they
had acquired in European laboratories included
Henry Pickering Bowditch, who had trained with
Carl Ludwig and Henry Newell Martin, a student of
Michael Foster and Thomas Henry Huxley. Bowditch
founded the first physiologic laboratory at Harvard
in 1871. Martin emigrated from England to Baltimore
and founded the earliest organized American physiology laboratory at The Johns Hopkins University in
1876, which also has been cited as the first physiologic laboratory in the United States.[14]

Pathology and Instruments:

Studies of morbid anatomy and its relationship to
diagnostic signs reopened discussions of disease classification. The body was dissected to clarify and provide more details about the effects of disease shortly
before the period when diagnostic instruments began
to provide more details about the manifestations and
signs of disease. Therefore, morbid anatomy and
instrumentally deduced disease signs formed the
basis for distinguishing between diseases and naming
them. Some generalized terms previously applied to
diseases, such as fever and inflammation, were replaced or augmented by names signifying specific
aspects of disease usually involving tissue or functional changes.

A good example of the refinement of nosology
growing out of the refinement of diagnosis based on
technology is the separation of kidney diseases originally included under the term Bright's disease. The
range of tissue changes in the kidneys, urine, and
blood associated with kidney diseases was discovered
with the aid of microscopes and other equipment. To
understand how medical technology brought about
changes in nosology, we must begin with a brief discussion of the development of pathologic anatomy.

Erasistratus and Herophilus dissected the human
body in the third century B.C., but the accounts of
their work are lost. In the second century in his treatise On the Affected Parts, Galen had urged the dissection of the bodies of patients who had died of
disease, although his own anatomic descriptions were
based on the dissection of animals. The next dissections discussed in the medical literature are the autopsies performed on Italian plague and poison victims during the thirteenth and fourteenth centuries.
Within another several centuries, every important
anatomist was studying morbid anatomy by direct
observation of the cadaver.[15] Pathologists describing

the changes inflicted by disease on the tissues and
organs evolved rapidly in the eighteenth century. The
systematic study of pathologic anatomy began with
the publication in 1761 of Giovanni Morgagni's The
Seats and Causes of Diseases. Morgagni credited
earlier texts with pointing the way to his study of
morbid anatomy. He originally intended to augment
and bring up to date Theophile Bonet's Sepulchrum
anatomicum sive anatomica practica published in
1679, and he studied Schank and Grafenberg's Observations of 1665.[16]

Morgagni's book represented the culmination of
the evolution of morbid anatomy from an anatomy
relying only on the description of structures to an
anatomy grounded in interpretation of physical
symptoms and their linkage to anatomic lesions.
Interpretation depended on statistical correlations. A
lesion had to have been recorded in numerous instances of a disease to be considered an integral and
constant expression of the disease. Morgagni proposed the publication of a text relating the signs and
symptoms of diseases to their anatomic lesions. He
suggested that this book, bearing the title "Natural
History of Disease," would serve two functions:

So that if any physician observe a singular or any other
symptom in a patient and desires to know what internal
injury is wont to correspond to that symptom; or if any
anatomist find any particular morbid appearance in the dissection of a body and should wish to know what symptom
has preceded an injury of this kind in other bodies; the physician, by inspecting the first of the indexes, the anatomist,
by inspecting the second, will immediately find the observation which contains both (if both have been observed by
us).[17]

From the correlation of diagnostic signs with postmortem anatomic lesions evolved a clinical concept
of disease relying on physical methods of examination that increased the type and amount of information to be used as diagnostic criteria. Physical diagnosis may be said to have been formally launched in
1761, the year in which Morgagni's text appeared.
Leopold Auenbrugger published the Inventum
Novum, which reintroduced the ancient procedure of
locating thoracic lesions by percussion of the patient;[18] however, Auenbrugger employed a special
instrument called a pleximeter for the technique. Percussion was not generally applied to diagnosis until
after 1806 when the French clinician, Jean-Nicolas
Corvisart advanced the procedure.[19] To implement
his convictions, Corvisart urged that a text be prepared with the title "On the Seats and Causes of Diseases, Investigated by Diagnostic Signs and Confirmed by Autopsy."

Laennec, one of Corvisart's illustrious students, was the first to take up his teacher's challenge in his famous treatise on diseases of the chest in which he introduced the stethoscope and furthered use of the percussion hammer.[20] Other anatomists who contributed to this anatomic tradition included Philippe Pinel, Francois Xavier Bichat, John Hunter, and Matthew Baillie in the early nineteenth century. Instruments and laboratory procedures provided an unparalleled means of recognizing diseases at an earlier stage and comparing information obtained from the external appearance of diseases (signs and symptoms) and the end products found after death (lesions of morbid anatomy). After it was possible to delineate changes among cells, in addition to the changes that appeared on the surfaces of organs and tissues, the anatomic approach became vitally linked to physiologic and pathologic investigations.

Complementing the discoveries of the anatomist was an investigative method that advanced the understanding of the morbid process by expressing the normal and abnormal functions of the organs in numerical terms, which was launched in the English language by the original studies of Stephen Hales in the early eighteenth century. Hales' investigations of the vascular systems of animals revealed how "the relating of the dimensions and the geometry of the structure of an organ to its functions"[21] could be done. Gathered into tables, Hales' measurements brought attention to the value of numbering bodily functions so that they could be distinguished and evaluated. It was important to invent instruments to obtain information in this form. In 1793, Baillie, among others, recognized the significance of Hales' approach to functional changes when he stated: "It is very much to be regretted that the knowledge of structure does not certainly lead to the knowledge of morbid actions although the one is the effect of the other. Morbid actions are going on in the minute parts of an animal body excluded from observation."[22]

Among a host of physiologists and pathologists who realized the need to relate these two types of studies and be aware of their relationship to diagnosis was Johannes Mueller. In 1834 he claimed: "Pathologic anatomy continues to offer us a large amount of observations but their comprehension advances all too slowly. It is carried out only for correction of diagnosis and not for the aim of advancing pathology."[23] Mueller stressed that physiologic and anatomic investigations were to be combined with autopsy findings, a goal achieved by his student, Rudolf Virchow. As Paul Klemperer has observed, Virchow introduced "a new scientific approach to

the comprehension of the nature of disease through analysis of structure. Through Virchow the microscope became a reformatory instrument, not a mere diagnostic tool; in short, he is the creator of anatomic pathology, the morphologic discipline which inquired . . . into the mechanisms by which disease is provoked."[24] Virchow used the microscope to create a new discipline, which inspired contemporaries such as W. S. Greenfield of the University of Edinburgh.[25]

Measuring, testing, and probing the internal organs and their environment from the onset of illness to its termination was better accomplished with devices to compare and record chemical, cellular, and other physical changes throughout the course of an illness. Permanent records obtained from the diseased body became essential in documenting the history of a disease. Organs were made to draw graphs of their functional alterations when they changed their muscular rhythms (heart beat) or their use and disposal of chemical substances (urine, blood, glandular products) or their intake of oxygen and release of carbon dioxide, as well as other changes. Similar instruments were used in a variety of settings as the investigator improvised in his effort to uncover new types of data. Electric devices that amplified weak body signals and monitored chemical reactions demanded special skills to apply and interpret the results they provided. Those skilled enough to apply the new medical technology became medical technicians. Medical technology led to new professions and the evolution of pathologic anatomy from morbid anatomy, as well as clinical pathology from anatomic pathology.

THE PROFESSIONAL PATHOLOGIST:

Physicians studied basic laboratory procedures in courses on microscopy and histology as medical students. In classroom laboratories such as the one at Cambridge University organized by Michael Foster, microscopes with mounted specimens were placed on a conveyer and sent to each student's desk. Manuals and texts on the functions and uses of the microscope for physicians and histologists were prepared by the second half of the nineteenth century. Students were encouraged to purchase their own inexpensive microscopes by the end of the century. These microscopes were adequate if they possessed good lenses with a range of magnification between thirty and three hundred times the diameter of the specimen and if they were color corrected or achromatic. Steadiness, easy adjustment, and portability were other desirable qualities. Prominent manufacturers of microscopes for students included the London makers R. & J.

Beck; Ross; Powell; and Leasand; Swift; Crouch; Collins; Baker and Browning; the Parisian makers Hartnack and Verick; and Zeiss of Jena. Ladd and Pillischer, and Salmon Highley of London introduced special student models circa 1854 that sold for under ten pounds.[26]

Pathology was cast in a new mold resulting from techniques and disciplines that included the study of disease by anatomic, microscopic, functional, bacteriologic, chemical, experimental, and clinical methods in a planned and consistent program. Each of these areas had been explored earlier, but had not been combined to solve a specific disease problem before the end of the nineteenth century.[27] E. B. Krumbhaar observed that "the student of disease [by the end of the nineteenth century] whether working primarily in the pathological laboratory or in the clinic, must be equipped to study or direct the study of his problem by physical, chemical, mathematical and experimental methods, as well as by the older methods of anatomy or bedside study, as the case may be."[28] It was impossible to reach a high level of competence in each of these areas; therefore, researchers had to specialize in one or two areas and learn to depend on others who understood and could carry out examination techniques in the remaining areas. Cooperation between the diagnostician and the pathologist was not automatically arranged, nor necessarily conducive to improved medical diagnosis.

One consequence of increasing the technology employed in studies of physiology and pathology, as well as the competence of those who used the technology, was to separate the laboratory physician from the medical practitioner. When diagnostic confirmation was no longer the only aim of pathology, the individual who performed pathologic tests and the person who diagnosed and treated disease were no longer the same individual.

The future for an applied pathologist was not very promising in the mid-nineteenth century. His salary was no greater than that of a hospital house surgeon or house physician. Consequently, a pathologist usually remained on the hospital staff long enough to gain experience or until he could obtain a post as a physician or surgeon. A. W. Robson, Fellow of the Royal College of Surgeons, and others argued for improving the salary and prestige of pathologists, so that qualified individuals would plan to make pathology their profession.[29] Experience with laboratory procedures sharpened the pathologist's skills and increased the chances that he would master all types of laboratory techniques.

Finding a method to pay for pathologic examina-

tions was one step in providing an adequate salary for the pathologist. The alarm caused by epidemics had forced municipal and county governments to support laboratories and their staffs who examined human and animal specimens for the detection and control of infectious diseases. To raise the money to pay the pathologist who examined specimens for other than infectious diseases, Robson suggested that the general practice of providing low cost or free medical services to the poor and charging the wealthy patients for those same services be extended to pathologic examinations. The income from those procedures could then be used as a source of funds for those who conducted the tests. Private patients would pay for more elaborate tests in less demand, such as a biopsy for tumor detection or analysis of a test meal to understand the nature of a digestive disease, and benefit from the additional information these tests provided. For those lacking money to pay for these special tests, free hospital clinics were to be established with the understanding that the clinic would not compete for patients who were financially able to consult a private pathologist, in the manner in which hospitals refrained from competing for patients who were able to pay for their medical care and thus consulted private physicians.[30]

In the last quarter of the nineteenth century, pathology laboratories with the primary responsibility of analyzing specimens sent to them by clinicians were founded. They were established by a variety of sponsoring institutions, including medical schools, hospitals, medical societies, municipal authorities, and profit-making groups composed of private individuals. One of these laboratories, as it functioned in Edinburgh in the last decade of the nineteenth century and first half of the twentieth century, is reviewed in John Ritchie's *History of the Laboratory of the Royal College of Physicians of Edinburgh*.[31] In its first year, the Edinburgh laboratory examined 167 specimens for practitioners "and thus the most delicate methods of determining the nature of diseased structures and morbid secretions were carried into the everyday work of the Practitioner of Medicine."[32]

DEVELOPMENT OF DIAGNOSTIC PRACTICES:

The medical historian Charles Newman has divided medical practices since the Renaissance into three phases of development.[33] During the first stage when the Humoral Theory of Disease prevailed, the symptoms described by the patient were made the foundation of treatment growing out of this theory. The second stage began in the early nineteenth century, when diagnosis was based on physical examination of the patient and subsequent treatment of structural abnormalities. The last phase, beginning later in the nineteenth century but still being developed, relies on diagnosis from laboratory tests and concomitant treatment to remove the cause of the disorder. Newman considers the second phase to be the most revolutionary, since for the first time the physician depended on his skill with a device to probe and understand his patients' diseases. Newman believes this was the most important phase because it changed medicine from a theoretical to a science-based practice. His assessment is open to further discussion, especially related to the causes of this change and the implications of the change for medical practice. Some of the discussion appeared in the medical literature published over the past century and reveals that the social and institutional changes during the past century and a half were pivotal factors in the development of medical practice. Society guided the physician in his use of technology and offered opportunities for the improvement, as well as the stagnation, of the medical process. Instruments contributed to all aspects of diagnosis from the classification of diseases to the designation of specific signs by which diseases are distinguished from each other. Some of these changes in diagnosis are discussed to indicate how they were developed with medical technology.

CLASSIFICATION OF DISEASE:

Diagnosis of disease is directly related to the recognition and the classification of diseases. While diseases have been classified since antiquity, there were only sporadic efforts to change ancient categories of diseases, until the annual Bills of Mortality made it obvious that diagnoses of diseases were becoming inaccurate and obscure by the eighteenth century.[34] British reformers including John Fothergill and Thomas Percival made special efforts to enlighten the medical community to the advantages of periodically discarding obsolete disease names. Benjamin Rush's opposition to all disease-naming systems was shared by other American physicians with the consequence that American efforts to change disease classification came belatedly.[35]

Modern nosology (from the Greek terms for disease and discourse), or the full hierarchic and carefully defined arrangement of diseases, originated in the eighteenth century, partially as an extension of Linné's binomial system of classification of animals and plants,[36] and also, as an extension of the method of separating diseases into discrete entities distinguishable from each other and the hosts that expressed them. Robley Dunglison, who prepared medical dictionaries for American physicians, in 1848 listed a number of celebrated nosologists who had proposed modern systems of classification.[37] Others proposed partial systems, such as those limited to afflictions requiring surgery or those based on diseases affecting specific parts of the body such as the eye, ear, or brain.[38] William Cullen's system was preferred by British and American physicians, some of whom had studied in Scotland where they were first exposed to the system. James Currie was convinced that "since the introduction of scientific arrangement into medicine, diseases have been much reduced in number, and their nature has been more clearly understood."[39] One disease category demonstrating the pruning effect of Cullen's nosology was continued fevers. Cullen reduced continued fevers to three types, namely, Synocha, Typhus, and Snyochus. Cullen divided all diseases into four classes based on (1) the body temperature they induced, (2) the anatomic structures they affected, (3) the chemical changes they brought about, and (4) the topography or locus of the disease. Each of these effects of disease were best, although not invariably, described with the aid of instruments and devices suitable for measuring each change at it occurred within the body of the disease victim.

American physicians made an organized effort to classify diseases under the auspices of the newly formed American Medical Association. One of the resolutions passed at the meeting of the Association in 1846 established the formation of "a committee to prepare a nomenclature of disease adapted to the U.S., having references to a general registration of deaths."[40] Persistent efforts by the association resulted in a more reliable registration of the cause of death. Diseases were grouped according to their signs and symptoms, and therefore, as these were changed and augmented, new classification schemes were developed.[41] In some instances, the diagnostic instrument introduced previously unknown criteria for classifying diseases. This new evidence of disease included body sounds, changes resulting from mixing bodily fluids with specific chemicals, electric discharges of muscle fibers, rate of motion of substances passing through the digestive, respiratory, or circulatory systems, and others, all of which led to a reclassification of diseases. In the period when instruments offered new criteria by which to describe diseases, Linné's binomial model was rejected. To classifiers, the relationship between diseases became less significant to the identification of each disease than the objective data indicating the presence of disease that was available through the use of instruments and laboratory tests.

The assimilation of a disease category by the practitioner occurred at several levels. One level was explained as growing out of the physician's past experiences, which led him to recognize a disease by intuition. Up to the era of medical instrumentation, diagnosis by intuition was among the most highly regarded skills that physicians attributed to each other. Accounts of eminent doctors who appeared to recognize a disease almost spontaneously upon observing a patient continued into the twentieth century. Eventually, diagnostic intuition was attributed to those who could observe and recognize disease without employing any instrumental aids.[42] In some instances, the physician claimed to have developed his unusual skill by having used instruments to develop his observational faculties to the degree that he was able to rely entirely on his unaided senses. The physician's progression from instrumental to unassisted diagnosis was a goal set by some of the most respected nineteenth-century clinicians, including the British practitioner and cardiologist, James Mackenzie. A challenge to the tradition of ascribing diagnostic skill to intuition and instinct was codified in the popular American medical text by Jacob M. DaCosta of Philadelphia, entitled *Medical Diagnosis; with Special Reference to Practical Medicine.*[43] Introduced in 1864 and revised in later editions, the text eliminated the possibility of diagnosing by intuition and substituted a series of instrumentally derived signs and other observations from which operative diagnosis in the United States was to flow over the next century.[44]

SIGNS OF DISEASE:

Delineating the signs of diseases forms a special branch of medicine called semiology, which has been studied since antiquity. However, the signs of diseases remained fairly constant until instruments and physical methods of diagnosis enlarged the study of signs because of the new signs revealed through technology.[45] The patient's signs were placed within a disease category based on a series of physical manipulations. To confirm the presence of specific disease, the physician employed direct observation, with or without the aid of instruments; responses to simple and complex physical tests, such as nervous reflex and pupil response to light; laboratory analyses of bodily tissues and fluids; and exploratory surgery. The physician studied these data for signs of disease and decided a course of therapy to eliminate or arrest those aspects of the disease responsive to

treatment and most endangering the patient's life. Medical diagnosis emphasizing signs revealed with instruments and through tests has resulted in labeling the patient with a disease to the extent that the patient is often referred to as a "case" of the disease. Under this label, those aspects of the disease singled out with the various technologies of medicine have become the focal point of treatment and response to the patient. The terms *sign* and *symptom* have been used interchangeably, although these terms signify different stages in the disease process, which have become more obvious with medical instruments and the interpretation of diseases through the use of instruments. The semantic distinctions between sign and symptom rested on the actual demonstration of each of these disease markers. Rudolf Virchow recognized the displacement of the word *symptom* by the term *sign* and the term *disease* by both *symptom* and *sign* as the prime sources of diagnostic and nosological descriptions in 1881. He asked, as quoted by Cuming in 1884: "Can a diagnosis be made without a knowledge of symptoms? Certainly not. But, for the scientific physician, the symptoms are no more the expression of a hidden power itself, and endeavors to find where it is seated, in the hope of exploring even the nature of its seat. Hence the first question of the pathologist and of the biologist in general is, where? That is the anatomical question. No matter whether we endeavor to ascertain the place of disease, or of life with the anatomical knife, or only with the eye, or the hand; whether we dissect or only observe, the method of investigation is always anatomical."[46] An anatomic lesion was not only the source of disease, but also a sign of the disease. Those who questioned the belief that disease was anatomic queried whether the lesion caused the symptom or the symptom caused the lesion.[47] Whatever the position taken regarding disease and its location, a symptom no longer served as well as a sign, especially one uncovered with an instrument, in the organization, naming, and diagnosis of diseases.[48] It became acceptable to believe that "disease is an arbitrary designation," and that signs and symptoms would reveal more about the disease process to which the physician must respond than the name of the disease applied to this process. The process and the patient bearing the disease were summarily described as a case of the disease, not unlike the case of instruments employed to detect and treat the disease.

The diagnostic instrument assisted the physician to recognize anatomic changes due to disease by allowing him to distinguish physical properties of the impaired organ before they became morbid lesions. These included changes in tissue density and the ability of the tissues to conduct sounds. Walter Hayle Walshe of the University College Hospital in London explained in 1851:

So invariably do these alterations [tissue densities] bear a certain and fixed relation to the nature of the anatomical conditions with which they are associated, that the discovery of the former is conclusive as to the existence of the latter. And not only the nature, but the precise limits and the precise degree of these conditions are disclosed by the alterations referred to, which, for these reasons, constitute their *Physical Signs*. Interpreted by the observer, and not by the patient, . . . estimable . . ., often with mathematical precision, susceptible of indefinite refinement, . . . physical signs are . . . the true indices of the nature, extent and degree of organic textual changes, and may be regarded as instruments of pursuing morbid anatomy on the living body.[49]

The diseases of the respiratory, circulatory, and excretory organs were most likely to be diagnosed on the basis of physical signs.

The application of instruments and laboratory tests that resulted in the reclassification of diseases and resultant therapies is well illustrated in the delineation of diseases that affected the eyes and the kidneys. The ophthalmoscope made it possible to distinguish between a group of diseases formerly designated by the term *amaurosis*.[50] Chemical tests of the urine and microscopic study of kidney tissues enabled the components of Bright's disease to be segregated (see figure 7.1). Francis Delafield of New York in 1891 outlined the disease classification process prevailing in the nineteenth century by discussing the array of kidney diseases that were subsumed under the name "Bright's Disease." Richard Bright, a brilliant English clinician working at Guy's Hospital in London, in 1827 made the important discovery that dropsy, albumin in the urine, and inflammation were related to disease of the kidneys.[51] Three-quarters of a century after Bright's discovery, Delafield explained how a disease such as Bright's disease came to be subdivided into a number of diseases. To begin with, an astute observer noted instances of a disease that had not been previously singled out and given a special name. The physician's name was usually applied to this disease phenomenon. Other investigators then carried out microscopic and chemical studies of the diseased tissues, which revealed that the disease entity was, in fact, a combination of cellular, tissue, and fluid changes. At this time, the original name of the disease was retained but only for a few of the tissue

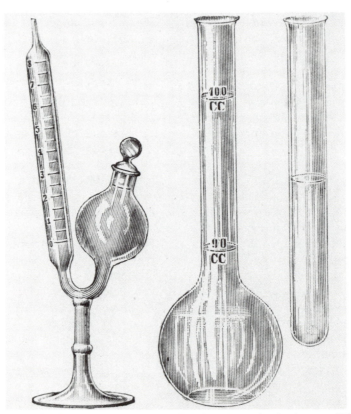

Figure 7.1. Urinalysis equipment circa 1893, from A. S. Aloe Catalogue, p. 626.

changes that appeared in the kidneys. In one instance, John Simon distinguished subacute nephritis from kidney changes due to Bright's disease on the basis of microscopic postmortem examinations, clinical observations, and hospital statistics. Simon proposed that Bright's disease be distinguished by the terms inflammation and scrofulous degeneration.[52] Further study led to more revisions in the signs associated with this disease until the name remained as a popular term but was abandoned by clinicians and replaced with other more precise words to distinguish a series of physical conditions based on cause, anatomic location, or specified morbid processes such as infection, tissue degeneration, and functional alteration.

Chemical tests of urine including the nitric acid test for albumin, Fehling's glycerine test for the presence of glucose, Gmelin's test for bile pigments, the Guiacum test for blood, and the Donné test for pus made differentiation between kidney diseases feasible. A complete set of test materials used in urinary examinations was prepared under the direction of Austin Flint, who presented instructions and the rationale for their use in his *Manual of Chemical Examination of the Urine in Disease*, published in 1870 and in six later editions (see figures 7.2 and 7.3).[53] Others who also provided instructions to the diagnostician using urinanalysis were Henry G. Piffard of New York in *A Guide to Urinary Analysis for the Use of Physicians and Students*, published in 1873, and Alfred Loomis of New York in *Lessons in Physical Diagnosis*, published in 1868 and later editions.[54] The equipment for these tests was advertised and widely sold by the New York firm, George Tiemann,[55] and by other medical instrument manufacturers and suppliers.

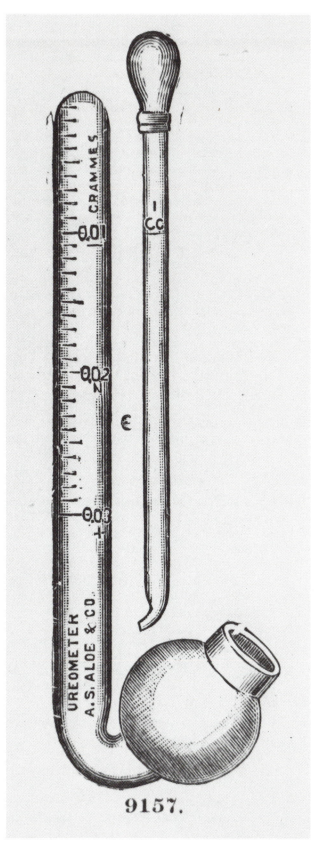

Figure 7.3. **Ureometer circa 1893,** from A. S. Aloe Catalogue, p. 628.

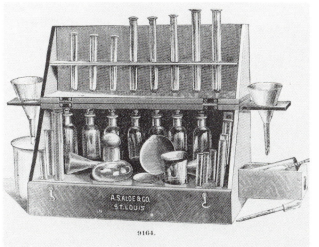

Figure 7.2. **Fehling's urine test set** from A. S. Aloe Catalogue, circa 1893, p. 629.

The next major diagnostic methods for distinguishing kidney diseases were loading tests or those in which an overdose of selected fluids was given to patients to test the functional capability of the kidneys to filter out specific chemical substances. Cryoscopy, or finding the freezing point of urine, a technique introduced by Von Korányi in 1897, was used to determine the molecular concentration of the urine and to measure the overload.[56] These functional tests for kidney disease were an extension of the program described by Ottomar Rosenbach (1851-1907) in his paper of 1878 on the investigation of stomach functions in order to diagnose its diseases. Rosenbach attempted to replace diagnosis based on anatomy with a functional diagnosis of each organ, which he described in his book *Grundlagen, Aufgaben und Grenzen der Therapie* in 1891.[57]

Increasingly in the nineteenth century, instruments in particular helped physicians determine what the parameters of disease were. It was noted with renewed interest that "disease itself contains no elements essentially different from those of health, but elements presented in a different and less useful order."[58] Instruments made it possible to detect and express more aspects of these differences in order to provide rational therapy for bringing the elements back to normal. Those factors impinging on or extracting from the body that could be measured and recorded with instruments have influenced the medical concept of disease in Western nations. However, not all rearrangements of physiologic functions and anatomic structures that might be associated with diseases appeared against the will of the afflicted person. Individuals were sometimes led to permit bodily changes that could be regarded as disfiguring but were acceptable for philosophical and theological reasons. For instance, all bodily mutilations and operations were not done to cure or ward off disease. Pierced ears and noses, scarified faces, tattoos, bound feet, and circumcisions are among the mutilations acceptable to some people and reflect the level of pain endurable to people for reasons other than cure of disease or maintenance of good physical health.

While the patient's tolerance for bodily changes is essential to the distinction made between diseases and health, the physician's observational acuity is important in finding the less obvious and obtrusive signs of disease. Michel Foucault offers interpretations of the change in the nineteenth-century physician's method of focusing on disease that explains the ability to recognize and locate disease in specific parts of the body. Foucault attributes a penetrating power to the physician's "gaze" or perception, encompassing all the senses—sight, touch, hearing, pressure, and taste.[59] He has found that

every great thought in the field of pathology lays down a configuration for disease whose spatial requisites are not necessarily those of classical geometry. The exact superposition of the "body" of the disease and the body of the sick man is no more than a historical, temporary datum. The space of *configuration* of the disease and the space of *localization* of the illness in the body have been superimposed in medical experience, for only a relatively short period of time—the period coincides with nineteenth century medicine and the privileges accorded to pathological anatomy.[60]

An excellent early example of discrimination was F.-J.-V. Broussais, who in his text *Examen de la Doctrine Médicale* of 1816 established the view that disease is not an entity but a series of pathologic reactions. Broussais relied on older theories of irritation and sympathy to describe those pathologic, disease-producing changes, which he would no longer classify as a local fixed phenomenon. His critics abounded, but an endorsement by J.-B. Bouillaud in 1826 summed up the impact of Broussais' discovery: "The medical revolution of which M. Broussais laid the foundations in 1816 is undoubtedly the most remarkable that medicine has undergone in modern times."[61]

To locate the Broussonian type of disease, it was necessary to track it down

by markers, gauged in depth, drawn to the surface, and projected virtually on the dispersed organs of the corpse. The "glance" has become a complex organization with a view to a spatial assignation of the invisible. Each sense organ received a partial instrumental function. Through touch we can locate visceral tumours, scirrhous masses, swellings of the ovary, and dilatations of the heart; while with the ear we can perceive "the crepitation of fragments of bone, the rumbling of aneurism, the more or less clear sounds of the thorax and the abdomen when sounded." The medical gaze is now endowed with a pleurisensorial structure. A gaze that touches, hears, and moreover, not by the essence or necessity, sees.[62]

Foucault's understanding of the nineteenth-century physician's approach to disease reflects Broussais' awareness of the physician's increased sensitivity to the patient's body. This awareness was soon enhanced by the application of diagnostic instruments. The effort to fix a penetrating "gaze" on the body's components in order to discover and reveal the path of disease was made possible by the joining of anatomy and pathology with the consequent blending of normal and abnormal functions and structures. The intense concentration on the physical body of the patient permitted the physician less time to search for external cultural forces that also contributed to disease. The human body became, in the gaze of the physician, more than ever an entity functioning within its own environment and under its own regulations. The reality of this attitude toward the body was brought to scientific eminence by Claude Bernard, who introduced the theory of the internal environment. Physicians could apply the internal environment concept of man in large part because they could decipher and describe parts of man's internal environment with the aid of instruments in ways never before imagined. It would take the next century and a half to discover the myriad interconnections within the body by using increasingly refined technology. While physicians were focused on these physical attributes, they ignored or minimized external factors or those relating to the culture, society, and economy within which humans lived.

Foucault summarizes these historical attempts to describe disease through the guidance of all the senses and the linking up of disease traces with postmortem lesions as a unique episode, which changed medical diagnosis and treatment ever after. Foucault believes that instruments, which made it feasible to magnify and extend the information gathered in by the senses, also placed a barrier to the physical contact between the doctor and the patient. The most dramatic demonstration of this thesis is Laennec's own admission that he designed the stethoscope to keep the physician's ear from the patient's chest by separating it with a cylinder of paper. However, internal body sounds, previously undetected or ignored because of their faintness were heard with the stethoscope when it was moved about the body surface, therefore making a greater variety of sound available to the diagnostician than would have been heard without the intervention of the stethoscope. Foucault's analysis of nineteenth-century linguistic nuances of medical diagnosis led him to conclude that by extending the sensorial "instrument" the physician was able to gaze into the body and see disease as it had never been seen previously. Foucault's position also suggests that when the physician was prepared theoretically for the particularization of disease and its multisensorial dimensions, a basis was laid for the application of diagnostic instruments that

would make more precise those signs of disease detected by the senses.

NOMENCLATURE:

Before physicians could discuss diseases in this period of constantly changing nomenclature and new physical criteria, a plan was decided on to standardize the names of the signs by which diseases were noted. At the international medical meeting of 1881, the clinicians met; Frederick A. Mahomed of the British Medical Association called for a committee to draw up a single code of terms to be used for describing the sounds heard in auscultation and percussion of the chest. Mahomed responded to Austin Flint's paper "An Analytical Study of Auscultation and Percussion" in which Flint tried to simplify the terminology of the physical signs associated with the lungs. C. T. Williams, one of the strong supporters of employing physical methods of diagnosis, ascribed the difficulty in finding uniform terms to describe the chest sounds to the instruments employed. The BMA president, Sir William Gull, proposed the formation of a committee, consisting of Ewart of Berlin, D'Epine of Geneva, Douglas Powell of England, Austin Flint of the United States, and Mahomed, to report to the congress in the following year with specific ideas for the project. The action the committee took was to have the British and American members draw up a list of terms in English, the Geneva representative provide a list in French, and the Berlin representative provide a list in German. After physicians outside the committee were consulted and lists exchanged, a synthesized list was published under three headings: palpation, percussion, and auscultation.[63] Austin Flint elicited interest among his colleagues by supplementing his prize essay of 1852 with another essay published in June, 1885 in the *JAMA*. Flint explained his studies of auscultation and percussion over the thirty-five-year interval.

My interest in the clinical study of variations in the pitch of sound did not end with the publication . . . of the prize essay. The conclusions at that time presented with diffidence were confirmed by further study, and together with additional conclusions, were submitted to the profession in my work on "Physical Exploration and the Diagnosis of Disease affecting the Respiratory System" published in 1856 [1st ed.] and in subsequent publications. My object in this supplementary paper, is to give a statement of the differential characters derived from the pitch of sound, in the signs obtained by auscultation and percussion, as applied to the respiratory system, especially insofar as knowledge of these characters has originated in my own studies, and to inquire how far the results of my studies are, at the present time, accepted by clinical observers.[64]

The first official *Nomenclature of Diseases*, which was not only based on physical diagnostic signs, was issued in 1869 and a second revised edition appeared in 1885. It was arranged so that diseases and their anatomic bases were cross-tabulated. "The horizontal line of the [disease] alphabet [was keyed to] the anatomical alphabet."[65] At the Ninth International Congress meeting in Washington, D.C. in 1887, uniformity in obstetric nomenclature was sought. Led by Alexander R. Simpson of Edinburgh, a committee of Miller, Simpson, William T. Lusk, and King was appointed to develop plans for achieving this goal.[66] Revisions of names for diseases and their symptoms and signs continued, especially incorporating the information collected with medical instruments.

DIFFERENTIAL DIAGNOSIS:

Instruments and laboratory tests introduced refinements into the diagnosis of abnormalities, which gave rise to a type of diagnosis of greater sophistication termed *differential diagnosis*. The term differential diagnosis was derived from the Latin term *diacritica signa* (signs by which one disease can be accurately discriminated from another.) Laennec introduced a preliminary form of differential diagnosis by calling attention to the variations among sounds occurring within the chest and the relationship of these sounds to postmortem lesions.[67] Austin Flint distinguished three types of diagnosis: direct, indirect, and differential in the last quarter of the nineteenth century. He based his distinctions on the ease with which they could be undertaken.[68] He explained that in direct diagnosis, upon superficial observation, sufficient and unequivocal evidence of disease was present. In indirect diagnosis, some of the expected signs associated with a particular disease appeared to be absent, and in differential diagnosis, a range of signs associated with several diseases were observed to be present for which testing, screening, and evaluation were required before the final diagnosis was made.[69] While differential diagnosis requires a multifaceted view of diseases and their signs, studies of the intricate tissue structures and the chemical components of fluids crucial to differential diagnosis became feasible after cell-, tissue-, and fluid-analyzing equipment was available including the microscope, spectroscope, electrophoresis apparatus, and other devices. These instruments became the basic tools of twentieth-century differential diagnosis.

The application of some physical diagnostic instruments to the differential diagnosis of disease was encouraged before the instruments had proven their value to the process. Sir Henry Thompson introduced Desormeaux's endoscope into the University College Hospital around 1863 because he thought it was desirable to test such devices in "a great medical school hospital" in the expectation that it might become an important diagnostic tool.[70] Twenty-five years later in 1888, an English surgeon evaluated the endoscope. E. Hurry Fenwick, surgeon to the London hospital and St. Peter's Hospital for Stone and Other Urinary Disease, explained, in response to the question, will the electric cystoscope (a form of endoscope inserted into the bladder) acquire value as a diagnostic agent?, "of its future importance in the differential diagnosis of the site of symptomless haematuria and pyuria, I have but little doubt."[71] Fenwick's monograph on the cystoscope and urethroscope, instruments designed and made by the physician Max Nitze of Berlin and the instrument maker Joseph Leiter of Vienna, instructed the English medical reader in the use of these instruments (see figure 7.4). Fenwick's book was praised, for "it will undoubtedly add to the reputation of the author and demonstrate to the profession that they have now within their reach one of the most valuable additions to our armamentarium of instruments for the purposes of diagnosis and direction of accurate treatment that have been introduced since the ophthalmoscope and laryngoscope."[72] By 1888, an important change was made in the instrument's illuminating source, which reduced the heat generated by the light bulb, thus enabling the physician to use it with less chance of injury to his patient's tissues.

Those diseases that were known to occur in multiple forms required the techniques of differential diagnosis to distinguish between them.[73] Diseases with multiple causes, which produced similar signs, such as an enlarged thyroid (goiter), were among diseases not easily diagnosed in the nineteenth and early twentieth centuries, but which prodded physicians to perfect their differential diagnostic techniques for recognizing the disease. Morell Mackenzie, the noted British eye, ear, nose, and throat specialist, discussed seven types of goiter in 1872. He noted that several forms of goiter could be treated successfully with the administration of iodine, which had been lacking in the patient's diet and which therefore, led to the mineral deficiency form of the disease. Mackenzie's recommendation to physicians was to treat patients with the signs of goiter conservatively, and partic-

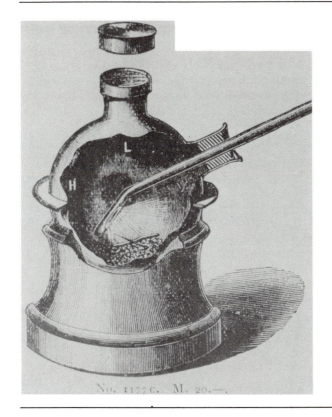

Figure 7.4. Nitze nineteenth-century cystoscope shown in simulated bladder to indicate its function from trade catalogue, *SI Photo No. 80-14529-13.*

ularly not to attempt to remove the gland unless there was serious functional impairment or a very enlarged tumor of the neck. Frequently, the patient urged his physician to surgically remove the gland because of the disfigurement in the neck and eyes that accompanied severe iodine deficiency goiter.[74] Lacking in Mackenzie's evaluation of the goiter which eventually would improve the diagnosis of this disease were chemical tests to determine the presence of thyroid hormones and iodine.

Recognized in the nineteenth century, tuberculosis was one of the four forms of phthisis including croupous, tubercular, catarrhal, and fibroid. Some of the diagnostic problems associated with tuberculosis were resolved by auscultation when phthisis, pleurisy, cancer, and abscesses were no longer confused with pneumonia and tuberculosis.[75] Disease surveys conducted among the medical profession in Britain and by life insurance companies in the United States were instituted to find the causes and most effective treatments for these diseases; instruments were designed and redesigned to aid in their diagnosis and numerous texts were published to teach their salient features. Tuberculosis as a leading cause of death was at the center of these strands of medical practice and spurred

increased research into the design of the stethoscope, which could be applied to diagnose differentially the forms of this disease.

The last quarter of the nineteenth century was a period of particular turmoil for many practitioners who tried to assimilate the explanations and diagnostic practices proposed in this period. Henry L. Byrd's refusal to accept contemporary explanations is not unexpected for an older physician or one with a limited medical education and provides an example of how the general practitioner responded to the new concepts and technology applied for the purposes of differential diagnosis. Byrd of the Baltimore Medical College could only cope with the torrent of new distinctions proposed for diseases by casting them aside. For instance, he preferred the older terms valued by his grandfather's generation such as sthenic and asthenic to distinguish a variety of diseases. He explained:

their peculiar fitness to occupy an enduring place in our nomenclature, and thus to keep the two widely separated and almost diametrically opposite states or conditions of the human organism in health and in disease, always prominently and perspicuously before the medical mind, a most important step will have been taken toward wiping away some of the flimsy drapery with which certain morbid conditions have been sought to be clothed by a few modern writers, and many of the hair-breadth distinctions between diseases, attempted to be made by others, bridged over or annihilated altogether.[76]

In the meantime, by the turn of the twentieth century, laboratory methods continued to be extended and applied to the diagnosis of a disease by those who studied disease assiduously. Richard C. Cabot of the Harvard Medical School emphasized the need to employ physiologic and chemical diagnosis before forming an hypothesis about a disease.[77] Cabot formulated a program for students and practitioners to follow that incorporated all aspects of disease studies and facilitated making a differential diagnosis. He called this method the Clinical Pathological Conference (CPC). The idea for Cabot's CPC originated in the Harvard Law School case study method, which Cabot had observed in 1903. He introduced the CPC into the medical school curriculum in 1906.[78] Cabot explained that to provide a set of rules to distinguish one disease from another was exceedingly difficult. Therefore, he designed a CPC routine to include testing all disease hypotheses by tissue and fluid analysis of cadaver specimens and correlation of the results with the disease signs and symptoms observed while the patient was alive. The clinician, medical student, and laboratory associate joined forces in evaluating a patient's disease, which was frequently chosen for the CPC on the basis of its unusual and difficult diagnostic features.

In 1912, Cabot made a statistical survey of the accuracy of diagnosis with which he was familiar. He was able to include 3,000 patients who could be followed up by autopsy to verify the causes of their deaths. His review of these patients' diseases and eventual deaths led him to conclude that a number of diseases including cirrhosis, acute endocarditis, acute nephritis, peptic ulcer, and others were relatively incurable at the time.[79] One of his purposes in publishing his study was to point out the common sources of diagnostic errors, so that physicians would become more attentive to their own limitations, and perhaps be able to eliminate diagnostic mistakes in the future.

Cabot hoped to classify a disease on the basis of the pathologic agent that caused it or the process that characterized it, rather than by the region or function disturbed by the disease, as was the custom. Accordingly, he classified 95% of 600 cases of heart disease into four major groups. These included those brought about by (1) rheumatic infection due to streptococci

bacteria, (2) syphilis, (3) arteriosclerosis, and (4) nephritis. A small percentage of heart diseases were not easily identified even though X-ray of the heart, the Wasserman test, and the "real test" for renal function were applied to the patient.

Sorting out the relevant from the irrelevant data was necessary to make a diagnosis that would suggest a program of therapy. Full knowledge of the disease depended on laboratory, microscopic, and chemical tests, while essential data or signs were crucial in making a clinical diagnosis.[80] To bring together in a concise format a basic core of twelve symptoms essential to the diagnosis of major diseases in Western countries, Herbert French of London compiled the first *Index of Differential Diagnosis* in 1912 to be used in conjunction with the *Index of Treatment* published in 1907. A second volume on differential diagnosis was published in 1914, which included nineteen more symptoms based on an analysis of the records of 317 patients.[81]

The terms applied to diseases became more restrictive in their meaning as the technology for uncovering disease signs became more extensive and specialized. Sign and symptom complexes in combination with disease complexes are the objectives of the most elaborate diagnostic procedures. Presently, the computer is the ultimate tool in helping the physician to match up all these variables, thereby reducing the chance of omitting any signs or misinterpreting them, which is a risk in differential diagnosis.[82]

W. R. Houston remarked in 1937, "The preferred diagnostic nosology is one which has 1) the greatest pragmatic power in the management of the individual patient, 2) the greatest utility in communication between the patient and physician and within the medical community and 3) the greatest efficiency in the explanation of phenomena and the formulation of theory. The semantic units of the diagnostic process are diseases . . ."[83] whose signs and symptoms are most definitely expressed in the terms arising from the use of a variety of instruments and medical technology.

IMPLICATIONS FOR MEDICAL DIAGNOSIS:

The most obvious expression of the changing concept of disease that grew out of nineteenth century medical technology was the greatly expanded group of names used to describe and differentiate diseases. These new disease terms arose from experimental and clinical investigations of diseases facilitated by instruments, devices, and tests. It would have been impossible without instrumental aids to segregate and provide detailed measurements and the interrelationships between body fluids and organs to the extent achieved in the nineteenth century. The isolation of disease within the smallest components of the body resulted from instrumental probing into body tissues.

Nineteenth-century physicians viewed, sometimes with alarm, the foremost task of the physiologist as selecting methods that employed special equipment to study bodily functions in increasing detail. For example, the circulation was divided into multiple phenomena including arterial and venous blood pressures, blood current velocity, contraction and relaxation of blood vessel muscular fibers, and the motion of the heart's valves.[84] The conscious efforts of physiologists to analyze through experiments the functions of the body led to a dynamic morbid anatomy in the early decades of the nineteenth century and a many-faceted differentiation of disease by the end of the century. The pathologist studies intensively the common components of diseases such as fever, inflammation, and catarrh.[85] The various phenomena associated with illness were discussed in anatomic and physiologic terms as gauged by instruments. Thus, the signs of disease derived from timing the pulse, measuring the exchange of gases in respiration, comparing skin colors and body temperatures, and other means were collected and related to both established and newly ascertained patterns of disease.[86] Methodical and accurate collection of data about disease when accumulated in large amounts revealed patterns that were of significance to the practitioner. For instance, the Collective Investigation Committee of Disease organized descriptions of diseases so that European and American physicians could contribute their personal observations to a central committee for analysis and study. Physicians were asked to answer prepared questionnaires usually requiring only brief answers. Thus, the general practitioner could add to the store of medical information by recording selected observations of his patients. Technical innovations facilitated data gathering by providing more objective and precise criteria for the physician to collect and enabled physicians to act collectively in a period when basic physiologic and pathologic data were becoming more significant.

Those diseases about which the most data were provided offered opportunities for further theory building. As was noted in Chapter Four, fever was among the earliest disease phenomena for which a large amount of precise data was gathered in the mid-nineteenth century. While fever had been a topic of importance since antiquity, the control and the mechanism of fever only became a subject of renewed intensive investigation by European investigators in the 1870s.[87] With reliable and readily available thermometers, and later, a continuously recording thermometer (thermograph), the temperatures of individuals during disease and in health were amassed, leading to various explanations of fever. Many attempts to explain the rise in body temperature were unsuccessful, but the ubiquitous presence of fever in so many patients demanded continued research to explain its cause, duration, and methods of control.

Theories of the cause and mechanism of fever abounded. Some of these were demonstrated through mechanical analogies and models. Rudolf Virchow theorized that fever was regulated by the nervous system, a view that was widely accepted.[88] Etienne Marey made the circulatory system, which had been linked to fever for centuries, the focus of his own research and speculated that a general relaxation of the vascular system of the external parts of the body led to warmer blood flowing into these vessels with a resultant increase in the temperature of the skin. Thomas Huxley provided a mechanical analogy that explained Marey's theory. Huxley compared the circulating blood to a hot-water heating system. Huxley's model explained that the blood distributed heat, remaining warmer within the body and cooler at the surface where the heat was easily dissipated. Temperature balance was disturbed when changes within the blood occurred, such as the amount of blood circulating through the vessels or the rate at which the blood flowed through the vessels.[89]

In 1887, Donald Macalister as the Croonian Lecturer of the Royal College of Physicians presented a theory of fever. Macalister coined three terms to designate the forces that seemed to contribute to the body temperature. The *thermogenic* force contributed to heat formation, the *thermolytic* force determined heat loss, and the *thermotaxic* force regulated heat adjustment. These forces stimulated appropriate nerves connected with the heat center and thus brought about the corresponding changes in body temperature. The thermometer did not reveal which of these forces was active or out of balance with the others, but it provided the net result of their interaction as an empirical and simple register of complex thermometric physiology and pathology.[90] Macalister insisted on knowing the source of fever and the physiologic causes of heat regulation in the body which, however, could not be discovered with the thermometer.

Nineteenth-century theorists and investigators reduced fever to a series of local and general causes and changed it from being classified as a disease, a category to which it had been assigned since antiquity.[91] Instead, fever was to be considered a sign or symptom of disease. Samuel Wilks, who studied the history of the clinical thermometer as well as being among the earliest to apply the instrument, understood by 1871 "that there is no more fever *per se* in typhus, typhoid, or scarlatina, than in a hundred other diseases; and we know also that under that vaguest of all terms, and one engendered in ignorance, 'common continued fever,' there had been included several totally different maladies, contagious and non-contagious. No term in the whole range of medicine (not excepting inflammation) has, I believe, wrought so much mischief on theoretic and practical medicine as the word 'fever'."[92] Wilks called for a concerted effort to educate the public, as well as physicians, into more of the intricacies of diseases to remove the confusion between fevers generated by an infectious disease and those due to other causes, and therefore, not to accept fever as a separate and distinct disease. One major step in the process of distinguishing the different causes of fevers as distinct diseases was the discovery of the specific pathogenic organisms which cause each type of fever and the unique signs resulting from bacterial invasion of the tissues. Richard Quain in the Harveian Lecture of 1885 emphasized that "no advance has been more important than that of the differentiation of the several forms of fever."[93] Along with his colleagues, he praised Sir William Jenner, president of the Royal College of Physicians, for recognizing the differences between typhoid and typhus fevers.

The British physician especially needed to be cautioned about the precise diagnosis of fever because of the consequences stemming from the treatment of infectious diseases by sending patients to segregated hospitals. By not distinguishing fevers on the basis of their causes, the physician caused all patients expressing a fever to be exposed to contagious diseases such as smallpox, typhus, and typhoid fevers. The patient could contract one of these dangerous diseases and become gravely ill, and perhaps, even die. *The Lancet* of 1872 carried two brief notices cautioning physicians to make an accurate diagnosis before sending a patient off to one of the contagious fever hospitals even though the dark, dirty, and confined rooms where poor patients often resided made it difficult to make the necessary physical examination of the patient. A tragedy had prompted medical leaders to call attention to the basic cause of recent deaths in a smallpox hospital, which they thought had been due to lack of segregation among contagious fever patients. Of sixteen patients sent to the London smallpox hospital, four individuals contracted smallpox within two weeks of admission and one of them died.[94] It was believed that the four smallpox victims had been unnecessarily exposed to the disease while confined to the hospital.

The thermometer led to an increase in the use of traditional therapeutic measures such as immersion in cold water baths, exposure to cool breezes, and so on to lower a patient's fever temperature. Less effort was applied to combat the other sequelae presented by diseases such as typhus fever and smallpox. It was accepted as it had been for millenia that if the fever could be reduced, the patient was apt to recover from the disease. With the thermometer to record slight changes in temperature, the application of cooling treatments became more precise. Physicians prescribed cold water baths in response to changes in body temperature indicated by the thermometer. However, W. H. Thomson, among others, in 1876 was concerned about the other components of the treatment of typhoid fever and insisted that "the physician should remember that the heat . . . is *not really the disease* to be combatted."[95] American physicians, with some exceptions, did not favor cooling therapy and generally lacked any specialized equipment to apply body cooling therapy. German ingenuity led to the invention of novel types of cooling equipment, including devices for immersing the patient in cold water, ice packs, and chemically induced cooling solutions, to treat fevers. Physicians who did not have ready access to such devices until the twentieth century emphasized the symptomatic nature of fever. Nelson Jones of Circleville, Ohio, for example, adopted the long-held view that fever was a natural defense against the invasion of disease and should be permitted to run its course. "For we are not yet sure," he claimed, "but, what a high temperature is one of the safeguards and efficient means employed by Nature to rid the system of an essential poison; and it is highly possible, indeed, that the febrile heat is one way in which the system reacts against the organisms that produce disease, in favor of health."[96] By the end of the nineteenth century, therapy to reduce fever included use of fever-reducing drugs. Antipyretic drugs, or those with the special capacity to lower body temperature, were synthesized in pharmaceutical laboratories. Aspirin was the most dramatic discovery among this class of drugs. Some other antipyretics, which were derived from coal-tar products, included creosote compounds, antipyrine and acetanilide which produced deleterious side-effects in the patient for whom the physician, anxious to eliminate the fever, prescribed them freely. Concentration on the elevated body temperature led to therapy that was concentrated and sometime dangerous, when it ignored or conflicted with other aspects of the disease.[97] (For a more detailed discussion of fever and the thermometer, see Chapter Four.)

INSTRUMENTS AND DISEASE:

From employing a relatively simple instrument like the thermometer to the use of complex timing and analyzing mechanisms, laboratory and clinical technology provided the major sources of information for the recategorization of diseases. Key by-products of physiology and pathology when explored with technology were diseases divided into numerous components, thus expanding nosology. Temperature and fever when measured precisely provided the basis for diagnosing diseases. Fever became one of a series of definitive diagnostic criteria which previously had included external body characteristics or those observed from outside the body.[98] Redefinition of diseases resulted from discoveries of the pathologic anatomist and the clinical pathologist, who were able to distinguish a greater assortment of details in the structures and substances of human organs, tissues, and cells. Rudolf Virchow singled out what he regarded as the best nineteenth-century example of an instrument (the ophthalmoscope) that enabled physicians to divide disease into some of its components. He commented at the British Medical Association meeting in 1873 that

disease is an unity only in an elementary organism—in a cell. It is always a compound phenomenon in a higher, in a compounded organism; and nobody will have perfect knowledge if he be not enabled to divide elementary components. This is shown by that branch of medical science which has now reached the highest degree of scientific surety—ophthalmology—whose methods make it possible to fix real elementary pathological alterations, and their continuation to compound diseases.[99]

Observation of the internal structure and condition of the eye enabled the physician to discover the beginnings of tissue and cell changes indicative of diseases not restricted to the eye.

As has been pointed out earlier, the stethoscope and microscope had served as the major sources of physical diagnosis. Each instrument introduced fundamental changes in the characterization of the signs and lesions of disease. Pathologists had speculated that functional diseases could be traced to physical alterations, even though tissue changes might not be observable. At the beginning of the nineteenth century, Xavier Bichat had classified diseases on the basis of the destruction of the tissues within the organs. Without a microscope to guide his observations (in fact, he rejected the microscope as unnecessary for studying tissues), Bichat divided all body tissues into twenty-one varieties. He set an example for the tissue pathologist Jean Cruveilhier and the cellular pathologist Rudolf Virchow, who did employ magnification to identify disease sites within the tissues. Tissue destruction continued to be refined as better lenses made these changes apparent to the many investigators who learned to use microscopes regularly in their study of pathological specimens.

William Seller of Edinburgh noted several basic changes in the classification of diseases, about which he cautioned the physician. During the transition period when the microscope was coming into use, the medical significance of what it revealed was not always self-evident and could be detrimental to the patient. Seller had no reservations about the future impact of instruments including the microscope in raising medical diagnosis to an accurate science, but he believed that the "distant harvest" had not yet appeared in diagnosing and treating disease. He noted that the common basic morbid anatomic terms, functional and organic or structural, generally applied to describe the results of an autopsy were being replaced by terms reflecting the finer distinctions observed with the microscope.[100] Microscopic data could be confusing to the physician who relied on the older distinctions as a basis for treatment. Seller explained that since antiquity, disease had been broadly categorized as functional or organic depending on the locus of the pathology. Those diseases described as functional were believed to be curable or at least more responsive to treatment, whereas diseases classified as organic in nature were usually considered chronic or even fatal[101] and often not amenable to treatment. Localized injuries to the tissues of an organ, which remained functionally adequate, were detectable with the microscope and sometimes with the stethoscope. By concentrating on changes revealed by these instruments, it was difficult to distinguish an organic from a functional impairment in the customary manner. This led to therapeutic measures not always in the best interest of the patient, in the sense that physicians tended to despair of being able to treat effectively any diseases diagnosed as being structural. An anonymous author in 1883 described the chief characteristics of a functional disease as one in which "the symptoms, although they may be the same in appearance, differ in nature and degree, and are characterized by being produced by causes which would not be followed by gross tissue change, by extreme *viability*, by their readiness to undergo change, and by the possibility of their sudden and complete recovery without leaving a trace of their existence."[102] Seller argued for making a further distinction between diseases based on different types of structural changes. Some organic changes were transient or confined to a few tissues within an organ. Other organic changes were permanent and could be discerned with the microscope. By adding this clarification, Seller hoped to preserve the accepted functional-organic or structural disease classification among diseases and to encourage physicians to employ treatment leading to a cure.[103] To Seller it seemed important to equate all new categories of diseases with the older categories, so that treatment would not be discouraged too often or without sufficient reason.[104] Seller was attempting to provide a practical solution to a dilemma posed by typing diseases as being functional or organic during the period before the microscope and stethoscope had made the issue critical by changing the meaning of these terms.

In time, greater perspective and experience with the diagnostic signs introduced by the microscope and stethoscope led to praise instead of dismay for the greater complexity brought into diagnosis with instruments. Edmund A. Parkes, a noted British hygienist whose medical career spanned the period of adjustment to several diagnostic instruments (1836-1876), reflected on the differences between instrument- and non-instrument-based diagnosis: "what a light the discovery of the renal and auscultatory signs throw upon the chaotic practice of earlier times. Our every-day work became at once defined; indecision, the most harassing of our troubles, was replaced by certainty; symptoms thought to be identical were suddenly separated; what had been deemed important was seen to be useless; what seemed insignificant was shown to be full of meaning."[105]

The significance of making a distinction between structural and functional diseases was again debated when further evidence of tissue destruction was revealed through yet another technique, that of chemical analysis. The structural-functional dichotomy began to appear even more arbitrary and unimportant for therapy. At whatever level of detail disease

signs and lesions were discernible, it became possible to expect that greater perfection of the techniques employed in locating disease loci would reveal more minute changes.[106] In the nineteenth century, knowledge of the nervous system seemed to offer a prime means of distinguishing between organic and functional diseases,[107] particularly when the ophthalmoscope was applied to detect traces of nerve deterioration within the eye, or the mallet was used to test simple reflexes by striking the knee or the elbow in the region of the joints. The difficulties introduced by applying instruments and chemical tests to separate structural from functional diseases eventually resulted in emphasis on their recategorization based on these distinctions. Functional disease may have been as severe as organic disease and have produced equal distress for the patient, although in the nineteenth century it appeared to physicians that diseases that primarily affected the function of an organ offered better prospects for the physicians to apply their medical skills in successful treatment.

Debating the structural and functional aspects of diseases brought out the similarities between the questions posed by physiologists and by pathologists. One striking discovery apparent to nineteenth-century investigators to emerge from the integration of physiology and pathology was the increased understanding of normal physiologic processes. Pathologic phenomena, even those of seemingly small import, could help unravel physiologic enigmas. The subtle recesses of disease uncovered by the pathologist sometimes provided a standard or limit by which to define normal structures and functions more useful than direct examination of healthy tissues. W. S. Greenfield of Edinburgh in 1881 provided two examples to illustrate the impact of pathology upon physiology. Waxy degeneration of the liver and deterioration of the spinal cord were among those pathologic processes revealing physiologic information and leading to changes in physiologic theories.[108] Fluids secreted by organs and tissues were reacted with chemical reagents to elucidate their compositions. Physiologists utilized the information gained by the removal of the liver or thyroid from an experimental animal and pathologists constantly relied on confirmed physiology for its parameters. These two sciences achieved their respective goals to study the normal and abnormal by comparing and contrasting their respective discoveries and observations. Michael Foster declared in 1880: "Physiology might be considered the watchdog against vagrant pathological theories."[109]

Laboratory and diagnostic instruments were essential in establishing the linkage between physiology and pathology. One of the first medical instruments to serve this purpose was the ophthalmoscope. Clifford Allbutt stated the reasons for its success in 1871 in his monograph on the use of the ophthalmoscope to detect diseases of the nervous system. Examination of the eyes for the purpose of finding clues to nervous disorders had preceded the invention of the ophthalmoscope, but with the instrument, slighter changes of a wider range became visible to the physician.[110] For this reason, Allbutt opposed narrow specialization in the application of the instrument to diagnose eye diseases. The ophthalmoscope he believed should be used to further broad investigations of disease. He based his assessment of the theoretical and methodical value of the instrument on the belief that it is

in these slighter deviations from the normal order, in spasmodic neuralgias, local tremors, transient suspensions of the senses, and such minor indications of lessened tension, and increasing instability that we shall ultimately find the explanation of the more typical forms of disorder. It is not by setting up opposition standards to the standard of health that we shall learn the modes of initiation of morbid changes, but rather by watching the outskirts of health itself. Before we can comprehend extensive changes, we must familiarize ourselves with slighter ones, and so take with us the clues to the larger mystery.[111]

The ophthalmoscope, like the microscope, introduced a precision into disease differentiation and description which trained the investigator's eye to "see many more new things before . . .[which had been] overlooked."[112] The instrument also "enabled the physician who mastered it to proceed with more confidence in [his or her] examination, and to speak more decidedly as to prognosis and treatment."[113]

Allbutt's views were not widely pursued and extended at first, because the early form of the ophthalmoscope was not an instrument that could be easily learned and applied. A decade later, Bradbury in a talk to the British Medical Association in which he reported on a variety of diagnostic instruments, had to remind his audience that the ophthalmoscope must no longer be regarded as an instrument of use only for the ophthalmic surgeon. To stimulate interest in its use, he mentioned some of the diseases the ophthalmoscope could be used to diagnose, which included tumors, syphilis, Bright's disease, acute tuberculosis, locomoter ataxia, and cerebral embolism.[114] Half a century after Allbutt's essay appeared, nonspecialist physicians still, too often, neglected the ophthalmo-

scope because it seemed impossible for them to learn to use within a reasonable amount of time. Teachers like the Philadelphia ophthalmologist, William Fisher, instructed medical students how to use the instrument by having them practice on a wooden model of the eye. Mastery of the technique of applying the instrument before approaching a patient was Fisher's aim. He advocated the most popular model of the ophthalmoscope, the electrically lighted Loring instrument, which contained a perforated mirror for reflecting light into the patient's eye.[115]

DISTINGUISHING THE NORMAL AND ABNORMAL:

Defining the abnormal or diseased and marking it off from the normal or healthy organism presented continued difficulties. Medical technology provided evidence to demonstrate that these two physical states of being could never be completely separated, no matter how their parameters were defined. Hermann Boerhaave reiterated the ancient view that "morbus est vita praeter naturam."(Illness is abnormal life).[116] This quotation was repeated by James Cuming in 1884 to support his own view that "disease was to be regarded as simply a perverted life-process and that there was an essential identity between physiological and pathological processes."[117] Discussion of the issues raised by contrasting the normal with those slight individual differences which, although discernible, were not classified as diseases spurred the growth of physiology and pathology and their emergence as major professions in the service of medicine. Thomas Huxley, whose aim had been to indicate the fundamental connection between pathology and physiology as branches of biology and to relate all these sciences to medicine, summed up the relationship between health and disease as he understood it in 1881:

Living matter is characterized by its innate tendency to exhibit a definite series of the morphological and physiological phenomena which constitute organisation and life. Given a certain range of conditions, and these phenomena remain the same, within narrow limits, for each kind of thing. They furnish the normal and typical character of the species; and, as such, they are the subject-matter of ordinary biology. Outside the range of these conditions, the normal course of the cycle of vital phenomena is disturbed, abnormal structure makes its appearance, or the proper character and mutual adjustment of the functions cease to be preserved. [These deviations] may have no notable influence on the general well-being of the economy, or they may favour it. On the other hand, they may be of such a nature as to impede the activities of the organism, or even to involve its destruction. In the first case, these perturbations are ranged under the wide . . . category of "variations"; in the second, they are called "lesions," "states of poisoning," or "diseases;" and . . . they lie within the province of pathology. No sharp line of demarcation can be drawn between the two classes of phenomena. No one can say, for example, where anatomical variations end and tumours begin; nor where modification of function, which may at first promote health, passes into disease. All that can be said is that whatever change of structure or function is hurtful belongs to pathology. Hence it is obvious that pathology is a branch of biology; it is the morphology, the physiology, the distribution, the etiology of abnormal life.[118]

French pathologists also interpreted their investigations according to the view that pathology was best conceived as an extension of physiology.

F.-J.-V. Broussais was among the first to propose a type of physiologic medicine growing out of his perspective, which eliminated making a clear distinction between health and disease.[119] The basic propositions of Broussais were translated into English in 1832 by Isaac Hays and R. Eglesfeld Griffith. These include "Prop. 67: Health supposes the regular exercise of the functions, disease results from their irregularity; death from their cessation. Prop. 68: The functions are irregular when one or several of them are performed with too much or too little energy."[120] Health was a matter of the body's equilibrium, according to Broussais's theory. The idea was amplified in Claude Bernard's concept of homeostasis. Bernard regarded the normal and abnormal as facets of each other. He believed that one instinctively sensed the intimate relation between extremes "au point de manifester constamment la tendance de faire découler les seconds des premiers."[121] Bernard pointed to past accomplishments to show that when progress was made in physiology, a corresponding advance was made in pathology. The assumption that the natural and normal physiologic state helped to define morbid conditions or pathology was given a quantitative basis after instruments were designed to make suitable measurements.[122]

Sir William Gull, fashionable West-end practitioner, upon his election as chairman of the London Clinical Society in 1872, perhaps best summed up the consequences of relating disease to health in his address to his colleagues: ". . . that disease is not an entity to be exorcised from the body but an abnormal fulfilment of the ordinary functions of the individual."[123] For some people, ill-health is as natural as sound health.

"In any case, we are to study the individual, to ascertain as closely as possible what his ordinary condition is, and to keep in mind alike in forming a diagnosis and a prognosis and in suggesting a line of treatment."[124]

George Murray Humphry, the Cambridge Professor of Anatomy and President of the British Medical Association section of physiology in 1873 reasoned that control of disease was possible through improved physiologic studies brought about by technology—a recurrent theme used to justify the physician's use of tools, devices, hardware, and the information they provided.[125]

ADOLPHE QUETELET:

Concern for individual differences among the bodily functions had been expressed in the medical literature for centuries. However, in 1836 Adolphe Quetelet, Belgian astronomer and statistician, was the first to issue a mathematical assessment of the biological variations among human beings, as well as indicating methods of measuring these variations to determine a biologically acceptable average that could be used for reference in the practice of medicine. Quetelet's conception of the average person was based on his belief in the regularity of the laws of nature. One aspect of Quetelet's program called for collecting data on the capacities and limits of functions of all the body's organs and systems.[126] One of the few instruments available for making functional measurements in an office setting was the dynamometer designed by Regnier. The dynamometer measured the force of the skeletal muscles, and although it was not precise, it was useful to compare the muscular differences between the sexes and the differences in the muscle strength of the arms and legs at various ages and during different stages of disease. Quetelet provided tables of data based on measurements he collected from which he concluded that a male developed his greatest muscular strength between the ages of 25 to 30 years, whereas a female was able to develop only two-thirds of this maximum limit.[127]

A related type of study encouraged by Quetelet was also suggested by Charles Babbage. The study included measuring the rate of various activities people performed during a unit of time such as how many steps could be taken, how many hammer blows struck, and how many strokes of an oar could be made in one minute. He then wanted to compare all of these figures to find the ratios between the constants in each instance. Elementary studies of this type were the forerunners of more complex measurements involving athletes during and after strenuous exercises and of individuals exposed to environmental stresses. Experimental physiologists adopted various instruments for measuring the processes of special interest to them such as respiratory rate, heart rate, venous pulse, and so on, especially after the kymograph of Carl Ludwig was developed for recording these functions over an interval of time on graph paper, which could be permanently retained.[128]

Quetelet concluded that "the consideration of the average man is so important in medical science, that it is almost impossible to judge of the state of an individual without comparing it to that of another imagined person, regarded as being in a normal condition, and who is intrinsically no other than the individual we are considering."[129] English physicians such as F. J. Gant in 1857 reaffirmed Quetelet's conclusion and remarked on its relevance to medical practice that

true it is that disease cannot be exactly defined by contrast with anatomy and physiology for structures and functions themselves vary within the limits of their healthy conditions. Perhaps no two individuals are precisely alike structurally or functionally, not to mention the modifying circumstances of age, sex, etc. Disease must, therefore, be defined by comparison with the healthy condition of the individual, or at least with due allowances for individual differences.[130]

This conclusion suggested a relatively simple action for all individuals to follow, which would assist the physician in gathering the pertinent data. Aware of the crude state of medical record keeping in his time, Quetelet advised all individuals to make and keep records of their bodily functions while in a healthy state, particularly the pulse rate, respiration rate, and body temperature. The records obtained while the body was functioning normally could then be used as standards by the physician to compare with the record of these bodily functions during an illness.[131]

In 1884, a proposal was made in Britain to collect statistics from among the general population to discover the normal-abnormal limits of many bodily structures and functions. A "Life-History Album" sponsored by the Committee on Collective Investigation of Disease and completed by Francis Galton after its originator's death, was designed to be used by laymen to record their own physical and mental statistics. The Life-History Album was to serve as an individual's physiologic and pathologic diary, which would be available to the physician during a disease crisis. Marketed by Macmillan and Co. in several sizes at a cost of three shillings six pence and four shillings six pence, the album included space to record

stature, weight, chest girth, muscle strength, eye color, hair color, evidence of unusual mental or artistic capacity, and other measurements or functions deemed valuable. By assisting the medical investigator in building up the necessary records of physiologic and anatomic measurements from birth, a broad spectrum of data would be accumulated.[132]

The concept of the average person, which represents an unobtainable reality, was criticized by physicians and physiologists. Xavier Bichat rejected the average because he believed that it eliminated variability, and Claude Bernard disapproved of masking the changing and rhythmic character of processes essential to living organisms by averaging these phenomena. Bernard also was skeptical of analyzing the bodily fluids for their chemical components because this information could not indicate how these fluids were used by the body nor how they would have to be altered to cure disease.[133] Bernard emphasized that the basic laws of chemistry and physics do not vary in the organism, whether in illness or health, but the body's continual efforts to adapt and alter its own physiologic functions eluded any explanation of these internal efforts in valid operative terms, especially by statistical analysis of many individuals.

PIERRE C. A. LOUIS:

During the period that Quetelet prepared his studies on biological variability, and instruments to measure some of these variables were designed and applied, the French clinician Pierre C. A. Louis introduced the method of statistically analyzing the effectiveness of disease treatments by comparing the responses to specific therapies in use at the time. Louis perfected the "méthode numérique or numerical method" in his publication of 1835 entitled *Researches on the Effects of Bloodletting in Some Inflammatory Diseases*.[134] From his observations on the curative effects of bloodletting upon pneumonia victims, Louis concluded that bloodletting was not as useful as it was assumed to be in treating this disease. His method demonstrated that treatment could be made more precise since the numerical method would compensate for the inevitable variabilities in diagnosing and treating diseases by organizing facts of sufficient resemblance to "deduce laws which everyday's experience verifies."[135] He claimed "that it is impossible to appreciate each case with mathematical exactness, and it is precisely on this account that enumeration becomes necessary; by so doing, the errors (which are inevitable), being the same in two groups of patients subjected to different treatment, mutually compensate each other, and they may be disregarded without sensibly affecting the exactness of the results."[136] His explanation of the mathematical subtleties involved in statistics did not convince all his colleagues. Opponents such as Claude Bernard contested that Louis was "invoking the inflexibility of arithmetic, in order to escape the encroachments of the imagination and to efface differences and therefore committing an outrage upon good sense."[137] To this logic, Louis replied that the calculus or numerical method does not remove differences "it supposes them." Louis understood the importance of accumulating data from many patients and making these data relevant and meaningful by quantifying their salient features. "If then there is a means of embodying the experience of the ages, it is the numerical method."[138] Medical technology would ensure the success of the numerical method, and eventually, raise the method to the highest level of medical practice.

Louis' contemporaries, who adopted his statistical method of recording the disease histories of patients, explained their conception of the method. W. A. Guy, the Cambridge professor of forensic medicine, in 1839 published a statement on what he termed the "instruments of calculation" or statistics applied to organized and unorganized matter. He summarized the main advantages of the numerical method: "first, that the errors necessarily existing in our observations and experiments (the consequence of our senses, or of our instruments) neutralize each other, and leave the actual value of the object or objects observed; and, secondly, that the extreme quantitative differences existing between the several things observed, compensate one another, and leave a mean result which accurately expresses the value of the greater number of the things so observed."[139] He continued:

The profession of medicine gives ample scope for the application of numbers. If we consider the health of large masses of men placed under different circumstances, and acted on by different influences, it is to the numerical method that we must look for accurate information as to the effect of these circumstances. If we would compare one human body with another in respect of stature, weight, muscular force, or the development of its several parts, we must also resort to the numerical method. If, again, we direct attention to the several functions performed by the human body in a state of health, we find that most of them can only be adequately described by the aid of numbers. Thus the amount of the injesta and egesta, the quantity of the several secretions, the products of the respiratory process, the fre-

quency of the pulse and respiration—none of these can be expressed without the aid of numbers.[140]

Guy believed that the inexperienced physician would benefit most from the numerical method. The statistical resumé of stresses and their symptoms would provide the inexperienced physician with accurate data concerning the chances that certain symptoms and diseases were present and the types of treatments most likely to be successful.[141]

The most important and distinguishing feature of the numerical method for medical practice was that it turned a theory into a practice. Guy illustrated the uselessness to medical practice of even the most celebrated medical theory—the circulation of the blood —when not determined or explained numerically: "What for instance, has the beautiful theory of the circulation of the blood done for medicine?" Guy asked.

It has not taught us the use of the lancet, for that was in requisition long before in the time of Harvey, and we treat inflammation now as we did in the days of Hippocrates. As an acknowledged fact, indeed, the circulation of the blood has had an indirect influence upon other medical theories, but what direct practical application does it boast? Where are we to find a measure of the state of the circulation itself? The pulse, the only measure we possess, scarcely gives more information now than it gave to Celsus, more than eighteen centuries ago. Its changes are still as difficult to appreciate, and not less difficult to describe; and though Floyer invented the pulse-watch, and Heberden strongly recommended its employment, how little has yet been done to bring to perfection this imperfect measure of the circulation.[142]

With this example Guy pointed out that it was essential to apply instruments to the body if modern medical theories and practices were to be correlated.

Organizing the measurable characteristics of normal and abnormal structures and functions became the next stage in the changing descriptions of physiologic and pathologic entities. After Louis, statistical comparisons of treatments were made primarily from hospital records accumulated both nationally and internationally. Many measurements were facilitated by instruments, especially when they were collected with devices that permanently recorded functions over a period of time, such as the kymograph, sphygmograph, and electrocardiograph. These instruments provided a means to apply the circulation of the blood concept to medical diagnosis and treatment, a challenge physicians had recognized since the seventeenth century.

English biologists, Francis Galton and others less well known such as Charles Roberts, who carried Quetelet's mantle to England, extended "Quetelet's observation that certain measurable human characteristics are distributed like the error function."[143] The biological and psychological variations Galton discovered by applying the Gaussian Law of Errors were not to be eliminated as they had been by other investigators. According to Galton, "these errors or deviations were the very things I wanted to preserve and know about."[144] The International Health Exhibition of 1884 in London provided Galton with an unusual opportunity to measure nine to ten thousand individuals and thereby collect the raw data that he needed to flesh out his theories on the relations of the normal and abnormal in the function of the sensory organs.[145]

In a room thirty-six feet long and six feet wide, seventeen different measurements were made of each visitor, including height, weight, muscle strength, breathing capacity, vision, and hearing, at a cost of under three pounds per individual. The immense popularity of this anthropometric laboratory encouraged supporters to expect that a permanent anthropometric laboratory would be established in a national hygienic institution, which, however, was never accomplished.[146]

Roberts substituted for the word *average* the term *mean* or *typical*, which were terms adopted by George Milbry Gould and J. H. Baxter in the United States.[147] These terms were applied to the small measurable differences in the function of an organ, and therefore, in effect broadened the limits of what was accepted as normal and extended the concept of normal to include a series of circumscribed measurements, rather than a single measurement.

INSTRUMENTS TO MEASURE ANATOMIC AND PHYSIOLOGIC CHARACTERISTICS:

Galton stimulated the production and use of a variety of specialized instruments to determine the individual variations he was seeking. Some of the instruments he employed to measure the structures and functions of muscles and bones and to make size and weight measurements had existed for centuries. (See figures 7.5, 7.6, 7.7, 7.8.) These included calipers for measuring the size of the head, a rule or tape for other bodily measurements, a scale for recording the weight, and introduced in the early nineteenth century, the dynamometer to measure the strength of an arm, leg, or finger muscle. These instruments could have been used by physicians at the time Quetelet collected his data from medical associates, but in fact, were rarely applied to the human body during a physical examination until late in the nineteenth century.

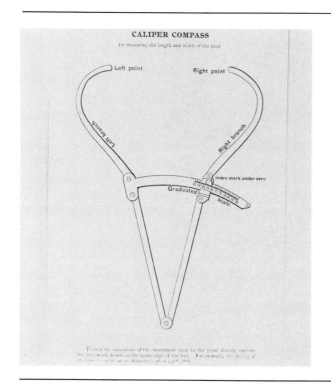

Figure 7.5 Caliper compass illustration from Alphonse Bertillon, *Signaletic Instructions Including the Theory and Practice of Anthropometrical Identification* (Chicago: The Werner Co., 1896), translated from the French under the supervision of Major R. W. McClaughry. *SI Photo No. 987928.*

MEASURING THE LENGTH OF RIGHT EAR (*b*)

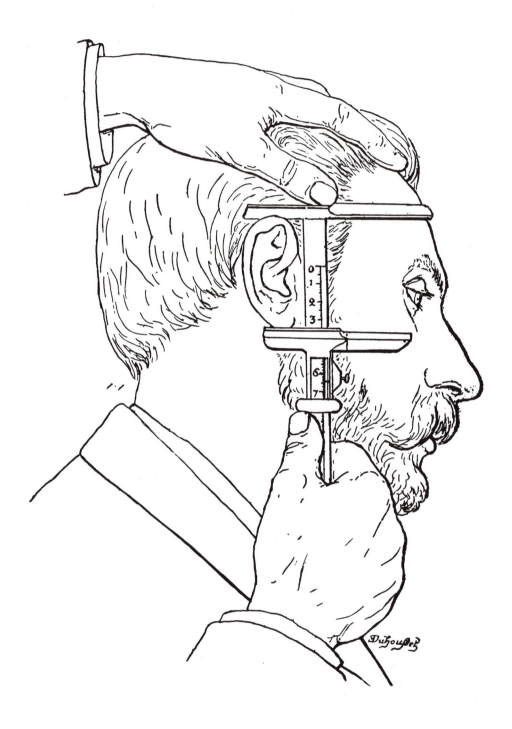

Special view for the study of the position of the fingers and of the instrument.

Figure 7.6. Measuring the length of the right ear. From Alphonse Bertillon, *Signaletic Instructions* (Chicago: The Werner Co., 1896). *SI Photo No. 78-7898.*

MEASURING THE LENGTH OF LEFT FOOT (a)

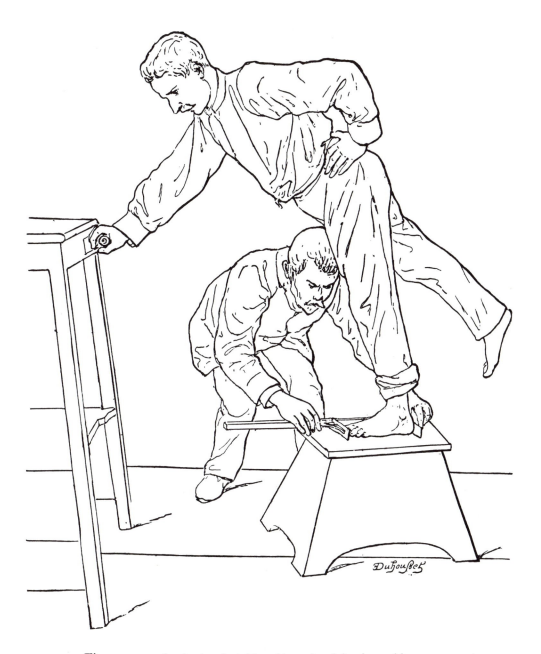

The operator, after having had his subject placed in the position represented above, presses the fixed branch of the instrument firmly against the back of the heel, taking care to have the graduated stem touch, if possible, the internal face of the heel and of the toe joint.   Then he gradually brings down the movable branch until it is in contact with the great toe, assuring himself by shaking the instrument a little that the movable branch has neither pushed back nor compressed the extremity of the great toe, and finally replaces the instrument, it necessary, and tightens it very slightly before reading the figure indicated (*Instr.*, p. 118).

Figure 7.7 Measuring the length of the left foot. From Alphonse Bertillon, *Signaletic Instructions* (Chicago: The Werner Co., 1896). *SI Photo No. 78-7920.*

MEASURING THE LEFT LITTLE FINGER (*a*)

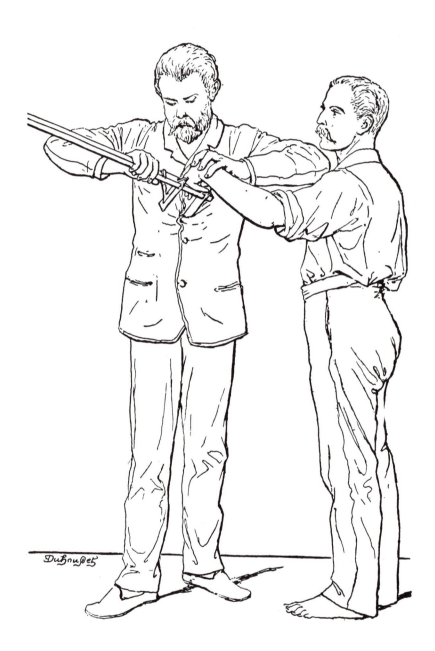

Proceed by analyzing the stages as in measuring the middle finger (*Instr.*, p. 125).

7.8 Measuring the length of the left little finger. Alphonse Bertillon, *Signaletic Instructions* (Chicago: The Werner Co., 1896). *SI Photo No. 78-7921.*

Finding the means to measure the characteristics deemed important in the quest for the delineation between the normal and abnormal led to an overlapping of goals between medical diagnosis and anthropometry. Anthropometry was viewed as related to physical diagnosis by some nineteenth-century practitioners. Charles Roberts considered physical diagnosis a type of practical anthropometry or measurement of humans. In calling for the teaching of the methods of anthropometry to medical students, Roberts discussed the method's value not only to define disease conditions but also to discover the influence of external agents on growth and development of the body and its organs.[148] "In its widest sense," he said, "diagnosis is anthropometry, for all our attempts at differentiation of diseases are measurements of either time or space, and all our instruments, whether for pathological or physiological investigation, are anthropometric instruments when applied to the investigation of the anatomy and functions of the human body."[149] Roberts reviewed the anthropometric instruments of value to the physician in 1878 and recommended that a basic set of instruments include boxwood calipers with a brass scale to measure from 1/5 to 20 or more inches, and a dynamometer manufactured by Coxeter of London. The

dynamometer consisted of a steel bar coiled on itself in the center with the ends left free to act as levers (see figure 7.9). Handles were attached to the levers and a graduated scale placed in front of the coil. The dynamometer could also function as a weighing machine when it was suspended from a beam or tripod by one handle with a stirrup or bar attached to the other for the person to hold while being weighed. Calipers, hand-rule, and measuring tape were fitted into a light case, which Roberts called a "physical examination case."[150] (See figures 7.10 and 7.11.) A decade later, Roberts expressed dismay at the large number of overly refined and sophisticated anthropometric instruments marketed by the Cambridge Instrument Company. He blamed Galton for the overabundance of instruments since he was the inventor of many of them. Roberts claimed that special instruments, such as the Galton whistle for detecting high frequency sounds, should not be advertised and sold as anthropometric instruments. Their intricate construction and complex function made them impractical for use during a regular physical examination (see figure 7.12). Diagnosticians became discouraged when confronted with a wide variety of instruments and stopped using all of them, including the basic instruments.

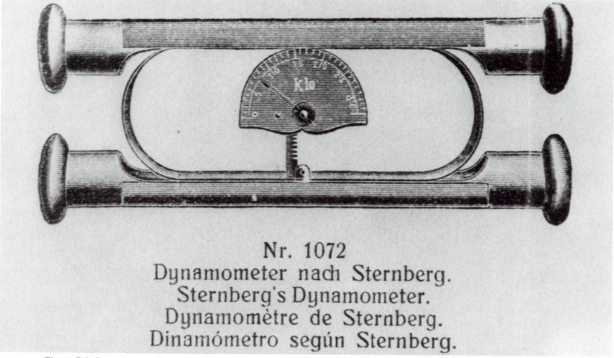

Nr. 1072
Dynamometer nach Sternberg.
Sternberg's Dynamometer.
Dynamomètre de Sternberg.
Dinamómetro según Sternberg.

Figure 7.9. Late nineteenth-century dynamometer by Sternberg sold by E. Zimmerman of Leipzig and Berlin. *SI Photo No. 74-6515.*

LARGE CALIPER RULE

for measuring the foot, the middle and little fingers and the forearm

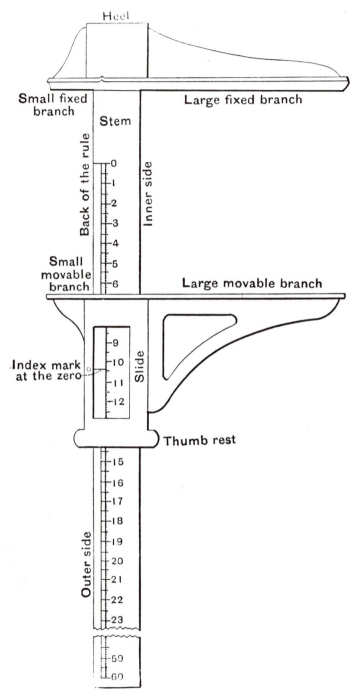

To read the indications of the instrument turn to the point directly opposite the zero mark traced on the middle of the left edge of the opening in the slide or thumb rest. For example, *the opening of the branches in the above drawing is about 10 cm 7mm.*

Figure 7.10. Large caliper rule. Alphonse Bertillon, *Signaletic Instructions* (Chicago: The Werner Co., 1896). *SI Photo No. 48-7916.*

MEASURING FURNITURE

showing arrangement of mural graduations

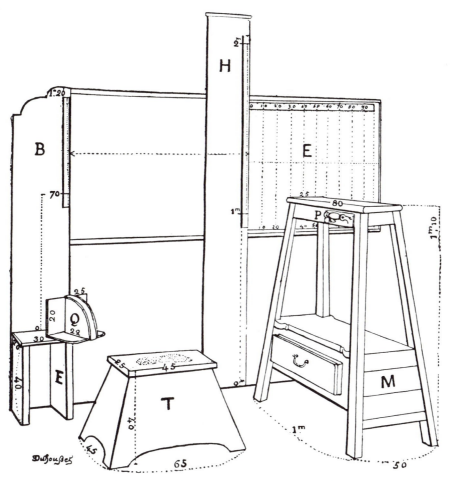

H. — Vertical rule one metre long for measuring the height (*Instr.*, p. 100).

E. — Graduations on paper or oilcloth for measuring the reach (*Instr.*, p. 103).

B. — Rule half a metre long for measuring the trunk or height of a man seated (*Instr.*, p. 105).

Q. — Portable square with double projection, used in measuring the height and the trunk.

E. — Stool used in measuring the trunk.

T. — Movable foot-stool to facilitate the measuring of the foot, of the cranial diameters and of the ear.

M. — Trestle specially intended for the measuring of the forearm, and affording a point of support (P) to the subject during the measuring of the foot (*Instr.*, p. 118).

Figure 7.11. **Measuring the furniture collection.** Alphonse Bertillon, *Signaletic Instructions* (Chicago: The Werner Co., 1896). *SI Photo No. 78-7900.*

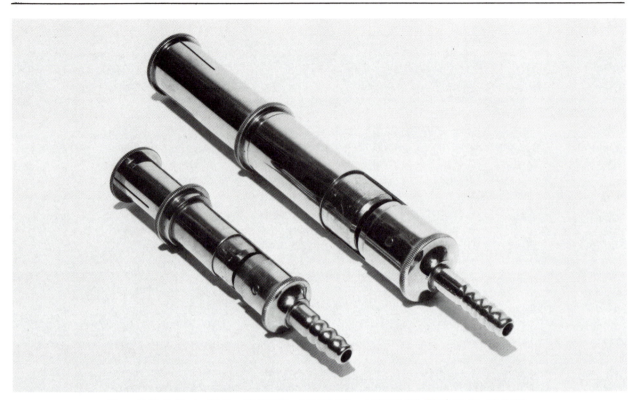

Figure 7.12. Galton's whistles. *NMAH No. 300427.196 and 300427.198, SI Photo No. 72-10707.*

At this time, a dynamometer was available for measuring the muscular power of the feet and the pulling and pushing forces of the hands and chest muscles. Some models provided a record printed on paper.[151] This instrument called a dynamograph recorded the length of time over which muscles could maintain tonic contractions. A more common application of the dynamometer in medical diagnosis was to indicate differences in muscular strength between the right and left hands, which generally registered on the dial of instrument as a fluctuation of less than ten degrees.[152] Roberts emphasized those measurements that could be easily consistently obtained. (See figures 7.13, 7.14, 7.15, 7.16, 7.17, and 7.18.) Above all, Roberts encouraged English physicians to become adept in anthropometry and to equal the skills of their colleagues in other countries. These skills included those of the Germans who used anthropometry to measure the physical differences between the races, the French physicians who used its methods to identify those who attempted to conceal or could not reveal their identity such as criminals and psychiatric patients, and American physicians who applied anthropometry to measure the effect of gymnastics and athletic exercise upon the muscles.[153]

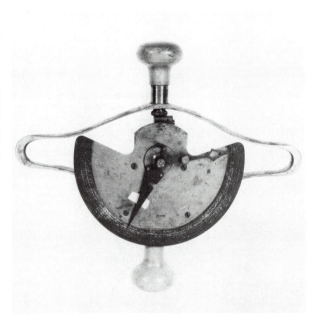

Figure 7.13. Dynamometer. *AFIP No. 285901, SI Photo No. 73-7213.*

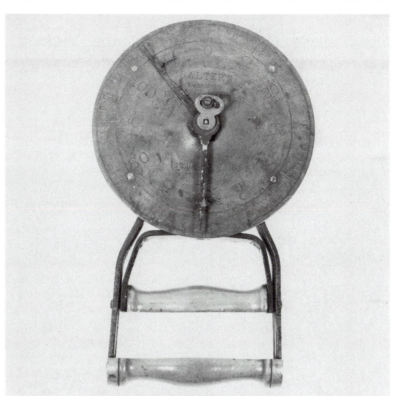

Figure 7.14. Salter Dynamometer. *AFIP No. 337589, SI Photo No. 73-7214.*

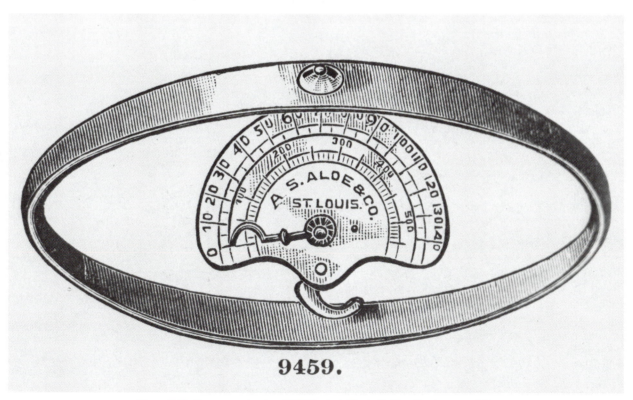

Figure 7.15. Dynamometer circa 1893 illustrated in A. S. Aloe Catalogue, p. 640.

Kny-Scheerer, a medical instrument supplier in New York, sold an acclaimed set of anthropometric instruments designed by Alphonse Bertillon of France, for examining criminals. This set contained various sized rules and calipers, nail scissors, a wedge for proving calipers, a metal plate, an ink roller, a tube of black ink, a dermatographic pencil, and a pointed rod for measuring the ear.[154] Manufacturers responded to the need to supply anthropometric instruments of acceptable standards and generated sales as physicians and biologists gathered physical measurements from numerous individuals in order to characterize the physical attributes of the "typical man." Anthropometric sets that were well organized and portable increased interest among physicians, who responded to the advertisements and promotional literature appearing in medical journals and books. This literature relied on testimonials given by scientific investigators. A. S. Aloe, medical instrument manufacturer of New York, advertised in 1893 that "in as much as a very essential part of anyone's physical education is based upon anthropometry, or the measurements of man, and as an important factor in anthropometry is the strength of muscles, it is therefore seen that all strength tests should be standards, so that at some time, if the various physical instructors will bring together the results of these tests, they will better serve to show the strength of the 'typical man'."[155]

Changes in the environment brought about greater frequency of accidents, which left more injured muscles and nerves, and thus, the physician was called on to employ anthropometric instruments to diagnose the extent of muscular damage and gauge the success of treatment. The practitioner became more experienced in diagnosing diseases related to nerve and muscular functions in part because he was confronted with an increasing number of patients who had received injuries resulting in paralysis and muscle weakness. The railroad and the factory provided the setting for a number of these accidents. Simple instruments that would reveal the extent of the injury as well as the degree of progress after treatment were in demand. The most common diagnostic methods in addition to visual inspection was manipulation of muscle complexes through special devices. Diagnosis of nervous system diseases depended on instruments that could measure two general functions: control of movement and sensibility to stimuli. To compare movement of selected muscles, the strength-measuring instrument of choice was the dynamometer. A variety of dynamometers for medical diagnosis were available by the last quarter of the nineteenth century. The simplest and the most useful dynamometer

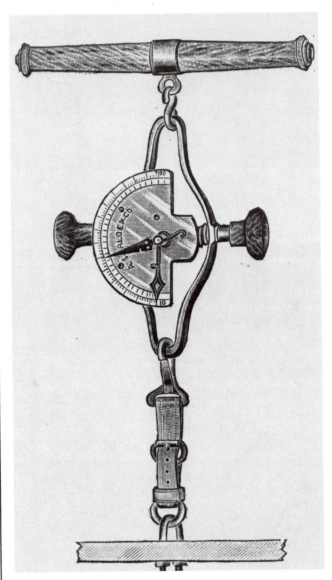

Figure 7.16. Dynamometer circa 1893 suspended from two supports, illustrated in A. S. Aloe Catalogue p. 636.

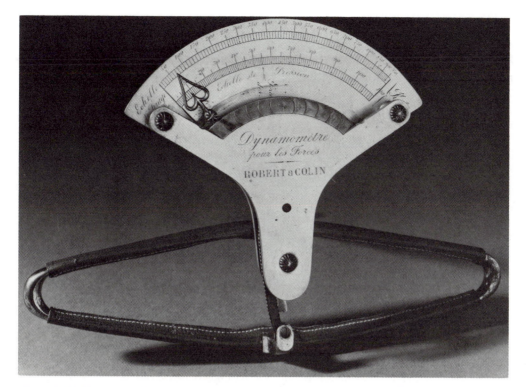

Figure 7.17. Mid-nineteenth century dynamometer made by Robert and Collin. *NMAH No. 78.0874.03, SI Photo No. 80-15209.*

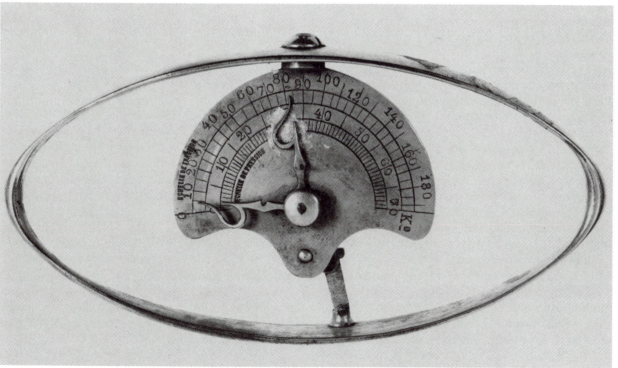

Figure 7.18. Dynamometer made by Charrière. *AFIP No. 337586, SI Photo No. 73-7209.*

for physicians consisted of an "elliptical steel spring which can be compressed in the hand or other parts of the body. Connected with it is a cog-wheel which moves an index-needle upon a dial, the index needle remaining where it is carried by the muscular effort of the patient."[156] The instrument was calibrated to read in pounds or kilograms of force, although physicians believed a measure of the degrees of force without regard to a specific unit was adequate for diagnostic purposes. The model produced by Emil L. Mathieu of Paris was among the most widely used. It contained a ratchet lock, which remained set at the point of maximum force reached by the patient, thereby allowing the physician time to read the instrument after the patient completed the test. With attachments to facilitate holding the instrument in place, this dynamometer could be used to measure muscle strength in various parts of the body.[157]

To measure the muscular force of the tongue and lips, specially designed pencil-shaped dynamometers were manufactured. The French firms of Charles Verdin and G. Boulitte sold the greatest variety of dynamometers, which were handsomely illustrated in their catalogues.[158]

By 1905, American physicians were being instructed in tests to use in the sudden loss of any of the five senses due to hysteria resulting from an accident and other causes. Among the more popular instruments recommended were the perimeter for detecting loss of peripheral vision, the tuning fork and Galton's whistle for testing deafness, Zwaardemaker's olfactometer for determining acuteness of smell, and an assortment of implements to test for sensitivity to touch and pain.[159] Measuring the sensitivity to touch appealed to the creative powers of those designing instruments for this purpose.

The aesthesiometer, which was named by Edward Sieveking in 1834, was the basic instrument for examining an individual's sensitivity to touch by indicating the minimum distance between two points that could be distinguished when the device was placed on the skin. The earliest model, designed by E. H. Weber, was constructed out of a long, straight piece of steel to which two movable points were attached in a cork shield.[160] In the 1840s, Weber and his brother constructed an aesthesiometer out of a compass, with one stationary end as in a shoemaker's rule.[161] Another popular form resembled a compass with an attached Vernier scale. Sieveking designed a model that was a modified ordinary beam-compass used by carpenters. Weber tested his instrument on many individuals and prepared a table of the distances to

be expected between the points of the aesthesiometer marked in lines or millimeters, and later, in inches, when placed on selected areas of the skin. These tables and a few others were widely distributed and consulted by physicians making the test on their patients. Weber concluded that "this distance varies in health between extremely wide limits, because some regions are abundantly supplied with sensory nerves and tactile corpuscles while others are not."[162] An instrument designed to test the distinction between pain and sensory nerve fibers was provided by Carroll. It had double points, one sharp and one dull on each of its legs. These points could be applied to the skin interchangeably and without the patient's knowledge of which one was being used.[163]

After Brown-Sequard increased awareness of the aesthesiometer among medical practitioners with his article in 1866,[164] physicians and surgeons used the instrument to measure sensory nerve damage resulting from deep wounds, bruises, shocks, and high fevers. Because there were differences among healthy individuals, critics like the English physician John W. Ogle believed the test for diagnostic purposes was inconclusive. E. Seguin explained that these differences were comparable to those differences to be expected in counting the pulse, the number of respirations, and so on. Ogle may have been persuaded by Seguin's explanation, for he exhibited an aesthesiometer and dynamometer at the First Annual Museum of the British Medical Association in Oxford in 1868.[165]

By the end of the nineteenth century, aesthesiometers were refined to be applied to a very small section of skin and for delivering a precisely measured amount of stimulus force (see figure 7.19). The most delicate instrument was developed by Von Frey of Leipzig, who made his instrument from hair that was attached to a short wooden handle, eighty millimeters in length. Single strands of hair varying in diameter from fine to coarse were obtained from the human scalp and beard, the horse's tail, and the hog's bristles. Lewellys F. Barker of Johns Hopkins reported on Von Frey's method of producing this delicate research tool and indicated the care with which these instruments were designed. Barker explained, "To test the stimulus-value of the hair, its area in cross section must be determined, as well as the weight which can be lifted by the hair when it is pressed with its cross section against one of the scale pans of a delicate balance. . . . with time and patience a set of such test hairs can be prepared varying in stimulus-value from .1 gram/millimeter squared to 300 grams/

millimeter squared."[166] Von Frey directed his mechanician E. Zimmermann to prepare a sample of this instrument which, he explained, "has the advantage that with a single hair one can obtain a large series of pressure-values at will. It consists of a long hair pushed through a capillary tube of very narrow lumen, much like that of a thermometer tube; the hair can be shoved through the lumen easily, but on pressure only the part of the hair outside the capillary tube can bend, and the force exerted is always greater the less the amount of hair outside the tube, and feebler the greater length of hair not inside the capillary tube."[167] Harvey Cushing demonstrated the instrument to colleagues and students in the Johns Hopkins wards in 1897. The instrument was applied to distinguish between loss of sensitivity to pressure and pain.

In a case in which ordinary slight stimuli appeared to call forth pain constantly, the idea had arisen that pressure sense was absent, the pain sense being very much exaggerated. It was easy with this instrument to show that the pressure sense was not abolished, though the threshold for pain was almost at the same level as the threshold for touch. With care, however, the pressure points could easily be made out. The significance of careful examinations in such cases is obvious, for it would be easy for the clinician to make the statement that tactile sense was destroyed in a given case in which in reality it was unaffected or but little affected. If such a case should come to autopsy, one might be entirely misled in interpreting the lesions found.[168]

A decade later, Alfred Gordon of Philadelphia devised a precision aesthesiometer, which he exhibited to the Philadelphia Neurological Society in January 1909. Neurologists were obtaining unreliable results in examinations for the several types of sensations; Gordon attributed these results to the difficulty in applying equal pressure on all parts of the skin tested. It occurred to him "that when the sharp end of the needle could be applied to the skin always with the same degree of pressure the results would be uniform."[169] His instrument, which could provide a uniform pressure regardless of how the instrument was applied, consisted of

one leg of an ordinary aesthesiometer . . . represented by a cylinder in which is placed a spring reaching about half-way of the cylinder. The spring is continued by a solid body (plunger), to the lower end of which a needle is attached. A micrometer screw surrounds the lower part of the plunger with the needle. By pressure on the plunger head the needle is lowered and protrudes from the cylinder. When the latter is done, the micrometer screw is placed by rotary move-

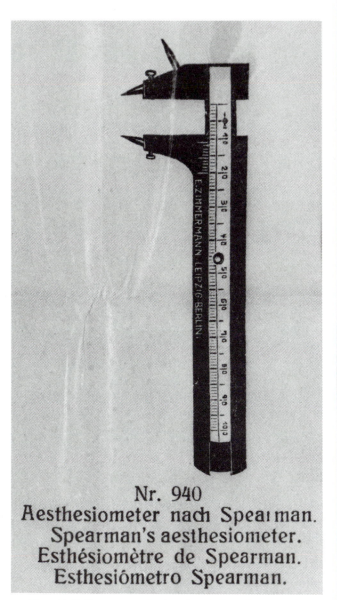

Nr. 940
Aesthesiometer nach Spearman.
Spearman's aesthesiometer.
Esthésiomètre de Spearman.
Esthesiómetro Spearman.

Figure 7.19. Spearman aesthesiometer. *SI Photo No. 74-6513.*

ments at the desired distance so that only a certain length of the needle projects. The exact position of the micrometer is then indicated by division lines immediately above. In this manner, no matter how much pressure is brought on the plunger head, the same amount of needle will protrude and the same amount of pressure will be produced with the latter on the skin.[170]

Gordon, an experimental psychologist, also applied the aesthesiometer as a physical foundation for his study of an individual's perceptual and observational powers. In addition, he developed other sophisticated equipment to measure variations in sight, color sense, pitch, and response to taste and touch. Many of these devices were difficult to apply correctly.[171]

Equipment manufacturers responded to the demands for specialized laboratory devices. The Cambridge Instrument Company of England, founded by Charles Darwin's son, Erasmus; Rudolph Koenig of Paris; and Max Kohl, R. Jung, and E. Zimmermann of Germany, among others, supplied instruments to experimental psychologists, physiologists, physicians, and anthropometrists. Often, on demand, they made special instruments to order. Some of this equipment served more than one purpose. Standard ancillary items like relays, timers, and electric apparatus were also employed in physics, chemistry, and biology laboratories, which encouraged producers to expect a continual need for these items.

Some physiologic and anthropometric testing equipment was improved and made easier to apply, which encouraged their use by laymen in the twentieth century. For example, J. A. Myers argued in 1925 for the installation of spirometers so that they would be available to all individuals. He claimed, "The time is at hand when all persons should know their actual vital lung capacities just as they should know their heights and weights."[172] He suggested that spirometers be placed in public places in the way that scales had been located for easy access to those wanting to know their weight.

Social and economic reasons have motivated municipalities to introduce body-measuring instruments into the community. For instance, since the Second World War, Scandinavian law restricted the use of alcohol by drivers. Therefore, instruments to test the breath for alcoholic content called Testo-Reaction Matares were installed at airports and in taverns, where for a small fee, they could be used to warn a driver if he had exceeded the alcohol limit in his system.[173] Recreation led to the use of dynamometers, which were installed in elaborate machines to attract the attention of those eager to demonstrate their

muscular strength at fairs and amusement parks in many countries.

The application of instruments did not close all discussions over the differences between normal and abnormal functions and structures, nor did instruments provide an acceptable range of variability for the poles of human health and disease for all diseases, so that some of the questions posed in the nineteenth century remained unanswered in the twentieth century. Nevertheless, closer approximations to individual differences were formulated as a result of the accrual of physical data. Primary sources of this data included the anthropometric measurements taken by Gould and Baxter from soldiers during the American Civil War and by other investigators studying other armies in later wars. Data were gathered from children in schools and inmates of prisons. Statistical analysis of anthropometric data, gathered and stored in insurance company archives, offered the possibility of "yielding a veritable treasure store of useful and conclusive information."[174] It was suggested in 1912 that a national anthropometric survey based on United States life insurance records be taken to provide data for answering questions concerning physical development including the rate of growth according to age and sex.[175] Some lamented that physical data, indexed according to race and nationality, had not been systematically collected at the time individuals passed through American immigration centers. However, this early investigative negligence stimulated interest in finding other sources of similar data later on. As a result of other twentieth-century projects employed to gather anthropometrical data, it was further confirmed that the finest of details separated physiologic and pathologic processes, which were explained as occurring on a cellular and molecular level.

EARLY TWENTIETH-CENTURY VIEWS ON THE NORMAL AND ABNORMAL:

The special powers of physical adaptation and variability common to living things are one of the roots of the physiologist's and pathologist's difficulties in establishing the limits of normality and abnormality for each individual. The standard of abnormality for function of an organ, which is determined by comparing and averaging a number of individual measurements, does not necessarily define a disease in the sense of lack of sufficient function. Extremes of mental and physical functions expressed, for example, by a very high intelligence or the excessive endurance and strength of an athlete's muscles is abnormal or above average but not classified as a disease. Generally, only those physical differences, however slight or excessive, that lead to pain and other discomforts, as well as the possibility of death, are considered diseases. Imbalance and disequilibrium between the organs and systems produce dysfunction, which becomes disease when the arrangement is uncomfortable and life threatening.[176]

Cultural factors are significant in determining the individual's reaction to changes within his or her own body. An impressive example of the extreme variability of a physiologic function and the care with which it must be studied is found in the level of hypoglycemia discovered in 1934 among black Africans by L. Pales and Monglond. Using blood- and urine-testing equipment, they discovered that Africans could function with glucose levels that would produce coma and convulsions in Europeans. Georges Canguilhem, a historian of the subject, summed up the implications of this discovery: "Ces états sont à la limite de la physiologie et de la pathologie. Du point de vue européen, ils sont pathologiques; du point de vue indigneé, ils sont si étroitement liés a l'état habituel du Noir que si l'on n'avait pas les termes comparatifs du Blanc on pourrait le considérer presque comme physiologique."[177]

Another biological phenomenon that seems to defy categorization in terms of a normal-abnormal dichotomy is the sudden appearance of an allergy to a substance taken into the body. Normally, antibodies are built up in the blood serum when an individual is first exposed to a foreign protein. These antibodies provide protection against future exposure except in some instances when a reaction develops, which is manifested as an over-production of the substance histamine. When this occurs, successive reactions may be so severe that a sequence of changes called anaphylaxis takes place, producing respiratory failure that may result in death unless an injection of antihistamine is immediately given to the patient.[178]

In 1930, Wilfred Trotter of University College Hospital in London stated that the knowledge of normal physiology was almost wholly due to the experimental method.[179] Consequently, he believed that the experimental method should be applied to all studies of disease. Thomas Lewis in the same year presented instances of clinical reactions, which he knew to be normal through his laboratory investigations, but which were considered disease signs by many physicians.[180] Greater concentration on human physiology by physicians offered a rich opportunity to make them more aware of the subtle distinctions between

health and disease. Yet physicians conversant with the issues raised by physiologic experiments were skeptical of the applicability of information derived from the laboratory in studies conducted on animals They argued that in the laboratory environment an artificial pathology was created that would have to be discounted in evaluating the results of the experimental study[181] and extending them to human patients. Lewis drew attention to a study of those engaging in physical exercise as a source of data that promised to provide other indications of the limits of normal physiologic responses. The physical limitations of the body under stress were important in selecting recruits during World War I, yet the effects of stress due to physical exercise on the human body were known to few physicians, according to Lewis. Instruments that could be modified to measure and record the body's functions during exercise and under stress were essential to this research program and eventually were provided in such tests as the Master's two-step test for cardiac stress levels. This test and others were incorporated into the diagnostic procedures administered in the physician's office.

The modern concept of biological normality has been extensively discussed by Georges Canguilhem in *Le normal et le pathologique*.[182] His definition of normal centers on the concept originally introduced by Claude Bernard under the term *milieu intérieur* and amplified in Walter Cannon's homeostasis doctrine. Canguilhem recognized that a unique equilibrium is established between the body and the environment. Normal physiology, however, is not, for Canguilhem, an objective that scientific methods can unravel. Rather, physiology is a collection of biological situations and conditions that are considered normal.[183] In a crisis in which good health is threatened or altered, the physiologic response results in a new level of equilibrium, which then becomes the "normal" for the individual involved.[184] This individual never recovers from the disease in the sense of returning to the physiologic status he or she possessed prior to contracting the illness. The geographer, M. Sorré, confirmed Canguilhem's view from among the relationships he noted between individuals and their environments. He concluded that "physiological constants are not absolute. For each function and series of functions there is a margin about which the functional adaptation of the group or species settles."[185] Health is the physiologic condition in which a body is normal relative to the fluctuation of its milieu.[186] Medical treatment often is rooted in the spontaneous effort of the body to dominate and organize its environment according to its own needs. Without being a science, medicine employs instrumentally and scientifically discovered facts to understand the body's normal functions, and then, describes them sufficiently so that unhealthy deviations may be treated with the available technology.

More recently, emotional attitudes and reactions to physical changes are considered additional factors, which have become embodied in the study and practice of psychosomatic medicine. The psychological contribution to the disease process has made the attempt to define disease even more difficult in a period when laboratory investigations and diagnostic tools have brought physicians closer to the physical determinants of disease. Even though the diseased cell, tissue, and organ may be carefully described, the cause of its malformation or its classification into normal and abnormal is not always clearly discernible, especially if it involves the human psyche.

MEDICAL TECHNOLOGY AND THE SPECIALISTS:

Instruments provided a bridge between specialists, who could more easily use data gathered with the aid of materials as a common language. The interaction between medical specialists shifted the treatments offered to patients, so that those diagnostic and therapeutic methods delivered by or with the aid of instruments began to dominate medicine by the twentieth century. The attitudes of medical specialists to each other were crucial to the use of instruments, and although supported by instruments, these attitudes grew out of social and economic factors. The image of medical technology in society could enhance or retard its use by medical practitioners, just as the recognition of a physical function could shift from normal to abnormal, depending on the cultural and social conditions in which the individual lived.

The bacteriologic origin of disease dominated medical practice beginning with the acceptance of the germ theory in the last quarter of the nineteenth century and encouraged new alliances among medical specialists. Success in treating bacteriologically provoked diseases with chemicals completed the successful clinical cycle.[187] Bacteriology brought the clinician and the laboratory scientist into a relationship of dependence to a degree previously unknown. The laboratory techniques could provide rapid and definite answers to queries regarding the presence of specific bacteria in a patient's fluids or tissues, which suggested specific treatment to the clinician.[188] Clinicians who had ignored or been skeptical of scientific

aid before they had become dependent on the bacteriologic laboratory in their daily care of patients increased their respect for medical investigators who sought the control of disease in the laboratory.

Clinical pathology emphasizing specialized treatments developed quickly at the end of the nineteenth century. For instance, vaccine therapy was instituted to treat boils, acne, lupus vulgaris, rheumatoid arthritis, and other chronic diseases. The practitioner adopted these specialized laboratory techniques when the standard drugs and surgery were unsuccessful. Distrust stemming from professional distinctions between the clinician and laboratory researcher was replaced by a partnership of mutual respect. The patient's willingness to accept treatment delivered in this manner encouraged the liaison among these professionals. The bacteriologist became the consulting partner of the physician who had referred his patients for vaccine therapy. With the increased responsibility of treating patients, the clinical pathologist-bacteriologist sought greater status within the medical profession. The delicate technique of preparing the vaccine from an infusion containing the infecting microbe, and then injecting it into the patient in specific dosages controlled by a complicated blood test became a practice unto itself. When many patients sought such treatment, inoculation departments were established in large hospitals in Europe to meet this demand. Private clinics also provided these vaccinations, which previously had been applied to prevent contagious diseases.[189]

Devices that conducted the shorter wavelength light rays directly to a skin lesion formed the basis of another disease treatment, which became celebrated in this period. The method and the technology was devised by Niels Finsen, for which he won the first Nobel Prize to be awarded in medicine in 1904. His large machine for treating six to eight patients, known as the Finsen light, was installed in metropolitan hospitals where the treatment was given. One of the instruments was given to Queen Victoria and is on display in the Wellcome Historical Medical Museum in London.[190]

PHYSICIAN AND SURGEON:

Another dramatic change in treatment that entailed much technology was the rise of surgery in response to anesthetic-antiseptic technology upon which basis the surgeon recast his operative techniques. Medical practitioners of the period were compelled to look upon the surgeon not only as a rival but also as a competitor for the first time in the history of these professions. J. Mitchell Bruce summarized in 1910 the loss of professional prerogatives formerly reserved to the physician:

One after another the great viscera in their pathological and therapeutical relations, as objects of treatment and of formal study and demonstration . . ., as objects of physiological investigation and interest in the clinical wards and hospital laboratory—have been taken over in good measure by him [the surgeon]. The graver diseases of the stomach, the duodenum, the liver and gall-bladder, the appendix, the colon in its whole extent, the pancreas, the kidneys, the lungs and pleura—even the heart, the brain and the spinal cord—have one after another been gradually passing out of the hands and experience of the physician.[191]

The physician lauded the surgeon for his curative powers and for the new information surgical exploration of the viscera provided on the functions of these organs.

Medicine and surgery had been rival specialties, with surgery being considered the inferior practice. One source of the new alliance between these specialties was the application of physiologic research to surgery. In particular, the microscope opened up new vistas for surgeons, which made surgeons independent of the clinical observations of their physician colleagues because the surgeon could turn to direct microscopic observation of the tissues.

As early as the late eighteenth century, the surgeon, John Hunter, had introduced laboratory investigation to the surgeon. According to W. Stokes, Hunter "brought the scientific method into the study of the practice and welded scientific knowledge with the lessons of experience."[192] Characterized in the nineteenth century by the German Von Langenbeck as the move "from physiology to surgery, and from the microscope to the resection knife," the barriers between medicine and surgery in Britain began to be removed[193] as surgeons came to rely on the same laboratory exploration to which physicians responded. The success of surgery in eliminating some of its previous hazards by the adoption of sterilization influenced physicians to acknowledge the benefits gained in analyzing tissues for the presence of microorganisms and to accept the usefulness of bacteriologic research for medical practice. Surgery as the most technologically based branch of medicine began to draw upon the techniques of physiology and hastened the introduction of the technology into general medicine. Technology in the service of medicine was not as appealing to the general practitioner except in limited forms, since the disease discovered by diagnostic instruments could not always be sorted out easily, whereas the surgeon who was skilled in segregating tissues and organs found it convenient to isolate disease with the microscope, as well as with his standard tool for the purpose, the scalpel. Pathologic surgery, or the excision of diseased tissues and organs, cemented the bond between surgery and anatomy.[194]

One important result for the physician induced by having to share what was considered to be the practice of internal medicine with the surgeon was the physician's search for other disease parameters, which he might take charge of without the surgeon's assistance. The physician henceforth studied more avidly the environment and the life-style of the patient. In addition to studying the details of an acute or chronic disease as expressed in body tissues and organs, physicians began to counsel their patients on the importance of understanding the differing aspects of their physical surroundings, including their professions, forms of recreations, diets, and the impact of all these parameters on the human body.[195] Although restricted and constrained in the control of internal diseases, the physician focused on the external environment and the hazards it posed to the human body. Postmortem studies supplemented with information gained through diagnostic technology were related to the hazardous elements of the environment. Technology employed throughout society was making continual and ever-changing demands on the body, which physicians expected to unravel and interpret for their patients. Interest in external causes of disease brought the physician ideologically closer to the public health movement to which only a few physicians had previously responded enthusiastically. Public health revived as a result of the conquest of bacterial diseases. Diseases spawned by technology added a new dimension to the concerns of physicians interested in public health. For instance, the health of those segregated in schools, asylums, and prisons caught the attention of medical educators and internists, who discussed these individuals' special problems and needs in the medical journals. Ventilation, illumination, sewerage, exercise, and food were among the topics scrutinized for their effect on the health of individuals in all of those institutions.[196]

The surgeon also responded to unique opportunities created by the impact of technology on specific labor groups like the railway worker. The surgeon specializing in railroad-related diseases and accidents treated those who sustained injuries in the course of building railroads and running the trains within the North American continent. In 1894, out of 147,704 miles of railroad in the United States and Canada, all but 17,088 miles were assigned to 5,466 railway surgeons, who were expected to respond to calls for assistance within their jurisdictions. A total of 1,767 surgeons belonged to the National Association of Railway Surgeons, which published a journal called *The Railway Surgeon*. These surgeons were trained to set broken bones, close wounds, and amputate mangled limbs, but by the end of the century, the need for other methods to treat other subtle types of disease, especially neurologic disorders, resulting from injury on the railroads was clearly apparent. The average surgeon was not sufficiently prepared to diagnose and treat these ailments and called on physicians for advice.[197]

PHYSICIAN AND LABORATORY SCIENTIST:

The relationship between the sciences and medicine, particularly physiology, pathology, clinical science, chemistry, and biology, oscillated in response to the technological changes that occurred in each specialty. As a new level of knowledge was reached, its implications for medicine were applied. However, none of the sciences continued to develop on the strength of its usefulness to medicine alone. Experimentation, whether on animals, humans, or in laboratory tests set up to isolate and intensify a particular phenomenon, was the hallmark of all these sciences. Experimentation at every level required special equipment and methods of recording processes over varying time intervals. As theory was tested in the laboratory or in an organism, tools, gadgets, and devices were invented and applied to isolate the phenomena pertaining to the theory and to mitigate inconvenience and danger to the test animal. Individuals who could use tools in the precise and careful manner required by experimentation were evaluated according to unique standards; thus, new criteria were established, which led to the formation of a new profession among those who could undertake these specialized tasks. When the number of individuals in each new profession increased, efforts were made to organize formally and distinguish the group from the larger medical community by both the methods employed and the goals sought. These changes in professional status and function introduced rivalries by bringing diverse goals into the processes of disease discovery and treatment.

Signs that technology threatened to divide the relationships between physiologists, pathologists, and physicians appeared in the early nineteenth century. Physicians had to be repeatedly persuaded that a knowledge of physiology and pathology was important for them in their daily confrontations with disease. Among those who publicly addressed the topic to inform general practitioners of the scientific roots of medicine was the professor of the practice of medicine, W. T. Gairdner of the University of Glasgow, on the occasion of his being installed for the second time as the president of the Glasgow Pathological and Clinical Society, which had been founded in 1873. He emphasized the dual name of the society and its relationship to its sister society, the Pathological Society of London, organized twenty-five years earlier.[198] The founders of the Glasgow Society took as their code that "the processes of disease [were] . . . one and the same in kind, whether they issue in the spoiling of a function, or of an organ, or, as most commonly happens, of both together . . . and the method of observation is the best which conjoins these two fields of observation, and adds to the study of organic ruins that of deranged vital phenomena."[199] Gairdner underlined the method of observation, collection of numerous patient histories, and careful descriptions exemplified in the records of leaders like Morgagni. Even though the contemporary methods employing new appliances, coupled with a "flood of new light from physiology and histological anatomy," were superior to the techniques used by Morgagni, his interest and conceptual role was unparalleled.[200] Morgagni's clinical acuity was impressive for "without him, we should probably have waited longer for Laennec, and might very probably have been at this hour without the stethoscope, and all that it has brought us."[201] The methods and appliances used in all the hospitals, which led to the triumphs of Matthew Baillie, the Hunters, Richard Bright, Astley Cooper and others, might not have appeared without the spur given by Morgagni. Gairdner confidently traced the rise of clinical technology to Morgagni and the development of pathologic anatomy.

Medical instruments and those employed in the laboratory sciences presented some problems for the medical student when he or she entered medical practice. Those most informed about instrumental and laboratory techniques have always cautioned the young physician about the limitations of physical examination techniques. Typical of this precautionary attitude was the view toward the application of one of the successful early tests for a major disease—the Wasserman test for syphilis. Fordyce in 1914 and C. F. Hoover in 1930 argued for combining the test with clinical observation to diagnose the malady. They insisted that if the laboratory test was questionable, the clinical experience was to be relied upon.[202] Albert Sterne cautioned in 1918 that "the Wasserman and other seriological tests are merely symptoms which, like other physical signs, may or may not be present. They are extremely valuable but not as determining as the objective clinical symptoms, notably when not definitely manifest. The laboratory is not a shortcut to diagnosis."[203]

Half a century after Gairdner's address, Thomas Lewis was invited by the physiological section of the British Association on 26 August 1920 to speak on the topic "The Relation of Physiology to Medicine." Among a number of subjects he reviewed were the difficulties arising in teaching a student to manipulate delicate and precise laboratory instruments, to prepare the student for applying crude instruments to examine and treat patients.[204] Technical competence learned in the physiologic laboratory did not prepare the student for the daily activities as a medical practitioner. Lewis insisted that the physician could not surpass the excellence of his or her own senses in making a routine examination of a patient and that the physician was actually handicapped by being taught to depend on apparatus for diagnostic information. Eliminating specialized tests and devices in general medical practice was an encouraging sign of progress and implied a growth toward maturity in medical practice. Others, like C. F. Hoover of Cleveland, acknowledged that "all laboratory tests and technical instruments have been devised to explain problems or to answer inquiries that have been raised by inquiring physicians,"[205] but admonished the clinician not to "resign his art in the face of instrumental devices."[206] For Hoover, a student of physics, chemistry, physiology, anatomy, and pathology only became a clinician after the individual had made many diagnoses in the clinic.

As the functions of the clinician and researcher diverged, each required different types of training. Based on the inherent differences in goals and methodology, Lewis and others argued for providing full-time research or clinical science positions, which would allow the researcher to apply his critical methods to questions without regard to other goals and to be free of the constant demands of patient care. The time had come when progress in clinical medicine would primarily result from intensive study of selected instances of disease, which was frequently undertaken with special instruments and appliances. Chance observation of patients had become outmoded as a source of medical advancement. The

practitioner did not have the special training necessary to proceed with intensive medical research. To bring medical research closer to the clinic and to supply the basis for clinical progress, Lewis envisioned a separate association of clinical medicine which "should have its separate scientific societies, should control its own publications, and should be able to confine its original reports to journals restricting themselves exclusively to original matter of proper quality."[207]

CONCLUSION:

Diagnosis, up to the nineteenth century, was primarily an oral and visual process unassisted by instruments. Exceptions existed to the extent that the practice of uroscopy can be considered physical inspection of urine. This analysis could be undertaken out of sight of the patient, however. The physician compared each patient with all of those individuals that he or she had observed in the past and had learned about in texts or from descriptions given by teachers in lectures and at the bedside in the hospital. To these traditional methods of teaching and learning about illness and its treatment, which have never been wholly abandoned, was added an expanded sensual dimension through the introduction of medical technology. Described as physical diagnosis because the physician makes direct contact with the patient, the method is principally characterized by the use of instruments and appliances. For a physical examination of a patient, implements are not essential, although instruments supplement and strengthen the faculties of hearing, seeing, and feeling in following the sequence of physiologic functions and the inspection of tissues.

The development of physical diagnosis in the nineteenth century captured the imagination and focus of medical practitioners and was immediately succeeded by a third form of diagnosis, in which laboratory analysis, primarily of a chemical nature, was the main component. Physical diagnosis and laboratory diagnosis when combined tended to dominate medical diagnosis and, in some instances, led to a lesser appreciation and reliance on visual inspection and observation without the assistance of mechanical appliances or chemical tests. The physician returned to the position of having less contact with the patient, when laboratory tests were used. This separation from the patient was reminiscent of the pre-physical diagnostic period when medical practice was almost entirely an intellectual process based on medical theories that the patient was not expected to understand.

Physiology and pathology, which evolved concurrently, were studies of vast importance to medicine. "The student of disease is interested in all physiological problems for the light that may be thrown on disease processes. The student of physiology is interested in certain problems of disease for the light that may be shed on physiological problems."[208] By the end of the first quarter of the twentieth century, it was generally accepted that in the words of Virchow, published much earlier, "each department of medicine must have its own field and must be investigated by itself."[209] Bacterial investigations for a period appeared to narrow the goals of medicine and reduce its rational components to those directly related to pathogenic organisms.[210] The laboratory methods devised to discover pathogenic bacteria were standardized and interrelated to include various types of bacteria. After the resurgence of all forms of physiologic and pathologic experimentation, new and complex techniques were devised. It became difficult to see the consequences of some of these techniques for medical practice. Physicians came to rely on laboratory tests extensively and sometimes abandoned or failed to use fully their clinical diagnostic skills. Ralph Stillman in 1935 reminded his American colleagues that "the laboratory is not a slot machine in which is to be dropped a tube of blood, a drop of pus or a piece of tissue and from which in return there is obtained a slip of paper upon which is typed a diagnosis."[211] This type of advice appeared early in the rise of the medical laboratory and continued throughout its history, stimulated by recurring instances of misuse and abuse.

Societal changes shaped the way in which refined diagnostic methods were applied in the nineteenth and early twentieth centuries. Physical examinations were mandated first for those seeking a job, joining the military forces, and later, as will be discussed in the next chapter, for purchasing life insurance. The requirements of each occupation determined the specific bodily characteristics the physician examined. For those applying for the police force and fire brigade, strength tests, similar to those discussed by Quetelet and Babbage, were found to be among the most valuable indicators in predicting fitness.[212] Life insurance companies, always seeking better indicators of long life, settled on definite limits for blood pressure, body weight, and body build correlated with age for each individual.[213] By the twentieth century, life insurance standards were more stringent in some

instances than those accepted by the medical profession. For instance, the blood pressure level measured by the sphygmomanometer was expected to be lower for an insurance applicant than what the general practitioner regarded as normal. In medical practice, blood pressure as one of many signs appeared to be of less immediate prognostic value than it was as a criterion of longevity.[214]

As will be discussed in the next chapter, another facet of societal pressures stemming from medical diagnosis was the dilemma posed by the apparently healthy individual who sought a physical examination to have early signs of disease detected and to avoid serious disease in the future. These individuals were somewhat reluctantly and haphazardly examined, especially when they seemed quite healthy. The standard of health and disease had to be more clearly distinguished and bolstered with more subtle indications for the physician to be able to determine who was expressing the earliest stages of disease. Investigation of the intricacies of physiology and pathology showed that not all measurable modifications of function or structure represent disease or need to be treated and changed. Culturally determined mores and habits occasionally permit individuals to adapt physically to emotional stresses that defy the usual laws and theories of medicine. At this point, the bodily standards developed from laboratory experimentation are of less significance to the medical practitioner. State and federal agencies through public health departments, in an effort to promote preventive medicine, prodded the medical profession into paying more attention to the general physical examination or "check-up."[215]

Medicine in the twentieth century included episodes of greater concern for preventive medicine. People were counseled to be more aware of the measures to take to preserve their health, as well as to note the early signs of disease. Popular medical publications alerted the literate public to their duties in maintaining good health.[216] Instruments were sold to patients who needed to keep a daily check on their blood pressure, or on the chemical composition of their urine if they were diabetics. Individuals were encouraged to keep up-to-date medical records. The goals of preventive medicine and medical practice coalesced into practices subsumed under the modern term, medical care, which includes a spectrum of patient participation and goals for remaining healthy, many of which are facilitated by medical instruments.

8

MEDICAL STANDARDS AND INSTRUMENTS

INTRODUCTION:

As mentioned in the preceding chapter, medical technology enabled physicians to examine more individuals who requested or required medical examinations for a variety of reasons including to acquire a job and buy life insurance, as well as to meet the medical requirements of an expanding population. Physical examination to diagnose and treat disease was a major motivation for developing instruments, tests, and devices, but in addition, new demands growing out of the structure of an industrial society further advanced the use of medical technology. Physicians were joined by institutions, including life insurance companies, the military services, and employers, in seeking to perfect physical examinations to provide information that would not only indicate the present physical status of an individual but also predict his or her physical condition in the future.

Life insurance companies attempted to strengthen the procedures for predicting length of life by encouraging physicians to devise accurate diagnostic tests for long-range prognosis. The most useful predictor of length of life by the early twentieth century was blood pressure and the patient's vital capacity or ability to take in and expel air, measured by an instrument called the spirometer. Physical standards set by life insurance companies based on their data compiled from thousands of clients were an important factor in establishing the basic measurable parameters of good health revealed by instruments and amenable to physical diagnosis from the mid-nineteenth century through the first half of the twentieth century.

In an effort to combine effectively the welfare of their clients and sound financial practices, insurance companies found that the most reliable method for determining the factors of mortality was statistical. Predicting longevity from statistics required large quantities of physiologic and pathologic data, which the insurance companies were in a good position to gather. However, a valid method and good sources of data did not always ensure meaningful studies or conclusions. For example, the report "Specialized Mortality Experience," prepared in 1912 under the direction of the American Actuarial Society, did not adequately distinguish inflammation, peritonitis, and appendicitis, which invalidated the conclusions reached about each of these diseases.[1]

Organization and interpretation of medical data required the talents of statisticians. Karl Pearson in his essay *The Chance of Death* displayed an immense ability to organize data pertaining to life, health, disease, and death. Of foremost value to insurance medicine was Pearson's assertion that the death rate was influenced 20 percent by the environment and 80 percent by heredity.[2] Insurance companies had relied heavily on longevity among close relatives in families to predict the length of life of life insurance policy applicants, a procedure which Pearson's conclusions largely confirmed. Inheritance was not measured by instruments and will not be further discussed here. To determine the remaining factors responsible for health and length of life, physicians resorted to measurements and diagnostic tests of applicants. The physical criteria became increasingly significant in selecting those whose heredity and family background were unknown or questionable and for confirming the expected degree of health based on inheritance. Physical diagnostic methods became critical to the determination of future health when other factors began to appear less certain and less under the control of the physician.

THE PHYSICAL EXAMINATION:

For millenia, physicians had learned to respond to those who became ill, but when called upon to uncover signs of disease before the individual felt ill or wanted to admit any physical deterioration, physicians found it expedient to employ sensitive and precise methods of physical examination. The need or desire for the physician to evaluate an individual's bodily functions through physical diagnosis when the person did not appear ill was an innovative medical practice of the nineteenth century, which emerged from a reordering of social factors and available medical technology. The reasons for obtaining a physical examination in the nineteenth and twentieth centuries were, in addition to responding to a patient's feelings of discomfort, to obtain life insurance, to enlist in the military forces, to obtain a job, to become eligible for a pension, and, to a lesser extent, to note the early signs of potentially serious diseases. For each of these purposes, a selective focusing of the examiner's techniques was required. Medical instruments expanded the range of criteria by which to judge the individual's state of health and provided new criteria for determining the presence of disease in its earliest stages.

The purpose of a medical examination determined the standards by which the physician selected the physical phenomena to be evaluated and the range of performance of each bodily function that would be considered normal. Physicians were hired by insurance companies, industries, the military forces, and government agencies to provide physical examinations for their clients and employees when physicians could manipulate a number of implements for the purpose of physical diagnosis, including the stethoscope, thermometer, endoscope, and spirometer, and in the last few years of the century, the X-ray tube.

One of the major targets of physical diagnosis for selecting insurance clients and those physically fit for employment were lung diseases generally subsumed within the term *phthisis*. Diagnosis by listening to sounds within the body was generally accepted to be the most effective method of revealing diseases of the chest until the end of the nineteenth century when chemical tests of bodily fluids and microscopic identification of invading organisms and diseased tissues also became important in the diagnostic process. In 1885, when lung diseases caused many deaths, E. D. Hudson commented that "it is accepted as a fact fully established that, by the application of acoustic laws, certain combinations of physical signs lead to an immediate and correct diagnosis in most cases of

pulmonary disease."[3] The nineteenth-century conception of phthisis was based on the conclusions of Adolph Piorry, who used percussion of the chest and René Laennec's auscultation of the chest, which incorporated the pathology of Gaspard Laurent Bayle and Pierre Louis. Phthisis and tuberculosis were considered to be hereditary diseases until around the 1870s when the role of bacteria and their toxins was identified and a new etiologic explanation was put forth for the transmission of the disease. Continental improvement in the diagnosis of lung disease was demanded by life insurance companies, who, apart from the government-sponsored commissions in Great Britain and a few citizens groups in other countries, were the major institutions encouraging specific measures to maintain the public's health on a continual basis and not only when an epidemic threatened many lives. The physicians who most satisfactorily diagnosed lung diseases were sought out by life insurance companies and rewarded with the payment of increased examination fees. The examining physician was guided by the insurance company medical director, who was a specialist in prognosis of the length of life. The medical director supervised those who administered the examinations and the director interpreted the results sent into the company. Medical directors practiced a type of medicine that placed the company's financial welfare on a par or even above the health of the insurance policy applicant. Medical directors interpreted the standards of the key bodily functions as they related to expected longevity, and therefore, encouraged life insurance examiners to use techniques that led to the adoption of instruments to measure these standards with the least possibility of error and subjective interpretation. The insurance company encouraged the physician to use reliable and simplified tools to measure the major predictors of a policy applicant's length of life (pulse rate, blood pressure, lung capacity). The physician who learned to use basic tools effectively entered the mainstream of American medical practice in the twentieth century.

Physicians who examined apparently well individuals had a wider latitude in interpreting the data they obtained. Published reports on the incidence of serious disorders among the patient population led the examiner to anticipate the appearance of some diseases among the individuals he examined, but it has remained difficult to select standards for deciding when to introduce treatment and of what type it should be in the pre-disease or non-acute stage of an illness. Instruments and devices have provided the main sources of information concerning the pre-disease condition. Instruments have been used to detect the presence of diseases including the chronic and noninfectious types, which may develop over a longer period than the acute and infectious diseases. Since physicians were able to measure the body functions more precisely than in the past, they noted the slight deviations characteristic of the earliest stages of disease and were forewarned of the disease's eventual full-scale attack on the patient's system.

PRECISION IN DIAGNOSIS AND THERAPY:

Precision measurement of the body's functions led to evaluation of the body in terms which the physician had not found useful or necessary previously. We have reviewed in the chapter on diagnosis the attempts to measure the functional capacity of the heart, lungs, stomach, and kidneys. One of the more unusual frameworks in which disease was to be interpreted with the aid of instruments was its relationship to the body's symmetry. Investigations revealed that the substances, as well as the form and structures, of the body's dual parts were alike. Disease appeared symmetrically (skin lesions, paralysis of the limbs) and was modified by the asymmetry of a deformed body. The tools to make the refined measurements for detecting the slight asymmetry in all organisms did not appear until the twentieth century (such as contour mapping of the body and X-ray sections), although the importance of symmetry to the concept of disease was predicted in the nineteenth century by James Paget.[4]

Precision in diagnosis was joined by precision in methods of therapy at the end of the nineteenth century. Traditional methods of treatment including hydrotherapy and physical exercise began to be administered in measured amounts much like drugs, which were prescribed in measured doses. For instance, the Brand Bath was designed to take advantage of the flexibility of delivering water under controlled temperature and pressure for a limited period of time. Applied in acute diseases, such as typhoid fever and pneumonia, and in chronic disorders including tuberculosis, rheumatism, and gout, the therapeutic functions of the bath were to support the nervous system, and secondarily, to reduce body temperature. Equipment for delivering the water under controlled conditions was installed in hospitals and spas in the 1890s, for "if precision in the technique be not observed and the patient exposed to lower temperatures or subjected to higher pressures . . . the results would be serious and discouraging."[5]

Equipment to carry out precision diagnosis was developed in response to physicians' demands and the standards established by special organizations created for the purpose. Diagnostic accuracy relied on precision instruments, which usually were standardized by the manufacturer and verified by a separate agency. Germany was the first country to organize effectively a national standards laboratory for testing and verifying the accuracy of scientific and industrial equipment. The Physikalisch-Technische Reichsanstalt was founded in Charlottenburg in 1887 and soon established standards for precision equipment including medically applied devices, which the world came to rely upon before other countries founded their own standardization laboratories. Before the twentieth century, Austria, Russia, and England had also set up instrument-testing centers to identify and certify precision equipment required by commerce and industry. Increased economic growth and commercial leadership amply repaid these investments in standardization laboratories. As was noted above, the National Bureau of Standards was founded in the United States in 1901, which, under its first Director, Samuel W. Stratton, was modeled on the Reichsanstalt. Among the first instruments to be calibrated by the Bureau of Standards were clinical thermometers.[6] With reliable equipment, physicians could practice a more precise medicine. Therefore, it is well to begin a discussion of some of the major contributing factors to standardization as applied to medicine.

Parameters for many types of physical diagnosis were expressed in terms of numerical standards. It was possible by the first quarter of the twentieth century to diagnose and confirm a number of prevalent and life-threatening diseases on the basis of data collected with instruments. Disease statistics, which helped to make this possible, had been gathered by medical leaders, who taught the application of instruments, and by institutions that had a financial investment in health, such as life insurance companies. These statistics provided a numerical framework within which to place an individual's physiologic and pathologic record. The role of Carl Wunderlich and others in measuring and establishing the relationship between normal and abnormal body temperatures has been discussed in chapter four. Now it is useful to discuss a nonmedical institution that collected other types of medical statistics generated by the development of physiologic standards in the period beginning at the end of the nineteenth century and early twentieth century.

LIFE INSURANCE MEDICINE:

INTRODUCTION:

Before discussing the standardization and instrument-related issues, it is well to review briefly the history of insurance medicine and some of the problems physicians faced in examining applicants for life insurance. With this background, the development of instrument-generated health standards and their role in insurance medicine can be placed in context.

The purpose of life insurance is to provide money for those left without economic support ensuing from death.[7] Life insurance "consists of a contract, whereby for a stipulated compensation, called the premium, . . . the insurer agrees to pay the . . . insured or his beneficiary, a fixed sum upon . . . death. . . ."[8] Men were primary purchasers of life insurance until the twentieth century. They were anxious to protect their wives and children in case of their own premature deaths. Up until the twentieth century, beneficiaries also purchased life insurance policies. The insurance company reduced the risk it faced by anyone dying before the company had been paid sufficient premiums on a policy by insuring a greater proportion of individuals who appeared to have a long life expectancy. In this manner, life insurance companies transferred the risk of an individual to a selected group of people.[9] So that those with the best chance of surviving into old age could be selected, life tables were constructed that could be used to predict the years of life remaining to someone at the age he or she applied for insurance. For William Farr, the foremost nineteenth-century British constructor of life tables, "A life table is a biometer; it gives the exact measure of the duration of life under given circumstances. It represents a generation of man passing through time."[10]

Thomas Laycock described the life table in 1864 as showing

out of an assumed number (say 100,000) born alive, the number living at every age for 100 or 105 years. . . . For commercial or financial purposes, the life table is invaluable. Although the duration of life of each individual is proverbially uncertain, that of 100,000 may be estimated to a fraction. But life insurers have this further security against loss, that while the Life Table they use is constructed on data drawn from every rank and condition of men, and under every possible condition as regards state of health, diet, occupation and the like, they only accept select lives, that is, persons in actual health, likely to live long, temperate in their habits, pursuing healthy occupations, resident in a healthy climate, etc."[11]

The life table remained the standard for predicting length of life until specific physical diagnostic standards offered more promise of predicting future diseases that were likely to shorten life.

Biometry, or the collection of statistical data on the inheritance of diseases and the effect of occupations, habits of living, and other factors, was reduced to a science applicable to life insurance through the efforts of investigators such as T. S. Lambert. Sophisticated evaluation of the medical factors began with the monumental statistical studies of Oscar H. Rogers, who studied all the records of the New York Life Insurance Company beginning in 1890. Rogers compared the records of individuals who had been accepted or rejected by the company over a period of twenty years and constructed a method of assigning a numerical value to each factor that directly effected health and length of life. Rogers' numerical method was incorporated into the company's method of selecting life insurance applicants in 1904.[12] When it became possible to define the function of an organ on a numerical scale, that organ's contribution to life expectancy was more readily evaluated.

MEDICAL EXAMINERS:

The earliest life insurance companies did not require that applicants receive medical examinations. Prior to 1820, the applicant signed a statement about the quality of his health.[13] Applicants continued to sign health statements into the twentieth century in addition to receiving a physical examination. Although as early as 1824 the physican was called upon to ascertain the presence of impediments that might shorten an individual's life, only many years later did medical examinations become a regular part of the procedure in selling life insurance. At first, the family doctor was consulted for an opinion on the potential health of the insurance applicant. Then, the insurance company employed its own medical examiners in an effort to receive more impartial medical advice, a procedure encouraged by William Farr.[14] A medical examiner was appointed by Equitable of England in 1858.[15] One of the largest American companies, the Metropolitan Life Insurance Company, set up a medical division in 1890, directed by a physician.[16] Insurance companies employed local physicians to administer physical examinations; many of these physicians had little insurance examining experience and frequently were the family physicians of those seeking life insurance. Medical examiners were paid a fee for each life insurance examination they administered. The insurance salesman, who wanted to insure as many individuals as possible, since he or she collected a commission on each policy sold, usually selected the medical examiner and could replace an examiner who rejected too many potential clients.[17]

Companies relied on the standard nineteenth-century markers of a shortened life, including ages of parents and grandparents at the time of their deaths and types of chronic diseases suffered by close relatives. Insurance company statistics confirmed the belief that inheritance was a major factor in achieving longevity.[18] In this period, when the theory of evolution and heredity was being debated, long-lived parents, grandparents, and siblings were considered a valid predictor of future long life.[19] The medical examiner was instructed to take a full family history.[20] An individual with long-lived forebears could expect to have the necessary resistance to survive the usual life-threatening diseases as long as he or she ate properly, abstained from alcohol, rested, and exercised normally.[21] Family susceptibility to phthisis provided essential evidence for predicting the applicant's likelihood of contracting tuberculosis, among the most dreaded diseases of the period. However, the information concerning the cause of death of parents and siblings could easily be falsified so that insurance companies did not always have a firm basis for using family history data collected by examiners.[22] Occupational hazards were increasingly taken into consideration before granting an insurance policy by the end of the century.[23]

The physician who became a life insurance medical examiner was expected to learn the economic basis of the insurance business. The medical examiner served to alert the company's directors that an applicant proposed for an insurance policy by an agent possessed certain liabilities, which could result in a shorter than expected life span. The examiners had to become adept at prognosis, a skill the physician was not particularly prepared to exercise after receiving the usual nineteenth-century medical education.[24] The medical examiner had to balance diverse factors. He had to appreciate the deceptive tactics of those applicants who tried to hide the precarious sides of their health,[25] to appease the agent whose commission would be forfeited by a rejected applicant, to diagnose without enjoying the usual privileged communication between patient and physician, and to be clear about the normal structures and functions of all parts of the human body.[26] A physician who was familiar with the applicant's health history was sometimes placed in the position of deciding between being loyal to the

applicant at the expense of the company. Doctors were sometimes criticized for their moral decisions, as well as for errors in physical diagnosis.[27]

By the end of the nineteenth century, insurance companies were beginning to question some of the medical examiner's decisions, including those that were based on physical examination. Insurance companies also were skeptical of the inexperienced physician's ability to select an applicant for life insurance, regardless of the methods he or she used to make the decision. Oliver Pillsbury, secretary of the National Insurance Convention of the United States, stated in 1873 that

to ask a medical man to give a correct physical description of a person, in answer to numerous and detailed questions, is a very different thing from asking him to give answers to a few indefinite questions, and a judgment upon the vitally important question of the insurability of the person. Almost any ordinary physician or average physician can do the former duty well; very few, and none without special study and practice, can do the latter.[28]

Company medical directors accepted their responsibilities in training the examining physician to be aware of the most crucial factors that were essential to predict length of life.

Insurance companies were constantly exposed to fraud. They frequently sold policies to individuals who suspected that their lives would be short. Fraud on the part of the agent, who received a commission for each policy sold, was another possibility. A third form of dishonesty arose when the physician was brought into the selection process. The tension between the physician, who wanted to give an honest but unfavorable report, and the agent, who wished to collect a commission by having the applicant accepted, continued as long as medical reports were transmitted via the sales agents to the company, rather than directly to the medical director from the examining physician.[29] Companies, in turn, developed unscrupulous practices such as covering up their financial losses in fear of losing clients, which sometimes resulted in bankruptcy and the loss of all the money invested by policy holders.[30]

Some companies deliberately operated on an unsound basis with the intention of defrauding their unsuspecting clients. Small industrial insurance companies adopted a practice of insuring all lives, including those of low risk, to collect the premiums, and then, at the time of death, reneged on the payment if the policyholder had died of a chronic disease. Physicians who were aware of these deceitful practices tried to satisfy the company's standards for payment to the family of the deceased policyholder by submitting a death certificate with an acceptable cause of death.[31] The practice of incorrectly stating the cause of death to satisfy the insurance company became so common in Lancashire, England by 1892 that the reputation of being a "good" doctor was earned by a physician who would supply a false death certificate and a "bad" doctor became one who told the truth about the insured person's cause of death and prevented the deceased individual's family from collecting insurance benefits. Being labeled as a "bad" doctor cost the physician connections in the community, and insurance agents boycotted him or her because such a physician prevented them from doing a lucrative business.[32]

To prevent fraudulent practices, the larger American life insurance companies organized themselves into an association called the Chamber of Life Insurance in 1874. Their goal was to obtain concerted action in all matters that tended to promote life insurance interests in the abstract.[33] One of their plans was to prepare a list of medical examiners, which all companies could consult for an unbiased and accurate medical report on a prospective client. The medical officers of insurance companies in England were advised to form an association in 1878 to discuss and promote their common interests.[34] In 1889, the Association of Life Insurance Medical Directors of America was formed to increase cooperation between directors of all companies.[35]

In addition to learning the role of the insurance examiner by practical experience, the examiner could study aspects of insurance medicine in a few metropolitan medical schools or through a series of articles published in the American medical journal *The Medical Record*. Medical examiners received information from this journal after 1873 in a special section devoted to insurance medicine. In this column the role, problems, and advancement of life insurance medical examinations were discussed. The insurance medicine section had been requested and was subsidized by insurance companies, which sent free subscriptions of the journal to medical examiners throughout the United States.[36] The life insurance medical department of *The Medical Record* continued until mid-1875, at the time when the journal changed from a bi-weekly to a weekly publication. Thereafter, related articles appeared sporadically until 1911 when a weekly insurance medicine column was reinstated. A highlight of the first series of articles was the publication in 1877 of William Detmold's lectures on

"Examination for Life Insurance," given to medical students at the College of Physicians and Surgeons in New York City. Concepts of disease as they related to longevity and insurance policies, as well as company-generated statistics related to disease, usually were not published in general textbooks of medicine, so the journal articles were especially valuable in this period.[37] Books on diagnostic medicine aimed at the life insurance company medical examiner began to appear in the last quarter of the century and would continue to be published into the twentieth century.

In 1891, a journal concentrating on problems of insurance medicine was established in New York City. *The Medical Examiner*, which later became *The Medical Examiner and Practitioner*, edited by George W. Wells, adopted the goal of presenting "topics of interest and importance to physicians and surgeons who act as Examiners for Life Insurance Companies, for the Army and Navy, for Government Departments, Railroad Companies, the Civil Service, etc."[38]

ECONOMIC ROLE OF LIFE INSURANCE MEDICINE:

Economic support of the American medical profession was increased by insurance medical examinations. By the fourth quarter of the century, American physicians outnumbered physicians in Great Britain, France, and Germany by at least three to one, although differences in population numbers were small. Thus, the increase in the number of life insurance medical examinations required in the United States provided American physicians with an income that would have eluded some of them in general practice. From a small beginning in the United States, when one hundred policies were issued in 1800, to over 56,000 policies issued in New York state alone just after the Civil War,[39] life insurance was sold in ever larger amounts to Americans.

By 1874, two hundred American companies issued more than half a million policies.[40] There was over a 500 percent increase in the insurance business between 1865 and 1905. The assets of all level premium life insurance companies were over five hundred million dollars in 1885 and by the end of 1905 had risen to almost three billion dollars.[41] Life insurance was believed to be primarily an American institution by the last decade of the nineteenth century,[42] and by 1920 more than three times as much insurance was sold in the United States as in the rest of the world. Three and a half billion dollars or 4 percent of the national income was invested in life insurance owned by 67 million policyholders. By 1932, there were more than one hundred different forms of life insurance combining the standard benefits with other plans for various security-threatening contingencies, including injury, disability, and loss of job.[43] It was impossible to know exactly how much money was paid to the medical profession for life insurance examinations, but it was accepted as quite considerable as early as 1875.[44] The fees physicians were paid for each medical examination of a life insurance applicant depended on the size of the company, the extent of the examination, and the economic conditions. These fees usually ranged from three dollars to ten dollars per examination. Extra fees were paid for special laboratory tests such as a urine test or microscopic examination.[45]

Growth of the American medical profession was spurred on by the development of the life insurance business, which depended increasingly on medical examinations for deciding at what cost and to whom policies should be sold. The ever-escalating insurance company demands for increasing the quantity and quality of physical examinations helped to shape the fundamental diagnostic components of American medicine. The volume of medical examinations requested by insurance companies in the twentieth century was staggering. By 1941, the number of examinations had grown to 1,310,257 for the Metropolitan Life Insurance Company alone. These examinations were carried out by 9,000 physicians who examined for this company in cities all over the United States.[46]

DENTISTRY AND LIFE INSURANCE MEDICINE:

Dental examinations and care entered life insurance company medical profiles shortly before World War I. Alonzo Nodine, a New York dentist, reported that one hundred insurance companies expressed interest in adding dental evaluations to the required physical examination for their prospective policyholders.[47] Nodine made it clear that

a septic, disorganized masticatory apparatus is a depot for harboring, propagating, and disseminating microorganisms, and the manufacture of toxins, ptomains, and other poisons it provides for their absorption into the blood and the lymph and their distribution to the structures of the mouth, accessory cavities, and the gastrointestinal and respiratory tracts. Defective dental conditions are known to produce effects on the nervous system, respiratory apparatus and digestive apparatus. . . .[48]

Proof of the effect of good dental care was provided by studies of institutionalized individuals. Dr. Key showed that, in the Saint Vincent Orphan Asylum of Boston, the number of infectious diseases decreased by 59 percent after the dental diseases of the 325 inmates had been treated.[49]

Of direct value to dentistry was the envisioned improvement in the image of the dental profession growing out of the standards imposed by insurance companies. "The institution of the dental examination for life insurance will do more than any other single measure to raise high the standard of dentistry in technical achievement and the just appreciation of its great field by the profession, individually and collectively, as it will equally and as surely raise high the appreciation of dentistry by the public."[50] The estimated cost to the insurance company of employing dentists to make the examinations and provide the necessary treatment was more than offset by the increased savings in not having to pay out insurance benefits to the relatives of those who had died prematurely.

Dentists needed to improve their public image because their mechanical methods of repairing decayed teeth were being blamed for the cause of many types of local and constitutional infections. Filling and capping teeth were procedures developed and primarily practiced in America, and they led, in some instances, to the creation of pockets of pus and decay in the tissues surrounding the teeth. Since it was possible to mask the areas of infection with gold and other metals used to restore and retain teeth that had been reduced by decay, the infection often remained undetected, and therefore, untreated until it had produced profound changes and sometimes major disease. An English physician, William Hunter, demonstrated the relation between oral sepsis and other diseases as a result of overlaying metal on incorrectly prepared teeth and gums.[51] Reforms were called for which combined scientifically based medicine and good mechanical dentistry. That dental health was included among the health parameters examined to obtain life insurance offered a strong stimulus to change dental procedures by making dentists more aware of the long-term effects of their methods.[52]

The economic, professional, and societal forces related to medical examinations undertaken for the purpose of determining life expectancy and the physical characteristics of value in establishing proficiency and adaptability to a job warrants more intensive study. Among the literature to be examined as a basis for this study are the texts prepared for medical examiners, the regulations and medical forms issued by insurance companies, company records, reports, and articles on aspects of life insurance and vocational medicine. These sources will provide the data for an evaluation of health and disease growing out of physical examinations and their impact on the development of American and European medical practice in the last quarter of the nineteenth and the first part of the twentieth centuries. Physical examination of the healthy individual was encouraged by institutions whose future success lay in the continuing health of their clients and employees. Periodic physical examinations of policyholders was promoted by insurance companies which, in some instances, paid for them. The Metropolitan Life Insurance Company began to offer free physical examinations in 1914 and sponsored national programs for encouraging every individual to obtain an annual physical examination. Increasingly, these examinations involved the use of instruments and laboratory tests to quantify the selected health parameters and to segregate the desirable from the undesirable insurance owners or to adjust the terms of an insurance policy to reflect the greater or lesser risks associated with each policyholder whose health parameters differed from the normal.

INSTRUMENTAL DIAGNOSIS FOR LIFE INSURANCE AND EMPLOYMENT:

Description, diagnosis, and treatment of disease formed the basis of the nineteenth-century medical curriculum, although a greater emphasis on recognizing a disease without being in a position to cure it was reflected in the young physician's practice at this time. The least time and effort was spent in preventing disease and improving health to avoid serious diseases since the techniques for these practices were not available. Laboratory tests and medical instruments enabled physicians to increase their knowledge of physiologic details applied primarily to diagnosis. Instruments made it possible to uncover disease in its incipient stages, which led to the possibility of earlier treatment and offered greater expectation of cure or arrest of disease. For those diseases, and there were many, such as defective heart valves, muscular degeneration, bacterial invasion, nervous disorders, and so on, for which no cure or effective treatment existed in the period, recognition of the earliest signs was not satisfying to the patient or the physician. Practitioners were intimidated by learning these early signs and saw no real purpose in knowing them since they could not recommend effective treatment and halt their progression into acute, chronic, or fatal disease. However, one compelling reason for increas-

ing sensitivity to the diagnosis of fatal disease, which was increasingly presented to more physicians, was the challenge to improve the methods for predicting the life expectancy of an individual applying for life insurance and seeking affiliation with other institutions with specific health requirements.

The physical examination an insurance applicant could expect to receive during the latter part of the nineteenth century emphasized listening to his or her chest and heart sounds and measuring the girth of the chest and the respiratory capacity of the lungs. Chemical tests of the urine were often required as well. Heart, lung, and kidney diseases were considered the major illnesses that shortened life in this period.[53] Auscultation with or without a stethoscope and percussion with or without a pleximeter were the primary diagnostic procedures an insurance company medical examiner was expected to undertake in an effort to discover the early signs of serious heart and lung diseases. Auscultation was the earliest, and remained the most commonly applied, diagnostic technique used in life insurance medical examinations. In the twentieth century, medical texts on physical examination for life insurance continued to stress auscultation above all other techniques. The sounds to be interpreted were kept to a minimum, for the majority of medical examiners could not be expected to use the stethoscope with finesse and great skill in this period. By the end of the nineteenth century, many clients were tested for kidney diseases on the basis of urinalysis employing various chemicals to reveal the presence of albumin, blood, and other impurities that indicated poor kidney function. Physicians and insurance agents were reluctant to subject the applicant to extensive procedures because physical examinations were unfamiliar and sometimes threatening to the layman. A physical examination was especially unfamiliar to those who had remained healthy. Physical examinations required a special skill on the part of the physician to execute them in an uncomplicated manner without causing embarrassment to the insurance applicant.[54]

In 1877, Professor William Detmold of New York City, who taught a course in insurance medicine, emphasized that the proper way to examine for an insurance policy was to use simple procedures and not attempt to perceive the fine distinctions in the results obtained. The examiner had to be able to recognize the normal heart and lung sounds, since he or she could then reject candidates who expressed other than the normal sounds in these organs. Detmold emphasized that it was unfair to expect a country practitioner, who was often engaged as a medical examiner, to provide a "highly scientific diagnosis."[55] Sixteen years later, Charles Dennison of Denver echoed Detmold's view that most physicians would not be able to make precision diagnoses. Dennison claimed

We must accept human nature as the past has shown it. . . . The great bulk of mankind do not care to be accurate, and the average medical practitioner is no exception. That physicians who examine for life insurance . . . can be relied upon for a refined diagnosis in the case of a man not seriously ill, is at least problematical. Many of these men started out in life impressed with the importance of auscultation and percussion, but have gradually come to give less and less time to all but those acutely ill. The experience of a medical director for more than twenty years shows that busy and skillful practitioners will not take the time to fill out a complicated chart, either for their patients or a company.[56]

The type and amount of insurance determined the extensiveness of the physical examination. Term life insurance, which provided protection for a limited number of years, demanded a less rigorous medical examination than a full-term life insurance policy.[57] Policies that paid small benefits did not require as much care in the medical examination as did policies paying large benefits since the loss to the company upon the premature death of the insured individual was less.

Simplicity in diagnosis gradually was replaced by sophisticated examination techniques as the desire to issue more insurance policies increased. The philosophy of the insurance company matured as society recognized a greater responsibility for those unable to support themselves. Insurance companies began to insure as many individuals as possible, not only to increase the companies' income but to allow wage earners to act responsibly by providing for the care of their families after their deaths. As insurance examiners became more business oriented, they began to accept the double role thrust upon them of recognizing poor risks, but equally important, of encouraging potentially long lived individuals to buy life insurance. Among the most difficult applicants to classify were those who presented suspicious heart sounds, which required sensitive instruments to hear and interpret. The sphygmograph, which was introduced by the mid-nineteenth century in European communities, was used to record heart and artery pulses in various parts of the body simultaneously. The instrument was recommended to diagnosticians for sepa-

rating structurally from functionally induced heart changes and distinguishing chronic or acute heart disease from transient heart anomalies. One of the American proponents, A. B. Isham of Cincinnati, Ohio urged that life insurance examiners use the sphygmograph in 1882.

[The] graphic method in diseases of the circulatory apparatus has within the past few years made positive additions to our means of arriving at certain conclusions in regard to valvular affections of the heart and calibre changes in the principal arterial vessels that no physician who has to deal with such conditions should content himself to rest in ignorance of the method and its results. It is of particular importance that examiners in life insurance should know what cardiosphygmomagraphy has accomplished, and should be competent to avail themselves of the advantages which it offers in clearing up doubtful cardiac physical signs. Without the graphic method the examiner cannot determine whether the sound be structural or functional. On the other hand, an examiner, by the aid of the graphic method, conjoined with other means of investigation, may base his opinion upon the functional or structural significance of a murmur with almost as much certainty as upon a mathematical demonstration.[58]

Precision through instruments became an elective procedure, which the physician applied to the most perplexing applicants. Edward Henry Sieveking in the several editions of his outstanding text on life insurance medicine published in 1875 and 1886 advised examiners to watch for "the process carried on within [the chest] by the stethoscope and by percussion, by the spirometer and by the sphygmomanometer, with results that amount to almost absolute certainty" (see figure 8.1).[59] The examiner had to employ his arsenal of diagnostic equipment selectively, for

in the ordinary inquiries necessary for life insurance, it is scarcely practicable to bring all these methods of research to bear upon every candidate for insurance. But there can be no doubt that, were we not afraid of frightening the customer, or were time no consideration, a more careful application of the various tests of pulmonary capacity would prevent many lives from being passed as normal, that now become claims at an earlier period than the medical examiner and his Board of Directors had reason to anticipate.[60]

It was generally accepted that, among the visceral organs, the lungs were amenable to the greatest variety of physical methods of examinations. Tuberculosis was the leading fatal respiratory disease during the period of rapid growth of the life insurance business. Insurance company directors argued for diagnosing

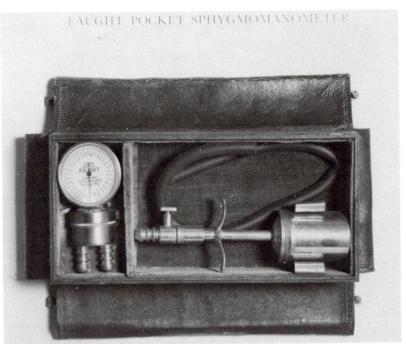

Figure 8.1. 1918 Faught pocket sphygmomanometer made by the George P. Pilling Co. of Philadelphia. *From the Philip Reichert Collection. SI Photo No. 63367-G.*

its presence as early as possible, which in turn, spurred the invention of various lung-testing devices that would provide data about the presence of the disease. Through measurement of chest size and the movements of its walls, in addition to percussion, auscultation, and application of the spirometer, the physician possessed tools to gauge quantitatively and qualitatively the function of the lungs (see figure 8.2.).[61] The spirometer was offered as an effective instrument in detecting the early or latent stages of consumption: ''Although it may not afford positive certainty, yet it challenges a renewed and more careful examination.''[62] The applicant was asked to exhale as much air as possible in one continuous forced expiration into the instrument, which measured the column of air expelled. This air was called the vital capacity of the lungs. The vital capacity was calculated for a number of individuals in each category based on height, weight, age, and sex; the resultant calculations became the ''norme.''[63] The vital capacity increased between the ages of fifteen and thirty-five years and decreased thereafter.[64] Following the first thorough discussion of the rationale and measurement of lung capacity presented by John Hutchinson in 1846, many versions of the spirometer were de-

signed and continued to be manufactured throughout the rest of the century. Containers made from metals, rubber bags, and cloth were sold. Some of these included those designed by Barnes, Shepard (nickel-plated), and Marsh, and the standard wet model composed of a zinc tank with brass tubes, resting in a galvanized iron body with iron brace and painted in dark red enamel (see figures 8.3 and 8.4).[65] Charles Dennison made a spirometer, as well as other instruments for measuring lung capacity, for use by the insurance examiner. His advice on the diagnosis and treatment of lung diseases was directed to the special concerns of the insurance company.[66]

Another important criterion for detecting lung disease was the size of the chest wall. Various instruments were invented for measuring chest size (see figure 8.5). After more than a decade of taking these measurements, Grahme Hammond, who had analyzed thousands of chest girth measurements, concluded that examiners had lost sight of the fact that they were, in fact, measuring the expansion of the lungs as they filled with oxygen and not the thickness of the chest muscles. Chest wall development was not essential to the condition of the lungs and had to be discounted when measuring the chest circumference for lung capacity. Hammond's studies revealed that the normal chest expanded only by an inch or so when filled with oxygen. Therefore, the instruments constructed for recording these changes had to be precise within the small range of an inch or so.[67] One instrument proposed for the purpose in 1881 was the cyrtometer, a scissor-like tool with an indicator at its distal end and aluminum strips that could be molded to the outline of the chest. It could be used to compare each side of the chest with the opposite side. To use the instrument, the physician

set the indicator at any given point, by means of the thumbscrew; place the strips tightly around the chest, and mould them to fit exactly the various depressions and elevations; loosen the thumbscrew on the indicator; open the scissorarms, and remove the instrument without displacing the strips; place the indicator in its former position and lay the instrument on a large sheet of paper; trace carefully all the curves of the strips with a lead-pencil, and the result will be an accurate outline of the chest wall.[68]

If the instrument were reversed end to end on the paper, the difference between the two sides of the chest would become apparent.

In addition to instruments for measuring chest size and capacity, others for pinpointing sounds originat-

ing in the chest were devised. A chest rule, or stethometer, to facilitate taking notes on the sounds heard over various parts of the chest was designed by Arthur Ransome in 1876. This light and flexible rule consisted "of thin narrow spring steel, so arranged as to form a rectangular parallelogram six inches long by three inches wide, and divided into eighteen squares of exactly one inch length of side."[69] With the aid of this rule, it was possible to mark in a diagrammatic fashion the exact position on the surface of the chest at which auscultation indicated the presence of a cavity or other disease signs. The rule permitted precision in auscultation and minimized the physician's need to memorize the areas over which he had detected certain sounds. Ransome introduced other instruments for investigating the complicated mechanism of respiration, including thoracic calipers, a goniometer for the ribs, and several forms of stethographs, in his book *On Stethometry*.[70]

Measurements of the chest remained an essential part of the life insurance examination into the twentieth century. Improvements in chest-measuring devices were based on an ideal instrument that would give accurate measurements of both sides of the chest simultaneously and each side separately and could be easily manipulated. The stethokyrtograph, designed

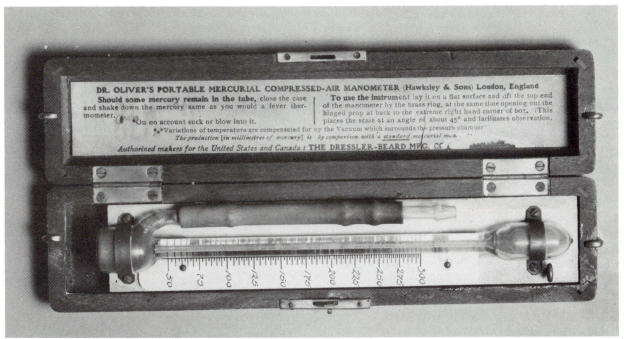

Figure 8.2. Dr. Oliver's portable mercurial compressed air manometer circa 1910. This instrument is an example of the effort to achieve convenience and portability, but at the sacrifice of accuracy and reliability. From the Philip Reichert Collection. *SI Photo No. 63367-E.*

by Richard Hogner of Boston in 1894, attempted to meet these criteria, belying its complex structure, which required delicate manipulation.[71] After the instrument was attached to the chest, it required three or four minutes to record three double registrations on paper, which could then be examined at the convenience of the physician. Occasionally, the instrument supplied information that cast another light on the diagnosis made on the basis of auscultation alone (see figure 8.6).

So that the earliest signs of lung disease could be detected, simple instruments were also invented. Edgar Holden in 1877 devised a soft rubber tube five-eighths of an inch in diameter and two feet long with metal tips. When the patient exhaled into the tube, forcing air through the tube, a rushing sound was produced, which when amplified by using the chest as a resonator, was believed to reflect tissue changes within the chest. The pitch and loudness of the chest sounds were changed when disease altered the density of the tissues.[72] Holden also invented a pneumatometer with the double function of a diagnostic and therapeutic instrument. It was used to measure the inspiratory and expiratory capacities of the lungs and to improve the chest capacity by forcibly opening the collapsed lung cells and those weakened by incipient disease. The graduated tube, which was manufactured by Shepard and Dudley of New York, permitted an individual's capacity for inspiration and expiration to be compared with previous measurements and recorded throughout the course of treatment.[73]

Mortimer Granville designed a pocket clinical pneograph, which John Weiss of London manufactured. It revealed the character of expiration by recording the process as tracings on paper, which could be analyzed at leisure.[74]

Mechanical gadgets to treat diseases of the chest were in vogue by the 1840s in Europe and the major cities of the United States. J. M. Howe of New York, a student of F. H. Ramadge of London, devised a container which could be filled three-fourths full of hot water, to which was attached a flexible tube with an ivory mouthpiece. The patient was expected to inhale warmed air coming from the container for periods of up to half an hour, one or more times each day until his condition had improved.[75] These early portable devices gave way to the large, heavy stationary units into which the patient was placed while being treated for lung diseases. Large pneumatic therapy chambers grew out of the technology devised for the manufacture of diving bells and were available to urban physicians in the 1880s. Experience with

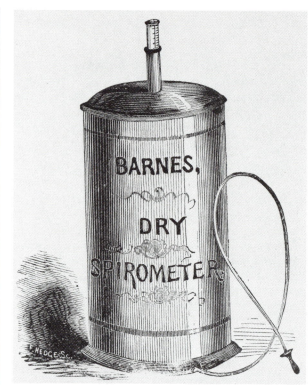

Figure 8.3. Barnes dry spirometer circa 1893 from *A. S. Aloe Catalogue, p. 640. SI Photo No. 78-4145.*

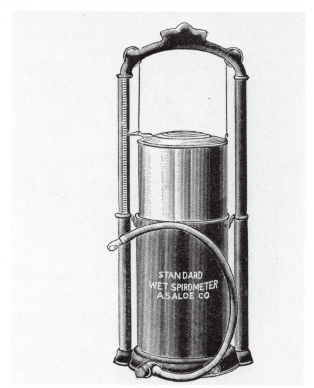

Figure 8.4. Standard wet spirometer circa 1893, from *A. S. Aloe Catalogue, p. 640. SI Photo No. 78-4146.*

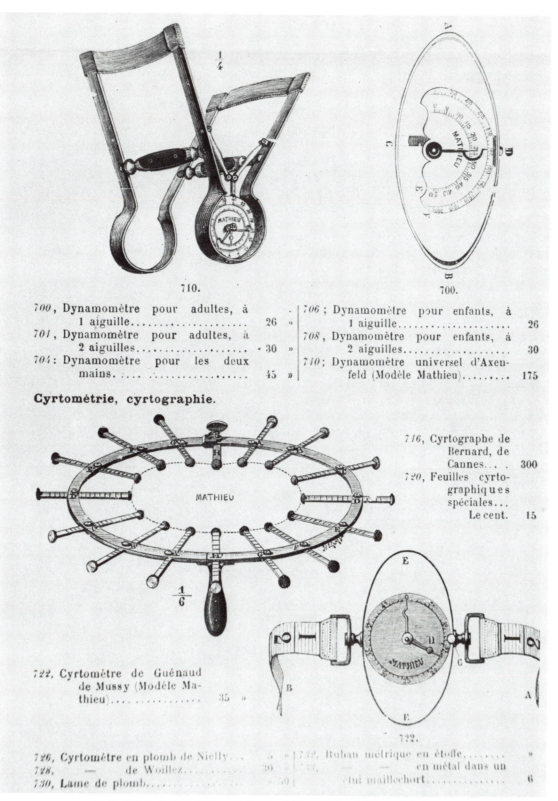

710.

700.

700, Dynamomètre pour adultes, à
    1 aiguille...................... 26 »

701, Dynamomètre pour adultes, à
    2 aiguilles.................... 30 »

704: Dynamomètre pour les deux
    mains. .... 45 »

706; Dynamomètre pour enfants, à
    1 aiguille.................... 26

708, Dynamomètre pour enfants, à
    2 aiguilles.................... 30

710; Dynamomètre universel d'Axen-
    feld (Modèle Mathieu)........ 175

Cyrtométrie, cyrtographie.

716, Cyrtographe de
    Bernard, de
    Cannes.... . 300

720, Feuilles cyrto-
    graphiq u e s
    spéciales...
           Le cent. 15

722, Cyrtomètre de Guénaud
    de Mussy (Modèle Ma-
    thieu)............... 35 »

726, Cyrtomètre en plomb de Nielly... 5 »

728, — de Woillez........... 30 »

730, Lame de plomb............. 50 »

742, Ruban métrique en étoffe........ »

743, — en métal dans un
    étui maillechort........... 6

Figure 8.5. Late nineteenth-century cyrtometer. *Mathieu Catalogue. SI Photo.*

diving bells since the sixteenth century indicated the dangerous symptoms leading to pain and collapse suffered by those who exposed themselves too quickly to pressurized and compressed air in order to go deeper under the water.[76]

Air baths and devices for artificially controlling the pressure of the air inhaled were widely used in medicine in the nineteenth century. Their therapeutic purpose was to increase lung capacity lost through disease by mechanically forcing more alveoli in the lungs to gather in oxygen than was possible in normal breathing, and to provide additional oxygen to the blood.[77] Air baths for medical purposes were encouraged as early as 1800 when the Royal Society of Harlaam in Holland offered a prize for an essay on the subject entitled "The Influence of Condensed Air on Animal and Vegetable Life."[78] Nothing came of this inducement. The first experiments with compressed air baths that proved practical were made in 1833 by Victor-Theodore Junod and improved by R. Taberié, C. G. Pravaz, and E. Bertin. Junod received a medal of honor, won the Monthym Prize twice and a cash award as late as 1876 for his method and devices.[79] Junod's pneumatic method of controlling the circulation (hemospasia), also a substitute for bloodletting, was supported by a galaxy of French physicians and physiologists.[80] In spite of this support and the fact that portable equipment could be used for Junod's treatment, it was neglected by those who had an "aversion . . . in adapting mechanical methods which are more laborious than writing prescriptions."[81] Among the earliest of the larger devices were the iron spheres that were large enough to hold from one to twelve people, which were employed by Tabarié, who "advised sittings of two hours' duration, with an increased pressure of from one-half to two-thirds of the atmosphere. A course of thirty to forty sittings were advised for radical cure."[82] Variations abounded in the amount of pressure and length of time to apply the chamber, as well as the diseases for which it was suitable. The safe amount of pressure was determined by A. H. Smith's study of watertight containers employed by divers. Smith

demonstrated that with an increase as great as fifteen to twenty pounds to the inch, no bad symptoms followed, either from the long immersion in the condensed air or the caisson or from the sudden transition to and from the external air. Not until a pressure of forty or fifty pounds or more super-added were the brain and cord engorged, or the possible introducers of nitrogen into the blood affected.[83]

The safe upper limit was rarely applied in treating lung diseases, although the ritual for treating emphysema and chronic bronchitis consisted of exposing

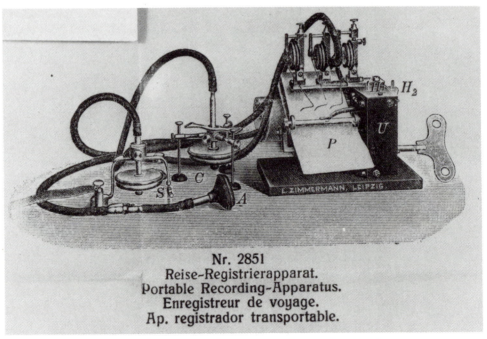

Figure 8.6. Portable recording apparatus. *SI Photo No. 74-6515.*

the sufferer to ten pounds of compressed air for two hours, of which half an hour was spent in raising the air pressure up to the limit, one hour in maintaining it, and half an hour in reducing inspiration of the compressed air.[84] The more usual air bath was typified by those prescribed for sufferers of phthisis and pulmonary emphysema at therapy centers in England. From 0.4 to 0.8 of an inch of compression was forced "into a neatly fitted metallic chamber, large enough to hold two persons, who may read, chat and sleep while their air cells are expanding and their tissues gaining strength under the dose of compressed oxygen."[85]

In keeping with the popularity of various types of mechanical treatments in Germany in the last quarter of the century, the smaller portable appliances were applied to force pressurized air into the lungs. These devices made the treatment accessible to patients in their own homes. In 1870, I. Hauke of Vienna devised the first portable manometer for condensing and rarifying air, which was perfected by L. Waldenburg of Berlin. Waldenburg's air pressure container was similar to a type used for storing illuminating gas. It was described in 1886 as containing "one cylinder, with an open end downward immersed in water, within a second and larger cylinder. By means of lateral uprights, with cords, pulleys, and graduated weights, the upper cylinder may at will be lowered and raised, and its contained air either condensed or rarefied. Tubing and a mouthpiece completed the apparatus."[86] Waldenburg's apparatus could be applied to administer four methods of treatment: "1. the inspiration of condensed air; 2. the expiration into condensed air; 3. the inspiration of rarefied air; 4. the expiration into rarefied air."[87] Waldenburg based the efficacy of his device on the results he obtained with its use. He claimed

inspiration of condensed air, as well as expiration into rarified air, increase permanently the vital capacity of the lungs (as shown by spirometry) and the power of inspiration and expiration as measureable by the pneumatometer. This fact appears to me of such paramount importance, that it alone leads me to consider the pneumatic method as one of the most important remedial agents of therapeutics.[88]

Otto and Reynders of New York imported several of Waldenburg's devices for sale to German physicians who had immigrated to the city and who brought these devices to the attention of the American physician A. Ross, who in turn investigated the history and use of the devices. Waldenburg's pneumatic apparatus was displayed in the South Kensington Museum in 1877.[89]

Pneumatic medicine, or the inhalation of gases to treat diseases of the lungs, was tried out a century before the increased pressure chambers came into vogue. Therapeutic inhalation of the gases including carbon dioxide, hydrogen, oxygen, and a few of the hydrocarbons was a form of therapy fostered by Thomas Beddoes and James Watt and encouraged by others of the Birmingham scientific circle. It reached a peak in 1796 when the portable apparatus for administering the gases could be purchased cheaply.[90] Pneumatic devices and the principle of these early investigations were combined later to treat lungs containing disease-causing bacteria. The apparatus was used to administer antiseptic medicinals under pressure. The treatment consisted "in immersing a patient in a partial vacuum, thereby removing to a sufficient degree the external pressure of the atmosphere, and at the same time supplying the lungs with air at its normal pressure, and to a greater or lesser extent impregnated with the substances which it is desired to administer."[91] The dilation of the lung cells is dependent upon the difference between the decrease in the external pressure and the pressure of air entering the lungs because "air charged to its utmost limit with remedial agents can be made to deposit its contents in cavities or other disease portions of the lungs under these circumstances."[92] Treatment of sixty-two patients suffering from various lung diseases were recorded. The majority of them received daily applications lasting from ten to thirty minutes resulting in thirty-four recoveries; most of these patients had suffered from bronchitis.[93]

The most popular device for administering bactericides was the cabinet designed in the 1870s by Joseph Ketchum and Herbert F. Williams of Brooklyn, New York.[94] This cabinet enabled the patient to inhale heated and medicated air at atmospheric pressure but with less pressure applied to the thoracic walls and the peripheral circulation of the body. The cabinet was described by Williams in 1876:

The cabinet is an air-tight chamber, in which the patient sits or reclines, breathing from the outside through a flexible tube . . . a small portion of the air is exhaust[ed] . . . causing a deep, easy and pleasant inhalation, filling every part of the lungs with the air or spray, producing a stronger and more regular circulation, bringing the blood into complete relation with oxygen of the air, and introducing the medication in every recess with ease. [This aids] . . . the patient to take a deeper breath than he otherwise could. . . . In this way . . . the same effect upon the lungs [is produced] that a dumbbell [produced] upon the muscles of the arms, for the effect is to exhale and not to inhale.[95]

The device permitted complete control over the movements of respiration to the extent of increasing or diminishing the force, frequency, and depth of each breath without the slightest effort or discomfort on the part of the patient. H. F. Williams described the benefit of the cabinet "as due to the reduction of congestion in the lungs by the air pressure within them, and by the increased expansion and movement of the lungs favoring their greater action and modifying their nutrition."[96] A large plate glass window enabled the physician to observe the patient. The pneumatic cabinet was manufactured by the Pneumatic Cabinet Company of New York and was exhibited and demonstrated by De Waterville in 1887 at the Annual Museum of the British Medical Association.[97] Cabinets were in use by 1886 in Brooklyn, Albany, Troy, Chicago, Cincinnati, and Jacksonville.[98] Sales Giron in 1858 showed that a medicinal could be carried into the most remote alveolus of the lungs and remain there to deliver its curative properties.[99] He constructed an apparatus for pulverizing fluids so that they could be inhaled; however, to reach the lung tissue, that fluid had to be vaporized and the temperature of the vapor containing the medicated particles lowered after reaching the lungs. Ketchum thought that it was possible to lower the temperature within the lungs; however, D. W. McCaskey of the Fort Wayne College of Medicine designed an apparatus for introducing "air at a comparatively high but accurately measured temperature, saturated beyond question with medicated vapor of definite composition, using either volatile or non-volatile agents; in order that the relatively cool mucous lining may lower its temperature and cause deposit of its suspended moisture."[100] The higher pressures reached with the pneumatic cabinet, combined with the vaporizing and heating treatment added with McCaskey's apparatus, provided a dual form of therapeutics "for the treatment of that class of pulmonary diseases in which increased intra-pulmonary pressure and topical medication is indicated for bronchitis and phthisis."[101]

The cabinet was also believed capable of providing evidence for some unsolved problems of pneumotherapy and for more accurate diagnosis. "For methods of diagnosis one application will frequently so change the physical character of the chest sounds that that which before treatment was obscure and indefinite can readily be appreciated and classified."[102] The Williams' pneumatic cabinet was available to physicians on a rental basis, which discouraged practitioners with small incomes from using it because the annual rental cost was high. Renting medical apparatus rankled some members of the profession. One spokesman complained, "No physician would wish to rent his pocket-case, his saddlebags, hypodermic syringe, speculum or obstetrical forceps, nor would he wish to pay the whole cost [of each item] in two years' rental."[103] Within a year, the manufacturer acceded to the request published in the *Journal of the American Medical Association* that the apparatus be sold rather than rented.[104]

Another stigma against use of the device by physicians was that the cabinet had been patented by a layman. The inventor tried to eliminate professional opposition on these grounds by seeking the counsel of a medical professional like Prof. Samuel G. Armor.

In accordance with his advice, which was later on thoroughly endorsed by Prof. Henry I. Bowditch of Boston and other leaders in the profession, an Advisory Board of Physicians has been invested with the absolute power of rejecting or accepting any application for the use of these cabinets. This plan has so far restricted the process to absolutely appropriate and trustworthy hands. For the last year of his life Prof. Alfred L. Loomis of New York has occupied that position. It is designed to add to this Board a representative physician from each of the prominent medical centers of the country whose more accurate knowledge of the physicians residing in his own community will enable him with greater certainty to accept responsibility for them when entrusted with the apparatus.[105]

Compressed air had also been used to enhance the effects of an anesthetic or other medicinal for surgery or other treatment of other parts of the body. Paul Bert in 1878 experimented for the purpose of learning the physiologic effects of varying the barometric pressure on gases introduced into the blood. One conclusion he drew was that the anesthetic, nitrous oxide, should be administered under increased pressure. In "a mobile pressure chamber constructed to accommodate patient, surgeon and assistants the patient laid himself down on the operating table, and the anesthetic agent was given him. He took it very quietly, did not struggle, and was soon insensible. . . . after the wound was sewn up, the compressed air was allowed to escape; the patient got up from the table, walked out of the car and lay down on the grass; he complained of no headache nor nausea, but said he felt just as usual. The car is on wheels and is carried about from hospital to hospital; the hospitals being under Government, the car is a public one, and is taken all over Paris."[106] The vogue for giving nitrous oxide and oxygen under pressure was short-lived. Bert wrote in 1883: "I have no hesitation in saying that this method of anesthesia as nearly as possible approaches perfection. . . . Unfortunately, the necessity for employing complicated and costly mechanical apparatus—cast iron chambers to withstand the pressure, pumps, steam engines—makes it possible for large hospitals only to use this valuable method. In Paris a very fine installation has been made at the Hospital Saint Louis; and I know of others at Lyons, at Geneva, in Brussels and in some German cities."[107] Bert stimulated Americans to emulate his research and its applications. J. Leonard Corning of New York also found through experimentation that "by far the most useful service derivable from compressed air is found in its ability to enhance and perpetuate the effects of soluble remedies (introduced hypodermically, by the mouth or otherwise) upon the internal organs, and more especially upon the cerebro-spinal axis. Some chemical affinity between the remedy employed and the protoplasm of the nerve cells is, of course, assumed to exist.[108] To intensify and localize the effects of remedies upon the brain and spinal cord, Corning had a cylindrical chamber, six feet in diameter and six and one-half feet high built and installed in his home. Weighing over two tons and built with the help of Cockburn Barrow and Machine Company of New Jersey, the chamber was used to compress the air to a pressure of thirty pounds per square inch for one hour while the patient remained seated inside.[109]

The manufacture and sale of large iron chambers as pressure treatment devices by the Pneumatic Cabinet Company had ceased by 1890 when those in stock were sold off for scrap iron, although some physicians continued to use their cabinets for years afterward. C. Quimby of New York claimed that 75 to 80 percent of his patients with localized tuberculosis were helped by the curative effects of the cabinet, which he thought acted on all factors of tuberculosis except the bacillus that caused it.[110] The simple substitute recommended by Charles Dennison to replace the cabinet was a large hollow toothpick or a small glass pipette, plugged at one end, used as an exhaling tube. Its inventor claimed that "the principle involved is the secret of a peculiarly successful form of respiratory gymnastics. The idea is to inhale freely and fully but to exhale with effort and with restraint or some obstruction to the outgoing air. Thus the den-

sity of the expansive air within the thorax is so much increased that it will work its way into areas of lung where otherwise some air cells would be unused but for this prolonged effect. This process is much like the natural stimulus of altitude."[111]

LIFE INSURANCE CHEMICAL TESTS:

Intensive concentration on the chest and lungs resulted in the neglect of other organs and the diseases to which they were commonly exposed. However, by the 1890s, life insurance statistics led companies to become concerned about the possible deaths of their policyholders from apoplexy, heart disease, contagious diseases, and Bright's disease. Among the most indicative and easily applied examinations were the chemical tests devised to reveal the functions of the kidneys, ureters, and the bladder by analyzing the urine for albumin, blood, and sugar and inspecting it under the microscope for the presence of bacteria. Albumin in the urine was accepted only as presumptive evidence of damaged kidneys by the last quarter of the century, "yet, it has so long formed the basis upon which the diagnosis of renal pathology has been constructed and, moreover, as an element considered with other symptoms it still holds, and is likely to hold, an important place at least in preliminary investigation of renal disease."[112] The flurry of tests devised for detecting albumin included those "exceedingly delicate in reaction as to detect the presence of albumin when the older methods, as by heat and nitric acid, failed to do so completely."[113] Indecision based on the fact that so many tests were available led Charles Purdy to evaluate all the tests in use by 1884 "to carefully inquire into the relative value and reliability of the newer, as compared with the older tests, with the view of assigning to each their proper spheres in the routine of daily work."[114] (See figure 8.7.) In 1896, W. L. Champion of Atlanta urged that physicians pay more attention to the kidneys in examinations for life insurance. He had discovered a number of individuals with kidney lesions who had just previously been passed as acceptable for life insurance.[115]

Instructions given to life insurance examiners were typified by the basic procedure, laid down in 1886 by the medical director of a Philadelphia company, to be followed when albumin was discovered during an examination.

Where the applicant is 1) a young person of good habits, 2) good family record and 3) physique, and the amount of 4) albumin is small and 5) specific gravity normal, . . . make

GENITO-URINARY.

URETHRAL.

SCALES OR GAUGES

FOR GRADING THE SIZES OF URETHRAL INSTRUMENTS.

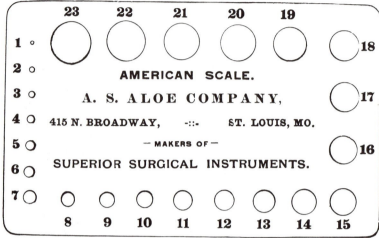

6636.—Face.

The American scale, introduced by Drs. Van Buren and Keyes, advances by diameters of one-half of a millimetre. The smallest size is half a millimetre in diameter, and is designated No. 1. No. 2 equals one millimetre, No. 3 equal to one and one-half millimeter in diameter, etc.

The American numbers and metrical diameters are stamped upon one side of this scale, the approximate French numbers on the other.

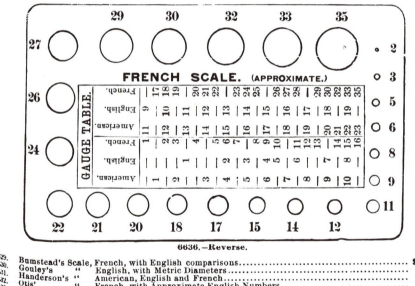

6636.—Reverse.

6629.	Bumstead's Scale, French, with English comparisons...	$	2	65
6630.	Gouley's " English, with Metric Diameters...		2	65
6631.	Handerson's " American, English and French.......................................		4	50
6632.	Otis' " French, with Approximate English Numbers............................		2	65
6633.	Thomas' " Adjustable Metric..		0	25
6634.	Van Buren & Keyes' Scale, American, with Approximate French Numbers, Steel, Nickel-plated,		2	65
6635.	" " " " " " " " Celluloid...........			10
6636.	" " " " " " " " Pasteboard, Gratis..			
6637.	Wyeth's United States Scale..		2	65

ALL INSTRUMENTS ILLUSTRATED ARE DESIGNATED BY BOLD-FACED FIGURES.

Figure 8.7. Scales for grading the sizes of urethral instruments circa 1893, according to the American and French systems from *A. S. Aloe Co. Catalogue, p. 395. SI Photo No. 78-4144.*

several examinations of the urine at . . . different times, to find whether the presence of albumin was accidental or not. In such cases, if it is proved that it is not a constant condition and due to renal disease, . . . a policy for small amount will be issued. If a large amount of insurance is requested . . . the company required a microscopical examination of the urine under such circumstances.

If the applicant is 1) past middle age, at the time when degenerative process begins, 2) has been a free liver or accustomed to luxurious habits or has undergone mental strain, 3) or had been overworked and closely confined to business, 4) with irregular hours, etc., the presence of the smallest amount of albumin in the urine [is] an absolute impediment to life insurance.[116]

It was necessary to remain cautious about the diagnosis to be made when albumin was present in the urine. Some physicians became convinced of the usefulness of the microscope in discovering kidney lesions among insurance applicants; this conviction led to an appreciation of the microscope for diagnosis of all their patients presenting symptoms of kidney disease. The insurance company paid an extra fee for examining the urine under the microscope but the physician was not always permitted to decide when this additional test should be made.

LIFE INSURANCE IN THE TWENTIETH CENTURY:

Analysis of life insurance company data eventually resulted in identifying those individuals who were better risks because they would live longer, and it permitted the company to devise a program of life insurance for individuals with some health impediments, who would pay a greater fee to compensate for their less-than-normal life expectancy. After the medical examination of applicants for life insurance was refined by the early twentieth century and the results combined with the development of sophisticated numerical methods for assigning insurance applicants to high-, average-, and low-risk categories, it became possible to sell insurance to almost all individuals who requested it. Douglas Powell in an address to the Society of Life Assurance Medical Officers in London in 1896 congratulated the companies for accepting some of the risks of impaired lives by selling them life insurance at calculated costs. His only objection was to the practice of ''loading'' or deducting a certain amount of money for each year that the individual did not live up to the calculated life expectancy,[117] but insurance companies replied that realistically they could not adopt a practice that would jeopardize their economic viability.

In 1900, S. Oakley Vander Poel in the United States studied the 12 to 15 percent of applicants rejected for life insurance between 1875 and 1890 because of their family history or physical disabilities and traced their subsequent histories. He found that almost all of these individuals could be accepted on a substandard basis, if not actually ill at the time of application.[118] This trend toward a more liberal medical policy of granting life insurance in the United States continued through the twentieth century. In 1924, the Prudential Life Insurance Company initiated a plan to insure all applicants regardless of their medical history.[119] In Britain by the third decade of the twentieth century, much insurance business was devoted to insuring impaired lives by charging these individuals appropriately higher premiums.[120] By 1934, many individuals were granted life insurance policies without a thorough medical examination.[121]

The life insurance actuary and statistician developed sophisticated methods of selecting policy holders in the twentieth century. One of these was announced in 1934 by the Joint Committee on ''Standard Mortality Ratios Incident to Variations in Height and Weight Among Men.'' The committee suggested a method of assigning a percentage valuation to each characteristic considered significant in determining the probable length of life. These were: (1) build (weight in relation to height), (2) family record, (3) occupation, (4) personal history, (5) habits, (6) physical condition, (7) habitat or residence, (8) moral hazard, and (9) plan of insurance applied for.[122] This method could be used to evaluate the majority of insurance applicants. The committee concluded that

the underlying principle in the numerical method of clinical selection rests on the assumption that the average risk accepted by a company has a value of one hundred per cent, and that each one of the factors which make up a risk shall be expressed numerically in terms of one hundred per cent, and that by the summation of them, or by some modification of their summation, the value of any risk shall be determined and expressed with relation to that standard. Everyone who passes judgment upon a risk carries out this process in his mind. The numerical method expresses each step in the mental process in terms of a definite standard and the final evaluation of the risk with comparatively few exceptions of material importance is the summation of these various items. All of these processes may be carried on by properly trained clerks, but where the numerical ratings as so determined bring a risk close to the borderline either on the standard or substandard side of the limit which the company fixes in advance, or where purely medical factors require more detailed analysis, the risk is then a proper subject for expert medical study.[123]

Thus, only in instances involving applications for large amounts of insurance, applicants with unusually dangerous occupations, or the need for answering special questions did an individual need to be examined in greater detail by a physician. The insurance company attempted to balance the number of high- and low-risk policies it issued and the premium charged for each in a manner to maximize its profits and minimize its losses.

The criteria used for selecting life insurance policyholders evolved from the discoveries of medical science in the nineteenth and twentieth centuries and the application of the principles of biometry combined with longevity studies, which resulted in the return to the practice of selling life insurance policies with minimal direct medical examination by the third decade of the twentieth century.[124]

Although the process of obtaining life insurance was streamlined and not tied to the physician's examination of every applicant, company statisticians continued to collect and analyze health- and disease-related data of policyholders. Two leaders in the program were Oscar Rogers and Arthur Hunter, who were employed by life insurance companies. In 1921, they compiled a list of the principal impairments of tens of thousands of individuals who had purchased life insurance policies. Among the more common disorders they found were: heart murmurs; overweight; albumin in the urine; irregular, intermittent, or rapid pulses; high blood pressure; sugar in the urine; asthma; pleurisy; middle ear disease; goiter; gall stones; syphilis; alcoholism; gastric or duodenal ulcers; and biliary colic.[125] Of these disorders, high blood pressure and diabetes were the most indicative of future serious disease and death and could be relied upon to indicate a shorter life expectancy for an insurance applicant.

Up to this period, clinicians had not collected massive amounts of data on disease[126] nor had they compared the healthy and sick population, which made Rogers and Hunter's analysis uniquely valuable. Analysis of disease was usually based on the studies of patients in hospitals, which meant that the health of the same individual was rarely followed for any length of time. Nonhospitalized patients often presented different medical profiles than those of acutely ill and hospitalized patients. Clinicians in 1880 had urged that medical records be compiled by the army, navy, life insurance examiners, hospitals, and schools for the purpose of uncovering idiosyncratic reactions to drugs.[127] General practitioners, in keeping records of their patients extending over a lifetime, added to

the type of statistics gathered in the hospital, but these records often were not brought together for comparison and analysis with the records of other physicians. Life insurance-derived health data was an important addition to the data gathered from the study of diseases and hospitalized individuals, which did not always reflect the physical standards of those who remained healthy, and who, of course, made up the major proportion of the population.[128]

Physiologic and anatomic data were also generated from individuals in other institutions. One of the most heterogeneous and cooperative groups from which bodily statistics were taken was school children. In the nineteenth century, physical data began to be collected from children attending school. Teachers were expected to make measurements of height, weight, chest girth, and similar traits, although taking these measurements and compiling the records was not always sufficiently encouraged to inspire diligence among those who collected the data. Although in 1876 Charles Roberts could find few physical or mental characteristics that correlated with a child's age within a three-year span, thirty-five years later a number of characteristics were found to be typical of children at each age. A sufficient quantity of measurements had been taken by the twentieth century to set up standards for the correlation between the physical and mental traits of children at each age and the expected normal development during each year.[129]

Some physiologic standards used to gauge length of life were not directly related to disease or its symptoms as noted by the patient or physician. More subtle signs occasionally could be detected with special instruments, and of these, the outstanding example was the sphygmomanometer (see figure 8.8). This instrument led insurance examiners to collect data on the pressure of the circulating blood, which resulted in the establishment of one of the most useful guides to physiologic well-being and incipient disease. Blood pressure statistics met the life insurance companies' goal of finding a correlation between the present state of health and future life expectancy. The technique was introduced in the nineteenth century and developed in the twentieth century. The application of blood pressure to insurance medicine was the most successful diagnostic technique developed to indicate length of life.

Blood pressure is an important physiologic function that can be demarcated on a numerical scale, which can only be precisely observed with the assistance of an instrument. The numerical data may be distinguished as normal or abnormal, although

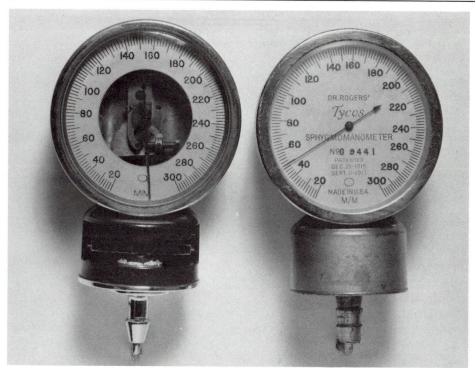

Figure 8.8. Dr. Roger's Tycos sphygmomanometer dials patented in 1915 and 1917. From *Philip Reichert Collection. SI Photo No. 63367-F.*

within narrow margins, based on other factors, medical insight is required to make the distinction. Blood pressure is "the pressure in the brachial or other arteries and it indicates the expansive force which the column of blood directs outward against its more or less elastic wall."[130] While it is possible to feel the difference between a very high or very low pressure by placing the artery between the figures, the quantitative differences are not easily judged in this manner.

There are two components to the blood pressure: diastolic and systolic. The diastolic pressure

is the constant resistance which the heart has to overcome before it can drive the blood forward, and is therefore the fundamental pressure as it represents: A- The constant pressure to which the arteries are subjected. B- The pressure which the heart has first of all to overcome. C- The constant strain which has to be borne by the aorta and aortic valves. Systolic pressure is the expression in millimeters of mercury of the intraventricular pressure and is subject to wide variations from physiological causes.[131]

An early attempt employing a device to display the differences in the force of the blood coursing through the surface arteries was made in the sixteenth century. Josephus Struthius, who was a pioneer in count-

ing the pulse, also applied weights to the artery in the wrist and distinguished the magnitude of the pulse by the amount of weight the arterial pressure would lift up.[132]

Stephen Hales made the first attempt to directly measure blood pressure quantitatively in 1709 at Corpus Christi College in Cambridge, England. He used a minimum of instruments. He needed a scalpel to open the crural artery and a measuring rod to determine the height of the column of blood. His method rested on the sacrifice of animals (horse, dog, deer), of which he recorded the height of the blood spurting from the punctured artery until the animal had bled to death.[133] Although Hales experimented in isolation, his important discoveries were very much part of the conceptual and experimental mechanical tradition in circulation research discussed by his contemporaries. Concurrently, Alphonse Borelli, the leading Italian proponent of iatro-mechanics, applied the laws of hydraulics to the study of the circulation. The first adequate formulation of these laws was supplied by Jean Poiseuille in 1828, which led to an avalanche of circulation physiology studies in living animals, and eventually in humans—studies dependent on ingenious instruments for their exploitation.[134] Instruments for measuring blood pressure without destroying the animal were devised in the nineteenth century. These measured the force required to overcome the pressure in the arteries by temporarily obliterating the vessel's diameter.[135]

Life insurance companies increasingly recognized the blood pressure as a good indicator of impending sickness and death when it reached certain levels.[136] Physicians adopted the measurement of blood pressure as a valuable signifier of future heart and vascular diseases after the insurance companies proved with their voluminous statistics that systolic blood pressure greater than 150 mm of mercury was a definite indicator of disease and a shortened life. Blood pressure as a factor in future disease increased in proportion as the pressure itself increased. Medical directors realized by the early decades of the twentieth century that insurance examiners and general medical practitioners were not interpreting or applying the blood pressure in the same way. Physicians doing research collected data on blood pressure recorded by the sphygmomanometer but these figures were not as meaningful to the general medical practitioner, who was concerned with the health of a patient at the time of an examination. Except for those blood pressure readings that were noted to be among the extreme values obtained, it was difficult to interpret the blood pressure in terms of a specific therapy or to warn the patient of impending disease. For many diseases, which produced a variety of symptoms, regulation of the blood pressure to a particular level did not appear to be a major or necessary part of therapy, nor was there an acceptable method of accomplishing this goal. Blood pressure measurement did not appear to provide information that was conclusive in determining the state of health and the expected progress of a patient or for deciding on the methods to deal with an acute illness.[137]

In previous centuries, therapeutic value had been attached to treatments that, in effect, lowered blood pressure, although their effect on blood pressure was not recognized nor used as a rationale for their application. Illnesses that were usually the result of excess fluid retention produced symptoms that could be relieved with the elimination of some of the body liquids. Before it was accurately measured, some of the symptoms of excessive blood pressure (ruddy complexion, headache, and dizziness) were regarded by physicians as significant disease indicators, which could be alleviated by lowering the volume of the blood and other fluids in the body. Various drugs, as well as bloodletting, had been prescribed to remove excess blood and fluids, thereby reducing the pressure of the blood, at least temporarily in the arteries. Body fluids also were eliminated by administering emetics and purges.

In the mid-1880s, Koerner and Oertal of Germany were hailed as creators of a new era in internal medicine with the announcement of a treatment for the regulation of blood pressure, which had the same effect as these older drug-induced methods. Their method had an immediate striking impact. They prescribed the "dry method" of controlling blood volume, which appeared to some of their contemporaries to be as sensational a therapeutic advance as the introduction of antisepsis into surgery. The treatment consisted of putting the patient on a water-restricted diet. Reduced water in the diet lessened the work of the heart, permitting the kidneys to rest and the blood pressure to be lowered.[138] Measurement of the blood pressure was not essential nor usually undertaken to determine when sufficient depletion had occurred. Progress in curing an acute disease, such as pleurisy, which was accompanied by excessive fluids in the lung tissues, helped the physician to decide when to stop the treatment. Statistics of those treated demonstrated the effectiveness of this method of therapy, which served well, until physicians learned to apply it more precisely by measuring the blood pressure on a numerical scale and correlating the data with other signs of the health of the individual.

Collection of data on blood pressure and correlation with specific diseases was essential before the sphygmomanometer could be applied routinely by the physician. Richard Shryock had pointed out that the invention of medical instruments had "made it less necessary to depend . . . on statistical data as a means of observation."[139] However, before this stage is reached, statistical correlation and analysis of the data recorded by the instrument must be gathered to determine the distinction between the normal and abnormal phenomena measured with the instrument. In order to apply the medical instrument and develop a valid therapy, standards had to be established, whether they were obtained in the form of numbers, colors, or descriptive terms. Sometimes these standards were discovered, as well as expressed, in the units in which the instruments were calibrated. To decide on the relevant units for expressing bodily functions required the observations of many individuals and their tabulation in statistical form. Samuel R. von Basch published some of the earliest studies of blood pressure measured in patients with a variety of diseases. These studies appeared in the journal

Zeitschrift fur klinische medizin, which was founded in 1880 by Frerichs and Leyden.[140] Pierre Carl E. Potain of France published the first extensive text on blood pressure and its limits in 1902, which was based on a study of 11,000 records taken over a period of thirty years.[141] In the twentieth century, others including T. C. Janeway, T. L. Brunton, and H. W. Cook joined Potain in collecting blood pressure statistics from smaller groups of individuals and arrived at varying blood pressure standards. The different types of sphygmomanometers used to record blood pressures contributed to some of these differences (see figure 8.9).

The insurance company standard or the normal limits proposed by Fisher were placed at 140-145 mm systolic pressure and 90-95 mm diastolic pressure. Fisher set a limit of 15 mm above the average for an individual to be an acceptable life insurance risk. Pressures above this level were called high blood pressure and the applicant with high blood pressure required further tests and evaluation.[142] The limits were accepted by American clinicians and heart specialists, including Walter Alverez, Morris Fishbein, Paul Dudley White, and others.[143] Other insurance company blood pressure statistics were soon accumulated. Over 18,000 readings were gathered between 1912 and 1914, which were published by Lewis F. MacKenzie of the Prudential Life Insurance Company of Newark, New Jersey in 1915.[144] Analysis of 36,104 recorded cases provided the basis for MacKenzie's conclusion that normal blood pressures had been determined within at least three millimeters' accuracy.[145] The definition of normal blood pressure that grew out of insurance company statistics remained unchallenged until 1952, when Arthur Master, Charles I. Garfield, and Max B. Walters provided new standards obtained from a statistical study of 74,000 unselected individuals, which raised the upper limit of the earlier established normal blood pressure standard.[146]

Before the clinical sphygmomanometer was perfected to the extent of providing reliable and consistent results, Richard Cabot of Boston prophesied in 1903 that "it seems to me likely that the charts of pulse rate will be supplemented before long by charts of blood pressure taken at regular intervals as a matter of routine."[147] Harvey Cushing made a similar forecast at about the same time.[148] Cabot realized that Oliver's hemogynamometer, in use at the time, might malfunction easily; yet even imperfect instruments were capable of yielding important information if applied to make comparative measurements

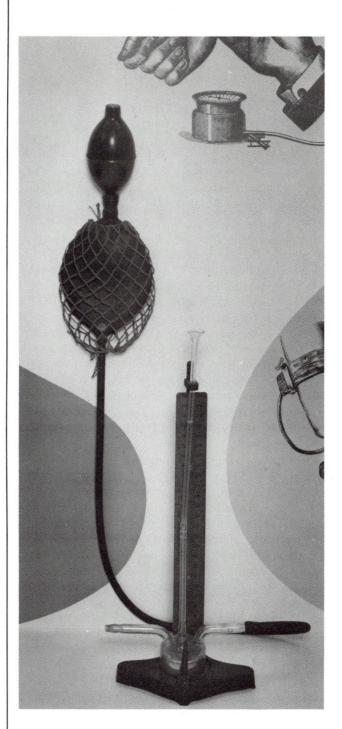

Figure 8.9. 1896 Riva Rocci sphygmomanometer. From *Philip Reichert Collection. SI Photo No. 63367-D.*

on the same patient, so that all elements of error remained constant. Within several decades, a number of other instruments had been invented and marketed. Von Basch described his sphygmomanometer in 1880 (see figure 8.10). It consisted of a "thick-walled glass tube containing mercury which opened out into a small knob connected to a membranous bulb filled with water. This 'pelotte' was placed on the artery until the pulse was obliterated."[149] Von Basch's device and other nineteenth-century sphygmomanometers remained research tools, since they were too difficult to maintain and apply in the course of a physical examination. The first aneroid manometer containing air was employed by Potain in 1889 to measure blood pressure. Substitution of an aneroid manometer, which used air instead of water to compress the artery in which the blood pressure was being measured, enabled the instrument to be made compact and portable.[150] The aneroid dial contained a magnified scale. S. Riva-Rocci in 1896 improved compression of the artery by using a thin rubber tube five centimeters wide, to encircle the upper arm, thereby giving a uniform pressure over a wider area.[151] In 1901, Leonard Hill and Harold Barnard attached in place of the mercury tube an aneroid manometer with a cuff, twelve to fourteen centimeters wide, which provided even more accurate readings. By 1920, the most popular portable manometer was one invented by Dr. Oscar H. Rogers, chief medical director of the New York Life Insurance Company.[152] R. Max Goepp attributed the popularity of blood pressure measurements as a routine clinical practice to the introduction of the easy to apply and accurate aneroid sphygmomanometer, of which Rogers' instrument was an outstanding example.[153]

A more effective method of correlating the pulse in the artery and the mercury level in the manometer was the auscultatory method, which employed a stethoscope to be applied in the elbow below the cuff to pick up four distinct sounds produced by the collapsing artery. The method was introduced by the Russian physician N. Korotkow in 1905.[154] He recommended that the systolic phase be recorded at the beginning of the first sound and the diastolic phase at the end of the fourth sound. Debate over which sound to use to distinguish the point at which the diastolic pressure occurred continued for decades. The Blood Pressure Committee, which was set up by the Association of Life Insurance Medical Directors, reported in 1921 that insurance company examiners and clinical teachers were not uniformly instructing physicians in the methods of recording the blood

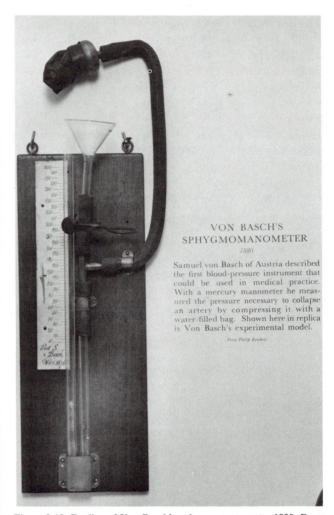

VON BASCH'S
SPHYGMOMANOMETER
1880

Samuel von Basch of Austria described the first blood-pressure instrument that could be used in medical practice. With a mercury manometer he measured the pressure necessary to collapse an artery by compressing it with a water-filled bag. Shown here in replica is Von Basch's experimental model.

From Philip Reichert

Figure 8.10. Replica of Von Basch's sphygmomanometer 1880. From *Philip Reichert Collection. SI Photo No. 63367-D.*

pressure.[155] A poll of leading clinicians was taken to determine the best method of recording the diastolic pressure. Among the teachers from Harvard, and clinicians from The Johns Hopkins Medical Schools and the Mayo Clinic, different methods were proposed. The committee recommended "the last loud tone at the end of the third phase as representing the correct diastolic pressure . . . and that those companies which have trained their examiners to report the end of the fourth phase, or the cessation of all sound, or which feel that this phase gives a valuable check on the examiners, should request both phases."[156] In 1939, the Committee on Standardization of Blood Pressure Readings of the American Heart Association, and of Great Britain and Ireland recommended that the time for recording the diastolic pressure be changed to the beginning of the fourth sound.[157]

The survey of medical teachers also revealed that other laboratory procedures were not being taught in a uniform manner either "so that it appears that different instructors in the same school and in different schools are teaching varying and often contradictory methods which may in part at least explain the deplorable confusion of both examiners and practitioners in regard to many simple and important clinical and laboratory procedures."[158]

Stimulation to apply instruments in the medical examination followed from the medical reports insurance companies demanded and the conclusions based on surveys of the statistics they had gathered, which indicated the most essential medical facts upon which to issue a policy and under what terms it should be issued. The Northwestern Mutual Life Insurance Company through its medical director, J. W. Fisher, was outstanding in promoting the use of the sphygmomanometer to measure blood pressure in the brachial artery in the first quarter of the twentieth century. Fisher claimed that "prior to 1907, little or no use was made of the sphygmomanometer, except in clinical cases." Fisher insisted that

no practitioner of medicine should be without the sphygmomanometer. He has in this instrument a most valuable aid in diagnosis. The sphygmomanometer is indispensable in life-insurance examinations, and the time is not far distant when all progressive life insurance companies will require its use in all examinations of applicants for life insurance.[159]

Three years later, he boasted,

Today, this prediction is practically fulfilled, and no up-to-date practitioner is without this very valuable aid in diagno-

sis, much of which has been due to the requirements of life-insurance companies in insisting on their examiners' using the sphygmomanometer in examinations for life insurance. I have received hundreds of letters thanking me for insisting on its use in examinations for the company and testifying to its very great value in private practice.[160]

Imperfect instruments contributed to the problem of standardizing blood pressure, especially the diastolic portion. An ideal instrument was characterized as being portable in size and weight, able to withstand rough use without loss of accuracy, and be available at minimal cost.[161] There were two main types of blood pressure instruments: the mercurial and the spring activated models. The mercury instrument was quickly spoiled with use since the mercury oxidized by sulfides, which made the substance stick to the sides of the tube. The spring form was delicate and required extra care to keep it from becoming out of adjustment. Edward K. Root in 1915 designed a spring manometer that could withstand greater shocks. He described it: "It has a diaphragm spring with a very much simplified multiplying device, by which the motion of the diaphragm is conveyed to the pointer and thus to the dial. The instrument can be made in quantity—that is to say in large numbers—probably for less than fifteen dollars —I think possibly for about twelve dollars."[162] To keep the cost of the unit down, Root suggested that life insurance companies buy the instrument

and sell it to their examiners, otherwise an instrument put upon the market and handled by the middle men and the trade generally, is bound to cost more, and in the nature of things will cost more. If the Association or any number of Companies in the Association choose to unite and put in an order large enough to any good maker,—for instance, the firm that made this, I believe they could get them very cheap and sell them to the examiners for cost. . . . I believe ordered in five hundred or one thousand lots, it could be sold to the Companies for anywhere from ten to twelve dollars a piece, and with the armlet and pump the total cost would probably be about fifteen to sixteen dollars.[163]

Although the instrument continued to need improvement, faith in the information the sphygmomanometer provided and its use for clinical evaluation of a patient or insurance applicant continued to grow. The Committee on Blood Pressure Tests, chaired by G. A. Van Wagenen of the Mutual Benefit Life Insurance Company, reported in 1915 "that both the sphygmomanometer and its use are now imperfect, and great improvement is to be expected in both; but even with the present form of instruments and manipulation, the results are of inestimable value to use, particularly in that class of cases which have defied our usual methods of insurance examination."[164] Following in the pattern of other laboratory tests and clinical examinations such as urinalysis, which was developed and perfected on data gathered over many years in the nineteenth century, blood pressure data were continuously gathered and the blood pressure standard was refined into the twentieth century.

A nonmedical consequence of measuring the blood pressure and other physiologic characteristics of a large segment of the general population was to use these standards in a social, economic, or political context. Some of these applications will be discussed in the next chapter to give an idea of their growth from and impact on American and British institutions and to suggest further studies in this important but neglected aspect of American and European medical history.

9

THE SOCIAL IMPLICATIONS OF STANDARDS

RISE IN PUBLIC HEALTH CONCERN:

Tests growing out of laboratory investigation and the invention of unique equipment and devices were important to the development of various physiologic and pathologic standards. Of equal or greater importance were the health goals promoted by political, social, and economic groups, such as life insurance companies discussed earlier, that depended on these laboratory standards for their formulation and achievement. Identifying the physical sources of normal and abnormal functions and structures enabled those with concern for the legal, moral, political, economic, and social aspects of disease to shape definite guidelines in each of these areas. Enforcing practices designed to minimize or prevent disease and its consequences became a multifaceted program, which ultimately rested on the test results provided by various mechanical devices and laboratory analyses of a chemical, bacteriologic, or microscopic type. The medical profession responded to society's leaders in setting up the organizations required to provide and apply the technical information. Other groups delivered technical services in response to governmental regulations, sometimes with limited guidance from physicians. Various reasons account for the desultory leadership of physicians in the disbursement of technical medical information and its practical consequences among the widest segments of the community. Not the least of these impediments were their own reservations about accepting the new medical technology, as well as understanding the disease consequences of all technology.

When technology employed throughout society began to affect the human body, physicians chastised themselves for lacking sufficient organization and methods to deal with all aspects of the impact of technology on human health. S. Weir Mitchell predicted in 1891 that "all the vast hygienic, social and moral problems of our restless, energetic, labour-craving race are, in some degree, those of the future student of disease in America."[1] One British observer in 1918 verified Mitchell's forecast and complained about physicians who were not meeting the challenge offered to them. Physicians were continuing to practice medicine much as they had in the seventeenth and eighteenth centuries when patients suffered from the diseases common to rural communities. The time had arrived when physicians must learn to expect and respond to diseases springing from schools, factories, mines, and urban living.[2] Furthermore, it was among the physician's duties to assist in setting up health-related job standards and to condemn unhygienic conditions in the factories, schools, and other city institutions. Physicians were expected to make recommendations and criticize environmental hazards, as had a group of physicians in New York City, who in 1878 had protested the noise generated by the recently installed Sixth Avenue elevated railroads.[3] Another hazard related to this new mode of transportation further substantiates how physicians responded to health problems created by technology with a technology of their own. The braking trains released hot flying metal splinters, which all too often ended up in the eyes of those who walked beneath the elevated railroad. Removing these foreign bodies from the eyes of pedestrians became so common that special devices were invented for the purpose.[4] Physicians in New York and other large American cities began to exert their responsibilities to public health in the last quarter of the nineteenth century.[5]

Physicians protested the unsanitary conditions of the public schools beginning in the 1870s. They objected to overcrowded classrooms, poor lighting, insufficient ventilation, and unsanitary water closets. The leading New York medical journal, *The Medical Record*, published many editorials supporting sanitary reforms in schools and other institutions such as reformatories. In the 1880s, the sanitation of the schools in Britain was credited with reducing child mortality by providing an alternative to the vitiated atmosphere of the children's homes and streets.[6] However, British schools were faulted for inflicting physical and mental damage to young students through excessive intellectual assignments, poor lighting, and unsatisfactory exercise periods.[7]

Architectural innovations could change a neighborhood into an unhealthy place to live. When tall buildings were first introduced in New York City, the resulting shade and restriction of airflow in the nearby streets drew scorn from physicians. Skyscrapers were called "abominations, and an unanswerable insult to the common sense of a plutocratically oppressed people depriving them of fresh air and sunlight."[8] Charles Wingate, sanitary engineer for the city was alarmed by the "draughts of sewer gas from the escape pipes of overtopping buildings into the windows, chimneys and light shafts of adjacent houses."[9]

Even more disastrous than environmental changes were catastrophes that resulted in loss of many lives over a brief period. Life insurance companies, which suffered immediate financial losses, and other institutions supported concerted action for improving public sanitation and encouraging regular physical examinations to reduce the possibility of a fatal epidemic. Among the opportunities for promoting health consciousness were public poster campaigns and hygiene museums in which exhibits displayed the fundamentals of community-based disease and its prevention. The health museum tried to impress the public with the vast differences in cost between preventing disease among a large group of people and treating illness after its symptoms had already appeared.[10] Another method open to all citizens and institutions was to insist that the state exercise its functions in promoting proper sanitation among its inhabitants. Failure to enforce sanitary regulations resulting in epidemics of smallpox, scarlet fever, and other serious diseases was a dereliction of duty that could be held up to the state and city governments.[11]

Assistance in detecting incipient disease and treating it before it became grave was offered to insurance companies and other institutions that required physical examinations when it became apparent to medical specialists, that, in the course of the examination, new medical techniques could be introduced to the public. As technology improved the capacity of medical specialists to identify and treat disease, these specialists saw an opportunity to attract new patients by making their specialty a part of the physical examination. Medical specialists argued that the savings to a group such as the life insurance companies would become greater if their specialties were included in the pre-policy physical examination. For instance, a New York dentist launched a campaign in the early 1920s to include dental inspection as one part of the physical examination required to obtain insurance. He emphasized the statement of Mr. Hyram J. Messenger, actuary of the Travelers' Insurance Company of Hartford, Connecticut,

that if the companies were to expend the sum of two hundred thousand dollars a year for the purpose of spreading the information in regard to personal hygiene and in cooperating with other agencies in health movements, also extending to policy-holders the privilege of frequent medical examinations, and if the result should show a decrease in the losses of the companies amounting to the insignificant sum of 16/100ths of one per cent, they would save enough to cover the cost. If this plan were carried out under good business methods, with all the companies working together, he would expect a decrease of one per cent of the death claims would result in the saving to the companies of $1,005,000, or seven times the amount expended. It is also the expressed opinion of an insurance man and newspaper editor that the institution of dental examination would decrease the losses more than two per cent.[12]

The dental examination did not become a standard component of the physical examination, although the fact that dental-related disease contributed to poor health was becoming more apparent in the period.

A major problem because it affected a large group of people resulted from the deterioration of vision due to aging. When office and factory jobs became common, the lack of ability to focus at close distances in those workers who were in their mid-forties or older required diagnosis and correction with spectacles. Recognition of these visual changes made it imperative to set standards in eye examinations and in the glasses prescribed to correct them.

The relationship between far-sightedness and office work was recognized by physicians like Frank Van Fleet, who in 1896 explained that

the cause for the increase of refraction cases is no deterioration of the eye, but increase in the necessity for correct vision. Farmers and people whose work is out of doors, calling for very little exercise of accommodation, do not, as a rule, require glasses; but the inhabitants of cities, where the occupations require prolonged and accurate work at short range, these are the people who require artificial aid through the medium of glasses. The tendency of population is toward cities, and here the demand for positions in which one can earn a living so exceeds the supply that defective vision places one entirely out of the race.[13]

Physicians were hard pressed to meet the spiraling demand for eye examinations and provide prescriptions for glasses. Consequently, optometrists and others not trained as physicians took the opportunity to provide vision examinations and prescribe glasses. They advertised themselves as glass fitters and were accused of not being able to differentiate between headaches, double vision, and other symptoms due to diseases of the eye and its lens and those eye conditions brought about by kidney disease, neuralgia, and nervous diseases, which could not be treated effectively by the prescription of eye glasses.[14] Van Fleet continued:

This necessity for perfect vision or for means where it can be obtained has brought about a revolution in the methods of examining eyes and of preparing lenses. It has also brought forward a class of people who, ill prepared to do that which they advertize to be able to do, work harm to the community, the evils of which can hardly be estimated. Here is a position in which the medical profession should take a decided stand. Not only do they owe it to themselves and to the future of the profession, but to the public which —as the showman said—delights in being humbugged. The ophthalmologist knows too well how many unfortunates there are who have lost time travelling from one optician to another for the relief of headache, neuralgia, nervousness, etc., until finally they came to the doctor in despair, only to find that during the time they have spent wandering about their disease has made such strides that death is inevitable.[15]

A revision in the laws that had allowed unqualified individuals to fit eyeglasses and other devices was inevitable. Furthermore, public demand for appliances to correct other bodily impairments led manufacturers and suppliers of the necessary devices, such as trusses and artificial limbs, to fit them to patients without the supervision of a physician. The physician had to learn to respond to the need for mechanisms to rehabilitate those whose bodies were left impaired by disease. Eventually legislation was required to ensure physicians the prerogative to supervise and control all aspects of physical examinations and diagnoses that resulted in the prescription of aids for the body.

DIAGNOSIS OF VISUAL ACUITY:

The economic impact of physical diagnosis became increasingly apparent in the nineteenth century. Major industries were directly effected by improved physical diagnostic techniques. One component of a diagnosis that illustrates this growing importance was diagnosis for eye diseases. The development and application of specific and simple visual tests were crucial to the growth of nineteenth-century industrial technology including the railroad system and factories, in which color discrimination and visual acuity were vital factors.

Many jobs that were introduced or expanded in the nineteenth century by new technologies depended heavily on possessing normal eyesight. The transportation industry reflects the increasing demand for workers with normal eyesight and the efforts of the industry to ensure that their employees met basic vision standards. Ships had been guided in response to colored signals, red on the port side and green on the starboard side, but it often was possible to find someone among the ship's crew to distinguish these colors if the captain was unable to do so. Trains also were controlled by signs and colored signals placed along the tracks, which had to be distinguished quickly by the engineer or signalman, although the engineer could also call upon other crewmen at times to help him distinguish the signals. After accidents began to occur that were attributed to misinterpreting a signal or not seeing it in time, visual acuity tests and color blindness tests were required for railroad trainmen. Earlier, British and American army recruits had been tested for visual defects, but privately controlled companies such as the railroads and others were slower to adopt and require specific visual standards for their employees, as well as the essential physical examinations for determining an individual's relationship to the normal standard of other bodily functions.[16] The early visual tests given to employees were not always satisfactory. In 1891, W. M. Beaumont explained that "the early days of railway travelling were the early days of ophthalmology, and the methods of testing the vision that were in vogue fifty years ago are quite unsuitable now."[17] Vision tests were developed and improved along with other methods of ophthalmologic diagnosis.

COLOR VISION TESTS:

The condition of color vision abnormalities, color blindness or Daltonism, named after the British chemist, John Dalton, one of its illustrious victims, was recognized at least as early as the eighteenth century.[18] Dalton, who was amused by his inability to distinguish red from green, published a detailed description of his condition in 1794. The occupational consequences of color blindness were first called to public attention by George Wilson of Edinburgh, who in 1855 stated the necessity of testing railroad employees and seamen for color vision. Working from studies undertaken by Seebeck in Berlin in 1837, the Swedish physiologist Frithiuf Holmgren of the University of Upsala designed color vision tests and successfully introduced them nationally in the last quarter of the nineteenth century. Holmgren's examination for color blindness was adopted in 1876 and given to all potential employees even before the rules and principles of testing for color blindness were codified into printed instructions.[19]

Holmgren based his test on the Young-Helmholtz theory of color. He proposed that a series of differently colored pieces of wool be presented to the prospective employee. The employee's ability to distinguish all colors was determined by how accurately he or she matched the color wool samples with their equivalents from a large collection of 150 variously colored wool pieces. The purpose of the test was "to discover the chromatic *perception* of the subject disregarding the *names* . . . given to the colors."[20] Color-blind persons often could name the color correctly, although they could not clearly see the color since they had learned to associate the correct term for what appeared gray or colorless to them.[21] Seebeck used colored pieces of paper and glass,[22] as well as Berlin wool, which also was preferred by Holmgren because

it can be procured in all possible colors corresponding to those of the spectrum, and each in all its shades, from the darkest to the lightest. Such selections may be found in trade, and are easily procured when and where desired. It can be used at once, and without any preparation for the examination, just as delivered from the factory. A skein of Berlin wool is equally colored, not only on one or two sides, but on all, and is easily detected in the package, even though there be but one thread of it. Berlin wool is not too strongly glaring and is, moreover, soft and manageable, and can be handled, packed and transported as desired, without damage, and is conveniently ready for use whenever needed.[23]

Holmgren designed a simple test that would reveal color blindness without giving a complete evaluation of the degree of the disability.[24] He was especially proud of his test, for he believed that it was one of

the rare instances in which physiology was of use to humanity "without the intervention of practical medicine."[25] Above all, Holmgren believed that he had attained his goal "of uniformity in the method of examination, in the classification and in the principles relating to the disposal of the *personnel*, [which] cannot be too highly estimated, for this is of consequence not only to science, and especially to statistics, but also to a purely practical end."[26] One man in every twenty-five or 4 percent were found to be color-blind, whereas one woman in 4,000 or 0.004 percent was similarly afflicted.[27] By 1918, color blindness was found to occur in 8.6 percent of men and 2.2 percent of women tested in the United States, while dangerous color blindness was found in 3.1 percent of males and 0.7 percent of females.[28]

The Pennsylvania Railroad Company of Philadelphia was a pioneer in the United States in requiring color vision tests by 1880 of their employees and a more extensive complete physical examination by 1885. Of its 50,000 employees, 10,000 needed to be able to distinguish between red and green lights in their jobs,[29] although this railroad line also used a system of white lights arranged in different patterns to use as signals to the engineers of the trains.

In the period before it was possible to discriminate with precision between the seriously color-insensitive individual and the partially color-blind person, simple color tests were developed that could be applied by nonmedical examiners. Among those devised were tests designed in 1880 by William Thomson, an employee of the Pennsylvania Railroad Company. "These instruments, together with rules for examining and recording the tests, were put into the charge of instructed lay officials, who made the examination and sent their reports to the surgical expert."[30] If a disability was detected from this screening process, a more extensive examination by a medical practitioner was recommended. Those individuals found unsuitable for tasks requiring recognition of signals were assigned to positions in which they could function without having to respond to colors. Four percent of 2,000 individuals were found defective in color vision. Although we have not discussed the methods of testing hearing acuity it is interesting to note that at this time 10 percent were discovered to be partially deaf or visually impaired by the first series of tests.

The color tests Thomson designed involved a further simplification of the Holmgren wool test. Thomson arranged it so that laymen could assist in the examination of 35,000 employees scattered over 2,500 miles of the railroad. The test was also arranged to determine visual acuity, as well as range and field of vision. Thomson described his apparatus for color testing at length and it is useful to note it here since it was a widely used method in the United States:

For the colour perception I have used an instrument composed of two narrow flat sticks hinged together at one end, and fastened by a catch to the other, between which are forty buttons attached to one stick, but capable of easy removal or transportation, and each one numbered from 1 to 40, the numbers being concealed by the second stick. To each button is attached a skein of worsted arranged on the following theory: Experience has taught me the 'confusion colours', for the three *test* colours viz. green, rose and red; and I have used in my arrangement only the real colours like the *tests*, and the 'confusion colours', omitting all the others and reducing the number from 150 to 40. The first twenty buttons have attached on the odd numbers various tints and shades of green, and on the even numbers the known 'confusion colours', grays, tans, light browns, etc.; and this half is for the diagnosis of colour-blindness. The second series, from 21 to 30, have the rose or purples on the odd numbers, and blues on the even; and the third from 31 to 40 have alternately reds and the proper confusion colours for red, viz. browns, sages and dark olives. A man is now placed before this instrument and told to select ten tints to match the *green* test, and if he has colour sense perfect, he promptly turns up over the stick the ten green skeins; a clerk than examines the numbers on the ten buttons, and he will find and record on a blank only odd numbers; the second, *purple* test is then similarly treated, and next the *red*, and if no defect is found, nothing but odd numbers are recorded. When colour-blindness is found, the confusion colours, with all the tests, are on the even numbers on the buttons, and a glance at the record enables an absent supervising officer to know that the man must be colour-blind, and to verify the examination by referring to a similar instrument in his own possession. No great skill, and no professional knowledge is needed to make this record, and the theory of the arrangement is so simple that a glance enables one to know, from the written report of the examination, the exact colours that were selected, and to decide if they were indicative of colour-blindness.[31]

At first both employees and employers, especially in England, were hesitant to evaluate an individual's ability to distinguish colors and decipher letters because some of the tests were considered faulty. Those who were inclined to criticize a basic test like the Holmgren test for color blindness withheld their comments out of fear that the examination would be abandoned altogether, since it had taken so much effort to get the British Board of Trade to apply the test routinely to all job applicants. Laborers whose jobs were placed in jeopardy by failing a vision test

soon enlisted local politicians in an effort to discredit the tests or the fact that they should be used as determinants of who qualifies for or retains a job. Nevertheless, visual examinations were continued.

The major criteria for vision testing adopted by the railroads in the 1890s included that the tests be administered by qualified physicians, that a minimal visual standard be established for each job, and that employees be reexamined regularly or at least once a year. Reexamination was crucial since failure of sight is often insidious. As Beaumont explained, "of all the senses it is the one most likely to change with advancing years"[32] and, therefore, requires periodic examination. The visual standards adopted by the Special International Committee appointed by the International Medical Congress in London in 1881 were that the

engine driver or stoker [possess] normal acuity of vision for form and normal refraction . . . and that vision for colours should amount to at least four-fifths of the normal. For other branches of railway services perfect vision for form was demanded for one eye only, while the other might attain to only half the standard. But colour vision of at least three-fourths of the normal was required. It was recognized by all that full acuity both for form and colour would be better, but the above standards was adopted as a minimum in view of the practical difficulties in securing a sufficiency of employees with sight perfect in all respects.[33]

Cooperation between railway authorities, ophthalmologists, and optometrists was needed to resolve the difficulties in the tests required for various jobs. Malcolm McHardy, an English specialist in ophthalmology rode the trains and observed from the vantage point of the trainmen to determine that "the visibility of railway semaphore signals ranges according to the state of the atmosphere, but almost as much according to the nature of the background against which they are seen, and which latter changes much with the seasons of the year."[34] He simulated "longsightedness," "shortsightedness," and astigmatism by wearing glasses with these defections, "for having become well acquainted with the signals, etc. on some eighty miles of railroad," he could see for himself how each of these conditions would handicap someone working on the train. McHardy thus demonstrated the weakness of "practical tests" when given under favorable conditions, especially those for distinguishing between red and green colors.[35]

Diagnostic tests for color vision were challenged in several ways by F. W. Edridge-Green, the noted British color authority, who devised yet another color vision test. He believed also that unless colored lights were presented under the varying conditions of fog, rain, hail, and snow that confronted the trainmen, the lights were useless as test objects. He criticized the Holmgren wools for possessing the defects growing out of the Young-Helmholtz theory on which the test was based. Furthermore, there was difficulty in obtaining correctly colored wools that did not fade and become soiled with use. The greens in particular were made more obvious by the changes due to handling them.[36] Asking an individual to name the color of objects selected at random was inefficient and uncertain. Testing for color distinction by asking the applicant to choose complementary colors was more likely to result in detection of the ignorant rather than the color-blind person, since color sense may be diminished but not enough to prevent a person from seeing complementary colors.[37]

One practical solution for meeting the needs of the color-blind individual was proposed by A. E. Wright in 1892, who adopted Hering's theory of color. Based on the concept that most color-blind individuals could see other colors, especially yellow and blue, Wright suggested that red lights be mixed with yellow hues and green lights mixed with blue hues, so that the person with color-deficient sight would be able to distinguish green and red.[38] Traffic lights continue to be manufactured on this principle.

By the turn of the century, the Holmgren color-blind test was the most universally applied test, although its inability to indicate less severe forms of the malady was acknowledged. Edridge-Green claimed that six varieties of color blindness could not be detected with the Holmgren test and that over one-third of those rejected by it, upon reexamination, were found to be normal for color perception.[39] The most obvious failure of the Holmgren wool test for those whose color sense had to function at great distances was a failure to test for this ability. Edridge-Green called this test and others of its type a test of "chromic myopia."

Thomas Bickerton of the Liverpool Royal Infirmary learned that the Holmgren test would not single out an individual with a slight degree of abnormal color sense; therefore, he sent one of his patients to the physicist, Oliver Lodge, who tested him with a spectroscope and discovered that the person could not distinguish slight changes in the shades of red. Bickerton concluded that "a person who loses the power to discriminate between colours at a distance, but retains it at close quarters, is clearly possessed of

a type of abnormal colour perception, which the Holmgren wool test can never discover."[40] He recommended that a quantitative test for color sight be instituted.[41]

A decade later, Edridge-Green revealed the success he had had in devising sophisticated color-blindness tests in the Hunterian Lecture, which he presented before the Royal College of Surgeons of England on 1 and 3 February 1911.[42] As a long-time student of the phenomenon, he recognized two distinct objectives of color-blindness tests: "those which are used for the purpose of ascertaining the special phenomena of colour blindness, and those which are employed when the inquiry is made for some special purpose."[43] The limitations of the tests included fixing an arbitrary standard and attempting not "to exclude a greater number than is absolutely necessary." Those with exceptional color sense also should be singled out "so that the captain might know on whom to rely in conditions of exceptional difficulty."[44]

Edridge-Green designed a lantern, which was manufactured by Reiner and Keeler of London and the New York-based company of Meyrowitz in its London plant. The lantern contained four discs; three carrying seven colored glasses and one with seven modifying glasses. Edridge-Green described it:

Each disc has a clear aperture. The other mechanical details are: an electric or oil lamp with projecting accessories, a diaphragm for diminishing the size of the light projected, handles for moving the discs, and the indicator showing the colour or modifier in use. The diaphragm is graduated in respect to three apertures to represent a 5½ inch railway signal bull's eye at 600, 800 and 1,000 yards respectively when the test is made at twenty feet.[45]

The inventor claimed to have constructed the test according to all the facts related to color blindness. He claimed to have obtained outstanding results with his test lantern. "I have never met with a single colour-blind person who has not been readily and easily detected with my lantern though I have examined many who have passed other lanterns and in some cases a number of other tests for colour blindness. In most cases, one turn of the wheel will be sufficient to make a color-blind person disclose his defect."[46]

Edridge-Green, unlike Holmgren, insisted that the individual being tested be allowed to indicate the colors presented to him by their names. There was no special test value in matching up one colored object with another, since everyone reacted to colors by the names that they associated with them. "The more an examiner has practical experience of colour blindness, the more will he recognize the fact that the colour blind are guided by their sensations of colour."[47] His lantern test picked up twelve out of 300 cases of color blindness among those being routinely examined, while the Holmgren test revealed only one in 300 of those being tested by the railroad companies.[48] The Edridge-Green lantern became the most acceptable instrument in the United States for indicating the dangerously color-blind individual, who could never distinguish between red and green, as well as those who were only slightly color-blind.[49]

Other tests Edridge-Green recommended were those for classifying individuals according to the degree of color blindness. These consisted of "four test colours and 180 confusion colours; 150 coloured wools, 10 skeins of silk, 10 small squares of coloured cardboard, and 10 small squares of coloured glass, representing the whole series of colors."[50] These colors were chosen for the purpose of presenting as much difficulty as possible to the color-blind person and as little as possible to the normally sighted individual. A pocket test, consisting of nineteen cards on which 112 single threads of wool were arranged, and a spectrometer, which could expose a portion of the light spectrum between any two desired wavelengths, completed the tests Edridge-Green thought were suitable and effective in testing for color blindness.

CLARITY OF VISION TESTS:

For the purpose of testing clarity of vision, a variety of examinations were proposed. The most widely adopted test, one designed by Herman Snellen in 1862, was based on the observation that in healthy eyes two points are seen separately when they are placed so that they subtend an angle of one minute. To make use of this fact, Snellen designed an alphabet of block letters with five component parts in the vertical and horizontal directions (see figure 9.1). Suggestions for improving Snellen's test included putting letters that are visually confusing on one line, i.e., O, C, G, and Q, using only certain letters (Oliver's suggestions) or differently shaped letters (designed by Charles M. Colver and James Wallace and published by Wall and Ochs of Philadelphia) and finally, using simple, constant geometrical figures. Edward Jackson chose an incomplete square arranged in four positions with the open end pointing in different directions. H. C. Boden and Co. published this test.[51]

To compensate for those individuals who might be

able to memorize an eye chart, in 1894 Edward W. Heckel of Pittsburgh, Pennsylvania, specialist in eye and ear diseases, designed a test chart with revolving rows of letters, including some printed in different type styles. The chart

consisted of a tripod upon which revolved a triangular box, presenting three flat surfaces, provided with grooves for the reception of strips of cardboard. There are nine of these spaces for the corresponding nine rows of letters from CC to X inclusive, on each side, thus giving three distinct surfaces which can be presented to view by simply turning the triangular box. The one in use [manufactured by Feick Bros.] is provided with ten distinct sets, including pot-hooks and German letters. This gives ninety rows of letters which when used, nine at a time, enables us to make almost an infinite number of combinations; enough, at least, to outwit the memory of our brightest patients.[52]

Another combination test card designed two years earlier to minimize the effects of memory was made by GaNun and Parsons of New York after D. W. Hunter's design.

The letters are arranged in rows, as on the ordinary test card, but instead of using a card, the letters are placed on revolving horizontal bars set in a frame, each bar having four sides. The bars are readily turned by buttons at the side of the frame. There are nine of these bars corresponding to the nine rows of letters from CC to X inclusive. As each of the nine bars has four rows of letters, one on each side, the arrangement provides for thirty-six rows of letters in the space of an ordinary test card, nine rows being visible at the same time. A quarter turn of two or three of the bars completely changes the appearance of the card, and the number of possible combinations of thirty-six, taken at a time, is almost endless, running into the millions.[53]

Improvements in tests continued apace, although for use en masse, sophistication in testing was limited by its cost. Elaborate tests for vision and the other senses such as those administered in physiology and experimental psychology laboratories of the period were too expensive to be used in screening prospective employees. Companies, which continuously hired new employees and retested older employees, required quick and cheaper tests. However, as employers assessed the investment they had made in their staffs, they found it economical to do some testing in order to diagnose and correct disabilities such as visual impairments, which lent themselves to adjustment by the use of spectacles.

Criticism of some of the sensory tests used on students and prospective employees included both the quality and design of the test materials. William S.

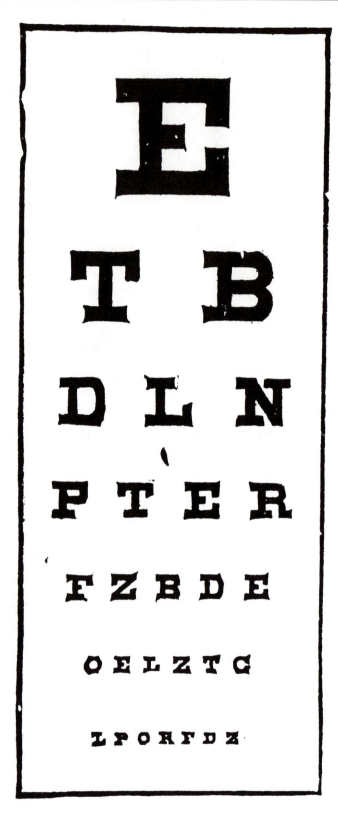

Figure 9.1. Snellen's 1862 eye test type for twenty-foot distance. From A. S. Aloe Catague, circa 1893, p. 192, *SI Photo No. 78–10552.*

Dennett demonstrated at the Ophthalmological Society of London in 1885 that the letters imprinted on vision test cards were not equally visible at the same distance. Although specialists had realized that some letters were easier to see than others (A, I, V, U, C were seen at the greatest distances and B and S at the least distance) the degree of difference had not been worked out carefully nor had a model been proposed for correcting the disparity over the several decades (1867-1887) since the test had been adopted. Dennett, therefore, designed according to mathematical laws letters that could be uniformly discriminated at specific distances.[54] Other visual defects brought forth an intriguing variety of tests. Astigmatism, which is a defect of the lens resulting in visual distortion of objects, was the most common eye disease detected (see figure 9.2). To test for this condition, William Little devised a system employing letters placed at a specific distance and position from the observer, which replaced more complex tests that used the ophthalmoscope, retinoscope, and kerotoscope. Underneath these letters, he placed the letters as they would appear to the victim of astigmatism. Both the words and combination of letters would appear the same to the patient who was astigmatic. For instance, FOOL

and PCCI would appear as FOOL to someone with astigmatism. Little's test, manufactured by J. W. Queen and Co. of Philadelphia, was one of a series of tests, including Dr. Pray's astigmatic letters and Dr. John Green's test diagrams for the detection and measurement of astigmatism (see figure 9.3).[55]

Vision examinations for those seeking disability pensions required awareness of other examination standards and techniques, for it was expected that a number of applicants would be imposters

who really have nothing abnormal about their eyes; they, in many instances having been induced by pension agents to add eye disease to their many other real or supposed infirmities, [or] . . . having slight disease or abnormal condition, which they greatly magnify, [or] . . . disease may have at one time existed and now have disappeared; but once having been on the pension rolls, they dislike to have their name stricken therefrom, [or] whose trouble originated prior to their enlistment, or subsequent to their discharge from the service, [or who] fancy themselves entitled to a pension on account of failing sight incident to age, and other factors which we know have nothing to do with exposure incident to army service, or have been stricken from the rolls, or rated too low, or never pensioned at all, because the medical examiner has either failed to detect existing disease, or underestimated its gravity.[56]

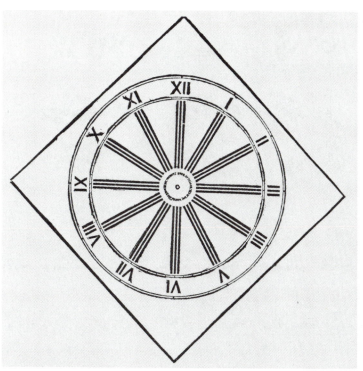

Figure 9.2. Green's astigmatic dial circa 1893, from A. S. Aloe Catalogue, p. 193. *SI Photo No. 78-10553.*

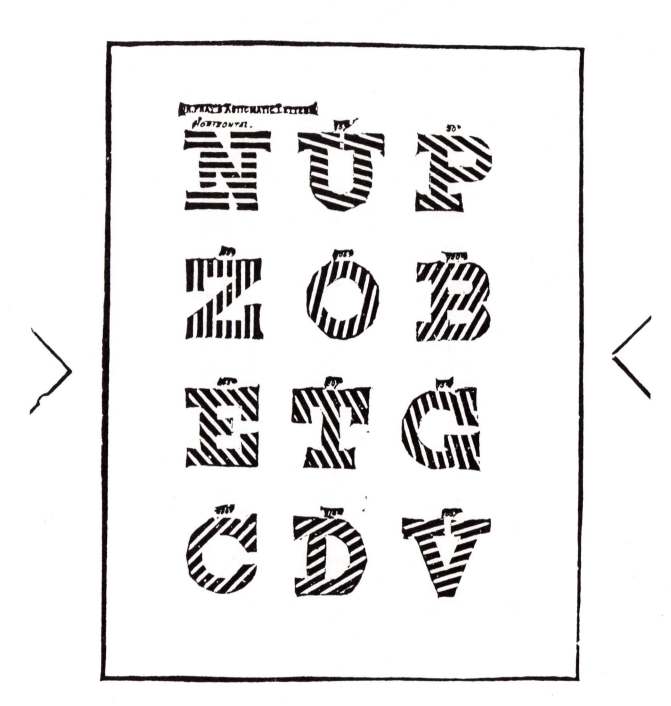

Figure 9.3. Pray's letters for testing vision, circa 1893, from A. S. Aloe Catalogue, p. 193. SI Photo No. 78-10555.

To determine if an anomaly of refraction (nearsightedness or farsightedness) existed, convex lenses of 1/42, 1/15, 1/10, and 1/5 diopters and concave lenses of 1/30, 1/20, 1/10, 1/5, and 1/3 diopters were sufficient, since finding out the exact degree of anomaly was not necessary for deciding on eligibility for a pension. A number of other aids and techniques were suggested, especially the use of an ophthalmoscope "as every disease behind the lens is a sealed book, objectively, without its aid." As we have noted earlier, the ophthalmoscope required "as much daily practice with it as it is necessary to the acquisition of a foreign living language."[57]

Industrial-sponsored physical examinations were eliminated when other dependable sources of health data were available. The excellent reputation of health standards adopted by life insurance companies as indicators in selecting policyholders spread through the rest of the business world. Firms did not require physical examinations of potential employees who had passed a life insurance physical examinations. Therefore, since those who had obtained life insurance policies could obtain jobs more readily, the number of individuals who brought insurance as adolescents so that they would be eligible for jobs increased, thus providing more income for the insurance companies[58] and increasing the role insurance companies played in determining health standards. Medical examinations given under the auspices of life insurance companies were viewed as models for other physicians to emulate. B. Joy Jeffries of Boston singled out life insurance companies for the care with which they chose medical examiners to test for color blindness by equating "examinations for life insurance [with] . . . a specialty."[59]

Physicians developed many diagnostic tests for understanding and predicting the functional potential of the body. Many of these tests were designed and evaluated by medical specialists, who examined each organ or region of the body and adapted their examinations to select for the unique physical requirements of each job or profession. Eye testing equipment provides only one example of the various types of aids and devices available to physicians by the early twentieth century. (See figures 9.4, 9.5, and 9.6.) National and international medical groups were formed to coordinate the myriad details involved in designing tests and testing instruments and to organize and evaluate the copious data generated by their use. Attempts by physicians to describe diseases more uniformly through the aid of technology and the data gathered collectively will be discussed to show how the intel-

lectual climate created by technology developed within medicine.

UNIFORMITY:

IN MEASUREMENT:

The society of physicians as society had to be strengthened in order to control and organize medical instruments and the data revealed by them. National medical societies through national and international meetings brought some of the technological consequences of medicine to the surface and spurred a cooperative interest in forming special committees to respond to the complex and ever-varying demands of society stemming from disease. The issues that spawned the earliest activity were related to the scientific and technological aspects of medical practice, since these had to be agreed upon and standardized to facilitate communication between all physicians. The campaign to bring uniformity into the practice of medicine was focused at the 1876 meeting of the American Medical Association and International Congress of Medicine in Philadelphia. This was "a world's Congress brought together for the discussion of general principles in medicine, general laws of disease, general methods of observation and study, and the general influence of climate, altitude, etc."[60] American leaders boosted the idea of uniformity in medicine and made it viable in this period, when international meetings were "in their infancy of usefulness."[61] Eduoard Seguin Sr. devoted his considerable talent at the end of his life to the organization of a committee for introducing uniform international medical standards essential to conduct international medical meetings where language differences and differing concepts of disease hindered effective communication among the participants. He pointed to the naturalists and chemists, who had created a standard nomenclature, including symbols and measurements, commencing at the end of the seventeenth century, for overcoming the language barriers in their fields and who served as examples of the types of standards for which physicians should strive.[62] Pharmacists were among the first in the medical community to seek actively a uniform system that applied to the measurement, naming, and dispensing of prescription drugs. They began to set up committees in 1865 at the First Pharmaceutic Congress in Brunswick. Although decisions were reached to use the metric system and the Latin language to describe drugs, an international formulary had not been produced by 1876, when

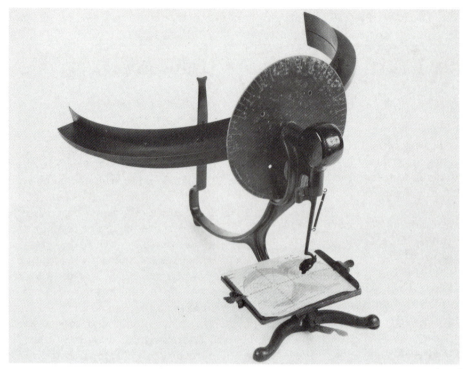

Figure 9.4. Self-recording perimeter designed by F. D. Skeel and manufactured by E. B. Meyrowitz of New York. Measures 52.7 x 55.6 x 38 cms. *NMAH No. M 7027, SI Photo No. 76-6504.*

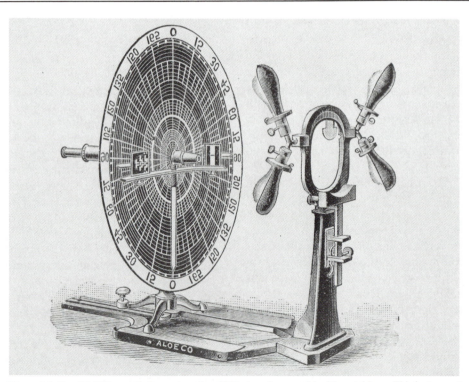

Figure 9.5. Javal-Schiötz ophthalmometer, circa 1893, American model with metal base. This instrument is intended for measuring the corneal curvature after the method described by Helmholtz in his text on physiological optics. From A. S. Aloe Catalogue, p. 171. *SI Photo No. 78–10549.*

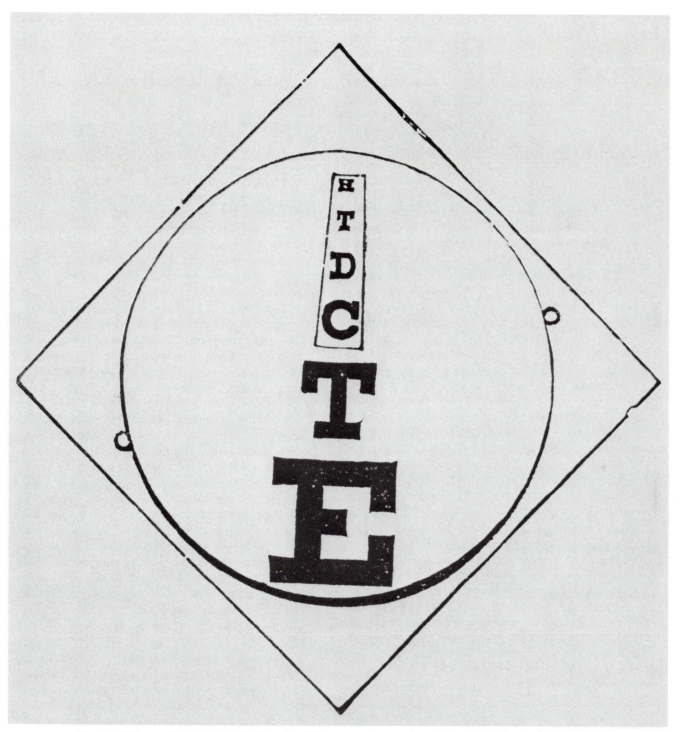

Figure 9.6. Thomson's interchangeable disc, circa 1893, mounted on pasteboard, from A. S. Aloe Catalogue, p. 193. *SI Photo No. 78–10554.*

physicians were invited to contribute to the committee preparing the standards. Adoption of the metric system continued to be debated for several decades among pharmacists and physicians. German pharmacists adopted the metric system in 1858, whereas the American and English pharmacopoeias were published in metric units for the first time in 1898. The adoption of metric units was hastened by the use of these units among scientists and by the fact that the metric system was less ambiguous. Laboratory equipment and other devices manufactured in Germany and France were calibrated in metric units. Since these countries supplied a large amount of medical equipment, it became necessary for all physicians to know the metric system to use the equipment. Primarily, two metric units were used by the pharmacist and the physician. These were the gram and the cubic centimeter, which presented few opportunities for confusion or misinterpretations for those unaccustomed to the metric system.[63] Papers were read in the sectional meetings of otology, ophthalmology, and pharmacy urging uniform measurements in these fields, primarily through adoption of the metric system, which was acceptable to those attending the sessions. Pathologists, clinicians, and others would soon follow in succeeding congresses with plans for standardization of the data and equipment employed in their special areas.

The American Medical Association appointed a committee to include Seguin, which would represent American physicians in Europe and advocate uniformity in clinical reports. At the International Medical Congress in Geneva in 1877, Seguin reported the following recommendations, which were adopted by the Congress: (1) that a universal pharmacopoeia be composed in Latin; (2) that all weights and measures be recorded in the decimal system and the Centigrade scale be marked on thermometers; (3) that a uniform nomenclature for chemicals be used (perhaps those of the Swedish chemist Berzelius); (4) that chemical preparations of determined strength and purity be prescribed and (5) that Galenic preparations be made as simple as possible. These five points reflect the effort applied over a decade to standardize drugs.[64] Adoption of the metric system in medical reports, medical texts, and hospital reports remained a goal in successive standardization programs. Seguin pursued application of the metric system in medicine at the International Medical Meeting in Amsterdam in 1879, and while traveling in Europe, he spoke in its behalf in Cork and Lyon shortly before his death in 1880.[65] Seguin's goal in medicine was supported by

the adoption in 1883 of the metric system in the scientific community and by the impetus of its applications in other areas, some of which were initially exhibited to the public at the Exhibition of 1851 in London.[66]

Physicians suggested various schemes for implementing the metric system. Some of these schemes combined features of the English and metric systems. George N. Kreider of Springfield, Illinois was among the group of scientists and physicians who encouraged use of the metric system by devising an "Americanized" metric system of apothecaries weights, which he suggested be printed on the back of every prescription blank. He drew up a table of conversions between grains, ounces, and grams.[67]

One impediment to the adoption of the metric system was that American pharmacists were not always familiar with the system and did not always have the properly graduated equipment to prepare drugs from prescriptions written in metric units. M. S. Buttle of New York reported a serious error on the part of the pharmacist who filled a prescription Buttle had written in metric measures. His solution to the problem he encountered was to stop using the metric system until pharmacists were required to be examined in its use and registered when competent and when they possessed adequate equipment to apply it.[68]

The rural practitioner had to find a method of ensuring the accuracy of drugs in identification, dosage, and quality. Simplified apparatus provided these physicians with the means to prepare their own prescriptions when they could not call upon a pharmacist to compound a drug. Robert M. Fuller of New York designed a simplified pill- and tablet-making machine in 1878 "for physicians practicing in the country, to whose use they are adapted by reason of their economy, dose-accuracy, compactness and palatable form for dispensing."[69] Physicians also were advised to prepare their own drugs when there was a danger that the pharmacist might alter the prescription because he or she thought it to be too potent.[70]

The American plan of uniformity urged by Seguin and others was proposed to tie the efforts of all specialists together. Medical technology provided a means to make the measurements for applying statistics or the numerical method and the concept of the average person to medical practice. Made more precise and practical by the invention of instruments of "positive diagnosis" including the thermometer, spirometer, and sphygmograph, the numerical method was "distinguishable by the broadness of its application to physic; being at the same time a principle and a method.''[71] Seguin expected that

the uniform application of the numerical method will render infinitely more abundant, accessible, readable, comparable and trustworthy, the observations on which the leaders support their theories or discoveries, and by which the country-practitioner will connect his mind with the medical movement, and eventually act his part in it. It is so that the records of each will be of service to all. . . . The diagnosis will become more and more precise and mathematical. The course of diseases will be more and more represented in figures or idealized in graphic traces. The action of medication on the organism, and the reaction of the functions on the treatment will be registered and reckoned as book-accounts.[72]

IN RECORD KEEPING:

The evolution of materials used to record the anatomic and physiologic parameters of a patient rapidly increased in the second half of the nineteenth century. For centuries, physicians had recorded their diagnostic findings in full statements or, to shorten their record keeping, in descriptive technical terms or an improvised shorthand. As the distinctions between the normal and abnormal became more specific and described in terms of numbers, colors, and sounds revealed through instruments and laboratory tests, specially designed and labeled forms to accommodate these terms were manufactured. A record of each time the pulse, temperature, blood pressure, or other parameter was measured was most easily read and interpreted when laid out in a graphic form or when several physical characteristics were compared in columns organized for quick inspection.

One complete physician's form called the "Visiting List" was distributed by Lindsay and Blakiston of Philadelphia and W. T. Keener of Chicago. Introduced in 1851, it came in several sizes to accommodate the record keeping for 25, 50, 75, and even 100 patients per week. It could be bought in six-month blocks or an edition with perpetually extending space. Among the useful information in the 1887 edition was a

ready method in asphyxia, a table of poisons and antidotes, tables of the metric system, a dose table rewritten to accord with the sixth revision of the U.S. Pharmacopoeia, a table of disinfectants, directions for the examination of urine, a table of standard reference books, table of incompatibles, a new table for computing the period of uterogestation, a list of new remedies for 1886-7, Sylvester's method for artificial respiration, and a diagram of the chest, besides the blank leaves for visiting lists, monthly memoranda, addresses of patients, nurses and others, of accounts rendered, memoranda of wants, obstetric and vaccination engagements, record of births and deaths, and cash account.[73]

Specialized tables, charts, and forms were constructed to meet the needs of each medical specialty. For instance, the application of the graphic method to hearing tests led to the design of a chart manufactured by E. B. Meyrowitz

to provide the otologist with a means of representing the results of tuning fork and other tests in a form more intelligible than that commonly used. In this chart the hearing power is expressed in percentages which are based upon the results obtained from the use of Hartmann's tuning forks, the acoumeter, the voice and the watch. The percentage line on each side of the central columns in numbered from 0 to 200, the 100 line being the line of normal hearing for all tests. The percentages employed are based upon the averages of a large number of tests made upon normal ears, and modified by comparing them with Hartmann's results. These averages have been printed . . . and a rapid calculation can be made from the percentage table which is printed on the back of each chart.[74]

This chart revealed at a glance the deviations from the normal of each patient examined and helped to organize the physician's thoughts in making a diagnosis of hearing acuity.

Temperature and diet charts were published by Wodderspoon and Co. in London. These low-cost charts were exhibited at the Annual Museum of the British Medical Association in 1887 and successive years.[75] Charts listing the instruments and appliances required for ordinary major and minor operations also were published. These were designed for the use of house-surgeons, junior practitioners, and surgical dressers, by Dr. L. Hepenstal Omsby.[76]

Outline diagrams of the organs were printed by Danielsson and Co. of London. These were designed to be filled in by the diagnostician for inclusion in a notebook or hospital report. They were provided with gum on the back for easy attachment to a report. Specially commended were those of the brain and spinal cord. They were exhibited at the Annual Museum in 1886.[77]

Dentists found it expedient to record on enlarged printed diagrams of the mouth and teeth the repairs and extractions they had made. One observer wryly commented that keeping these records necessitated "almost as much skill to properly record the operation in the diagram as to perform it in the mouth."[78] With this information correlated with a series of cards on file, which contained accounts of the diagnosis and treatment performed during each visit, the dentist was in a position to document his work thoroughly.

Insurance company medical examiners sometimes were unable to satisfy company medical directors with the reports of their examinations. One suggestion to help the physician organize the information sent in to the company was a printed form that brought together into a table all the pertinent facts. An example published in 1873 was a form designed to record family history. It contained columns for age, condition of health, age at death, length of illness, and previous health record of the parents and siblings of the applicant.[79] Major life insurance companies, led by John Hancock, supplied printed medical record forms that contained extensive questions for both the applicant and physician to answer. The list of ailments to be particularly noted included dizziness, diarrhea, delirium tremens, frequent desire to urinate, jaundice, lumps or swellings in any part of the body, open sores, back pain, swelling of the hands and feet, and stricture of the urethra. Questions to prompt the examiner included: "does he [the applicant] look older than the age stated; if so how many years older? Is there any indication that he is not entirely well?"[80]

Card files containing a patient's medical examination history were another form of recording and storing information. Robert Dickinson of New York recommended 6- by 6⅔- inch cards arranged alphabetically, which could be filed in a small box and carried about. Outline stamps of the organs and basic information printed on the card helped to organize the card and fill it up efficiently. The model for Dickinson's card was one used by the libraries in the Johns Hopkins Dispensary.[81]

Diagrams, charts, and various shorthand notations made graphic the records of the various sounds heard within the chest. R. C. M. Page of New York, who drew on the texts of the leading American teachers of diagnostic techniques (Loomis, Flint, DaCosta) suggested arrow-labeled diagrams be used to distinguish the respiratory sounds according to their duration, pitch, and other sounds produced when specific diseases are present. If one diagrammed normal respiration, expiration would appear shorter and lower in pitch than inspiration.[82]

Among the numerous nursing aids beginning to appear at the end of the nineteenth century were a slate and a printed form labeled with headings such as stimulants, diet, pulse, respiration, temperature,

sleep, and so on. These could be filled in for each patient by the nurse or physician. Fannin and Co. of Dublin produced the slate and H. Gilbertson and Sons of London published the forms.[83] (See figure 9.7.)

Printed scales and gauges such as those to be used with the various sizes of urethral instruments were made according to the standards adopted in the United States, France, and England. The American scale introduced by van Buren and Keyes increased in units of one-half millimeter beginning with the minimum diameter, designated by the number one, and continuing up to No. 23 or a diameter of 12 millimeters. The French scale increased by units of one-third millimeter. Thus, an instrument of nine millimeters' diameter was No. 18 on the American and No. 27 on the French scale. The English scale was irregular and differed between different makers and authors.[84]

The bookkeeping and accounting aspects of medical practice stimulated the design and production of special record books, provided by enterprising firms. Physicians' bills and receipt ledgers for the office, as well as to carry in the pocket, were copyrighted in 1887 by Henry Bernal and Co. of St. Louis, Missouri and advertised in *JAMA* of 1888. A diagram of the ledger book was displayed in the advertisement, "showing a condensed cash account with cash receipts from both 'regular' and 'transient' patients for each day in the year, besides four additional ruled pages for memoranda such as the 'address of nurses,' 'future engagements,' 'private consultation,' etc."[85] It was handsomely bound in Russian Bark and Corners with cloth sides and a spring back.

Seguin elaborated further on the practical consequences of records generated by instruments for all physicians.

Physicians are expected to no more write their prescriptions or [sic] borrowed slips of paper without keeping a copy, or on druggists' blank advertizements; neither to record their cases on pocket-books which contain the names of all the saints to be daily invoked to obtain a cure, instead of on books on which can be noted the physiological signs or aberrations of function which characterize diseases. The uniformity of the tables of observation used in private and hospital practice, will furnish the sure elements of medical statistics, not only in regard to the transitory population of hospitals, but to the families treated at home; it will present for the first time the true and full data for a history of health and disease.[86]

In recognizing the problems associated with improper and inadequate record keeping among physi-

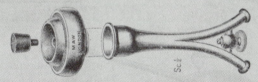
Figure 9.7. Charts advertised in 1897. Photo by author from *London Medical Gazette.*

cians, Seguin called attention to an aspect of medical technology that soon attracted a number of designers and manufacturers. Problems encountered in amassing large amounts of health and sickness data were alleviated by the appearance of simplified and well-organized data-gathering charts, lists, and other record-keeping units. Many types of charts were produced; however, few of these items ever became objects sought after by zealous collectors, so that our knowledge of the variety and extent of these items must largely be extracted from medical texts and journals and from among hospital records of the period. Seguin designed a few prescription and record blanks, which were manufactured by William Wood and Co.[87] Other charts, manufactured by George Charles Coles, superceded charts manufactured by Salt that were smaller and less convenient to use. Coles' charts contained columns for recording both the Centigrade and Fahrenheit systems and were relatively inexpensive; they cost one shilling for a book of twelve blanks or six shillings for one hundred loose charts useful in the hospital.[88] Salt and Son advertised pocket thermometer charts with Centigrade and Fahrenheit scales printed in two columns. Dotted lines traced on the charts showed the normal limits of variation between body temperatures. Additional space for notes on the urine, pulse, and respiration was also provided. These charts were sold in books of fifty and were perforated for easy removal.

IN TREATMENT:

In keeping with the trend toward exact measurement, forms of treatment other than the administration of drugs also were prescribed according to specified dosages in the nineteenth century. For instance, exercise prescribed for patients with cardiac disease was allotted in exact amounts, which were gradually increased. Max Joseph Oertel made maps of regions in Bavaria, which indicated in different colors the level, slightly sloping, moderately sloping, and steep paths his patients should take, depending on the severity of their illness. The trees were marked according to the colors of the map, so that each path could be easily identified. Benches were available for resting. Oertel believed that "by systematic practice on the easier paths heart and system are progressively trained and strengthened. Intelligent analysis may do the same work for cycling, horseback-riding and many other familiar exercises. In this way the dosage is practically reduced to a definite number of kilogrammetres in a given time, and a step has been taken in placing the prescription of exercise upon a scientific basis."[89] The design and production of numerous exercise devices by the Swedish gymnastic teacher Peter Ling and his followers, including Gustav Zander, advanced the program of prescribing specific amounts of exercise for all parts of the body. Machines to exercise the arms, legs, torso, head, neck, back, fingers, and other body parts were constructed and enabled the patient who could find a way to these units, to receive a daily, weekly, and monthly allotment of prescribed exercises.[90]

The diseases for which these mechanically applied exercises were prescribed were not restricted to the muscular system. Vibrations or fine shaking movements were applied for an enlarged spleen resulting from malaria and for other conditions such as ulcers, abscesses, fainting, and palpitation.[91]

Electricity was another source of treatment that needed to be measured. A. D. Rockwell of New York reviewed galvanic current dosage and concluded that "the human system reacts to no drug with such varying susceptibility as to electricity."[92] Electrosurgery required a "definitive expenditure of force," which Rockwell measured in milliamperes with a new meter that recorded from 0.1 ma to 500 ma. Although he could not claim any greater success in using electrotherapy when it was measured with a milliammeter, Rockwell believed a beginning electrotherapist "should no more think of attempting serious work without his indicator of current strength, than he should administer his drugs without his apothecary's measure."[93]

One other area in which standardization vastly improved the practice was dentistry. Some of the most detailed and rigid standards were required in the repair and replacement of teeth. The small size of the tooth surfaces to be rebuilt after the enamel was destroyed by decay made it imperative that the substances used to restore teeth expand and contract as little as possible so that they would remain within the tooth after it had been filled. To find the mixture or amalgam of metals that had these critical properties and also be resistant to corrosion, compatible with the body tissues, and attractive in the mouth required extensive testing on many patients. Greene Vardiman Black of Chicago perfected a process for making amalgams that were alloys of mercury and another metal, which for dental purposes was silver. After perfecting the amalgam, he taught metallurgists employed by dental manufacturers how to make and control the delicate balance of the metal mixture. Black made many of his own tools. He used a micrometer that was accurate to between 0.5 and 0.0001 of an inch, and he checked his measurements under a binocular microscope.[94]

Black developed a chart for mapping the teeth to record the site and extent of tooth decay, as well as the placement of each filling within a tooth. His aim in repairing teeth was to restore their natural contours and forms. Shunning patents and the possibility of extensive royalties on his inventions, Black received many encomiums from his dental colleagues and the medical profession. He is ranked as one of the most outstanding American dentists, in a specialty in which the United States has been considered unparalleled in excellence for technique and effectiveness since the mid-nineteenth century. The intense scrutiny of details enabled Black to establish the standards of filling teeth that brought this practice to perfection.

Keeping records of various aspects of disease was facilitated by the books, charts, graphs, and specialized tools and also by the leaders of medical societies, who arranged for the collection of information from all physicians who could be convinced of the need to report their observations on selected diseases. So that the collection of disease-related statistics would be useful to the greatest number of practitioners, all physicians were asked to fill out inquiry cards containing specific questions, which were collected, analyzed, and then published.

THE COLLECTIVE INVESTIGATION OF DISEASE:

Collecting data on disease through patient histories is fundamental to medical practice and has roots in antiquity. Physicians have supported their theories and descriptions of diseases with examples of those who contracted the disease and the subsequent experiences of the attending physician in evolving treatment. A new treatment or technique was introduced with an account of its use and effect on a small group of patients. These practices continued into the twentieth century.[95] An attempt was made to greatly expand the reports of experiences with diseases and their treatments in the nineteenth century. Medical societies began to sponsor projects for gathering clinical data from among their members and to explore unanswered questions about major diseases.

One of the most effective uses of the collective investigation technique in the nineteenth century was in the gathering of statistics to demonstrate the relative safety of the major types of chemicals used as anesthetics. Several fatalities among patients given chloroform alerted physicians to its potential danger

in the late 1840s and started the debate over its safety that would last throughout the century.

Although ether was the first anesthetic to be successfully used in an operation, the ease with which chloroform could be administered, coupled with the poor performance of the early ether inhalers and the lesser amount of chloroform required to produce deep narcosis, led physicians and surgeons to prefer chloroform as early as 1847. The announcement of the first fatalities after the administration of chloroform in 1847-1848 forced some French and Viennese surgeons to return to the use of ether or mixtures of the two gases. Others remained convinced of the benign nature of chloroform until it was statistically demonstrated at the end of the century that ether was safer.[96] Statistics were collected in a number of hospitals to document the number of patients who had died while under sedation with either anesthetic gas.[97] The Chloroform Committee Report of 1864 had alerted the British to the dangers of chloroform, but they only began to substitute ether after they were instructed by the American ophthalmologist, B. Joy Jeffries, in the use of the ether sponge. John Mason Warren of Boston in February 1847 had introduced the bell-shaped sponge for giving ether. It was applied directly to the nose and mouth or enclosed in a cone made from a towel, cardboard, felt, leather, or metal.[98] The sponge remained the major ether applicator throughout the nineteenth century in the United States.

In 1892, Ernst Julius Güerlt, surgeon and historian of surgery in Berlin, reported that he had collected on behalf of the German Surgical Society 24,625 reports of anesthesia administrations in 1890 and another 84,605 reports from sixty-two observers in 1891. In 1890, six deaths occurred, and the following year thirty-three were reported. Chloroform accounted for one in out of 8,431 cases.[99] These figures impressed the surgical profession, which then recommended ether or, on occasion, a mixture of chloroform and ether. Many provincial surgeons on the continent did not use any anesthetic until the last quarter of the century since they lacked both gases and the devices to administer them.[100]

The most comprehensive collective data-gathering program, which lasted from 1881 to 1887, was sponsored by the British Medical Association.[101] Leaders of the British medical profession spearheaded a national, and shortly thereafter, an international program to investigate collectively the cause, treatment, locus, predisposing factors, and sequelae of selected diseases. Some of the collected data involved the use of instruments, but since a good deal of the data did not require instruments, the program will be only briefly described here. It is the method and attempt to make physicians think about specific problems that was significant, but especially important was the fact that the type of information instruments could provide was brought to the physicians' attention. It should be noted that, although instruments would have provided a firmer basis for collecting data on diseases, they were used minimally, which indicates that many British practitioners were not expected or willing to use them during the 1880s when the most concerted effort was made to canvas physicians throughout the country. The association's efforts to collect disease histories reveals that physicians were aware of the need to organize themselves and their expanding information for the benefit of all practitioners. While much of the data collectively analyzed in this period was not generated by instruments, those studies that included instruments were regarded as more important and decisive. When the idea to gather data collectively was revived in 1926, the studies were concentrated on surgical operations.[102]

The Committee on the Collective Investigation of Disease (CICD) was organized in 1881 by George M. Humphry and most strongly promoted by its secretary, Frederick A. Mahomed, until his death in 1884. Mahomed, who designed a sphygmograph for use in medical practice, traveled to all parts of Great Britain to seek support for the collective investigation of disease.

Among the inquiries that were aided by the use of instruments were studies related to cardiac diseases. Secretary Isambard Owen, who succeeded Mahomed, suggested that a special study be made of cardiac murmurs, which were found to accompany many cases of chorea and rheumatism.[103] Dr. Tyson of Folkestone, another member of the CICD, proposed that a study be conducted on the prognosis of heart lesions, which were becoming easier to identify and describe with the stethoscope and sphygmograph.[104] This inquiry was undertaken in 1886, and the topic was placed on the program of the British annual meeting in 1886 under the title "Cases in which Disease of Heart Valves had been known to exist for upwards of five years, without causing serious symptoms."[105] Heart lesions also were noted in 1887 in the study of chorea. The data showed that heart disease followed a rheumatic attack that accompanied an episode of chorea. Heart murmurs appeared in 50 percent of the rheumatism victims, while only 35 percent escaped heart disease of any type.[106] The study, centered on

acute rheumatism, confirmed several uncertain points about the effect of the disease and its treatment. It was demonstrated that the most frequent recoveries from rheumatic affections were made by those who abstained from alcohol, that administration of salicylate or salicis was extremely effective (it only failed in 24 of 536 instances), and that 24 percent of rheumatic victims developed tonsillitis, a relationship previously surmised.[107]

At least one inquiry was approved by the committee on the condition that the data would be collected from physical diagnostic signs. A British physician, W. P. Herringham, in 1884 commented that pneumonia was a "bad subject, because its diagnosis is so difficult; but if it was decided upon, the committee could do no other than safeguard the inquiry as they did by a string of questions about physical signs. Without these questions we could not in this subject have relied upon the cases returned to us."[108]

CONCLUSION:

The collective investigation of disease was another attempt to add to the multifaceted medical information of the late nineteenth century. Although collective investigation was not as successful initially as some of its proponents had expected it to be, it was employed to find answers to specific questions of disease control, and was most conclusive about those answers contingent on physical signs determined by medical instruments.

One effect of even an aborted program of collective investigation was to enlighten physicians about the remaining crucial questions concerning the common diseases and to let them share their doubts involving possible answers. The communal spirit was enhanced for those who participated in the CICD-sponsored program. Having been prepared by participation in the disease observation and assessment process, physicians were apt to accept the suggestions for diagnosis and cure that grew out of these studies and those of laboratory investigators.

The inquiry cards in their early form called for minimal use of medical instruments. The goals of the CICD did not require the application of instruments. The absence of questions that would have called for answers in numerical terms obtained with an instrument (temperature was the one exception) provides evidence that medical practice for the majority of physicians was slowly absorbing medical technology. The thermometer, stethoscope, and microscope were the most commonly used instruments. By 1890, it still was not considered disgraceful to reject these instruments or to be endangering a patient's life if they were not applied.

Collective investigation provided a mechanism for uniting physicians in their thinking about common diseases by raising questions to which they could all respond, even if incompletely and unsatisfactorily. Organized nationally and internationally, investigations of disease increased the physician's awareness of the variability of diseases and impressed him or her with the need to think in terms of limits and standards. In the nineteenth century, physicians still were taught by a few teachers and among small groups of peers. As medical students and young practitioners, they examined few patients, so that the physicians' concept of the wider implications of disease and its manifestations among people of varying social, economic, and cultural backgrounds was limited or at least skewed. The variations within a disease are best understood by comparing large numbers of its victims, a goal which the Collective Investigation project sought. The project also prepared the physician to appreciate the need for quick and unbiased descriptions of the signs and symptoms of each disease. Instruments provided objective data, which could be summarized for large groups of observations. The moderate success and eventual cessation of the Collective Investigation project indicates that physicians were unable to build up standards and criteria for recognizing and treating diseases. Those who engineered the project and promoted its benefits were helping to prepare physicians to understand the importance of common methods of observation that could be obtained with instruments. Even if a physician did not have a desire to use an instrument in his or her own practice, there was a further stimulus when the physician realized how his or her observations could be added to create a large pool of data and made the basis of a greater understanding of disease. Setting up standards to recognize, describe, and alleviate disease was revitalized when instruments became an integral part of the methods used to gather and evaluate data. The reports of the Collective Investigation Committee impressed physicians with their common goals and the difficulties of attaining them. The demand of industry for laborers with specified physical capabilities such as normal eyesight and color vision encouraged physicians to adopt diagnostic tests and corrective measures that could be applied regularly to a large group of people. Technology would soon enable physicians to expand their collection of data vastly, and gain a new esteem for each other as members of an elite profession, which utilized special equipment unfamiliar to others. Instruments moved physicians into science and at the same time medicine became of more interest to the public intent on applying its new technology to social and economic problems. Physicians required more precise methods and instruments to deal with people who were not ill but whose physiologic functions needed to be measured and compared to a standard of value to society and for reasons other than those of the individual's health.

John Shaw Billings delivered the first address on medicine by an American physician as a guest of the British Medical Association in 1886. His theme centered on current aspects of American medicine that might be of value to the British, as well as the type of medical information American physicians could be expected to contribute in the future.

This is an age of machinery, of exchanges, of corporations, for all these correspond to one and the same fundamental idea. Men make machines to do what the individual cannot do; and they make them not only of brass and iron, but of men, for such an obvious source of power to the man or men who can master the combination is not likely to be overlooked. One result of such organization is seen in our encyclopedic works of medicine, whether these be called dictionaries or handbooks; another in the great medical journals; another in associations which seek to wield political influence; another in the comparatively recent attempt at collective investigation of disease. . . . it is by the combination of all these, with the efforts of individual workers, that substantial advance and improvement are to be effected.[109]

Billings was in an ideal position to assess the methods and long-range use of major collections in medicine, having spearheaded the establishment of the Army medical library and museum and the collection of vital statistics in the United States. His volume *National Medical Dictionary* (1890) presented tables of life expectancies based on life insurance data and tables of physical characteristics based on measurements of hundreds of thousands of individuals.[110]

10

CONCLUSION

INTRODUCTION:

Medicine reflects the economic, social, and technological enterprises of the periods and locales in which it is practiced. Medical practice in the nineteenth century demonstrates this relationship explicitly. As the Western world industrialized, medicine became a part of the Industrial Revolution by evolving into an instrument-centered practice. The goals, achievements, and failures of medicine during this period relate directly to the technological and sociological changes that swept through Western society. The most obvious changes within medical practice included the adoption of various instrumentally applied techniques.

The expanded social and economic horizons made possible by legislation that guaranteed medical treatment for more citizens, a greater public awareness and desire to remain healthy, and the need to identify individuals with special skills and good health provided physicians with more opportunities to practice medicine. Recently, the sociologists, Nöel and José Parry,[1] who studied nineteenth-century British medicine, concluded that physicians began to be recruited from among a wider segment of society, including the lower classes, as a direct result of the Poor Law of 1832. Another important stimulus to enlarging the scope of medicine and those who practiced it was the need for manual skills, which formerly wre disparaged by physicians. The new criteria for diagnosing and treating diseases encouraged individuals with special technologically related talents to qualify as physicians. Persons skilled in manipulating instruments and understanding diseases by the numbers, colors, sounds, and odors provided through the application of mechanical devices could become successful diagnosticians.

Instruments offered those with manual dexterity a chance to excel as physicians in a profession that previously had favored individuals with good memories and a penchant for theories (see figure 10.1). An extensive memory was not as crucial in examining a patient when methods for permanently recording sounds and other bodily measurements became available. Diagnosis became a more deliberate process. The aristocratic forces in medicine were weakened; democratization occurred to an extent formerly not possible in organized medicine. In addition, since few individuals possessed all of the skills associated with the technological details of instrument-centered medicine, the need for medical specialists who could master some of the many procedures grew along with developments in medical technology.

This new type of medical graduate flourished in the state- and health insurance-supported clinics and hospitals. Without technological aids and the institutions that they made possible, state-supported medicine would have developed more slowly and less efficiently. Certainly, it would have taken on a different character than it now possesses. The data supplied by laboratory tests and the instrumental measurement of physiologic functions and pathologic processes was entered more conveniently in the records of the numerous patients who were eligible for publically supported medical examinations and treatment. The systematization of medical reports depended on the use of technological aids to cope adequately with the greater volume of patients.

One problem introduced with the use of instruments was the increased intimacy and exploration of the body that instruments promoted (see figure 10.2). For the female patient, physical examination procedures could best be given by permitting women to be-

233

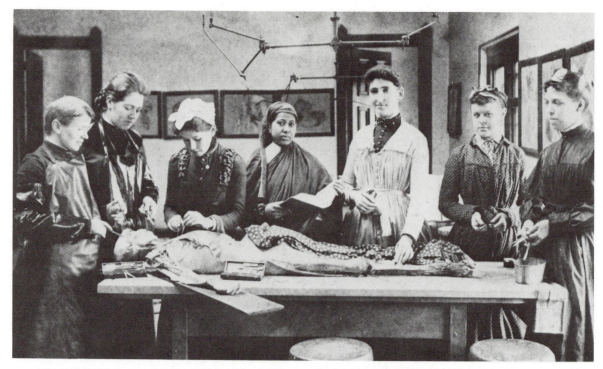

Figure 10.1. Medical students in 1892 dissecting a cadaver, at Women's Medical College in Philadelphia. Note small dissecting instruments used. From Elizabeth Ketcham whose mother is in the photograph. *SI Photo No. 75–10335.*

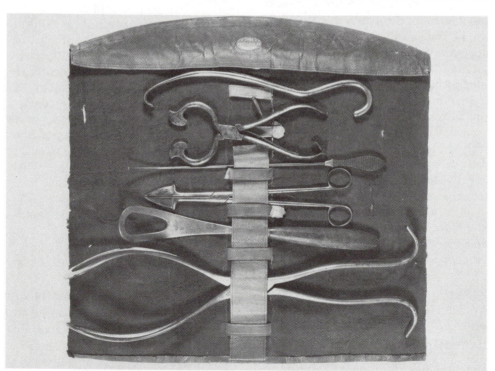

Figure 10.2. Nineteenth-century obstetrical kit used by Dr. Lewis Wolfley, Civil War Surgeon. *NMAH No. M-3132 SI Photo No. 63915.*

come physicians. Thus, in the period when instrumental physical diagnosis was introduced, the possibility that women could become physicians was defended on the grounds that they could examine women patients with less embarrassment to both physician and patient. Women physicians could also better understand the signs and symptoms of sex-related diseases. For those opposed to women becoming physicians, the innate qualification of women healers was used as an argument to restrict the types of medical specialties that women were expected to practice to gynecology, obstetrics, and pediatrics. These medical specialties encompassed the highest duties to be expected of most female physicians. Among the specialties not open to women were the highly respected fields including surgery and ophthalmology. Most women physicians served as general practitioners whose duties primarily centered on gynecology and obstetrics for all the women in their communities. In a study conducted in 1881 by the Womens' Medical College of Pennsylvania, 166 graduates who replied to a questionnaire querying them about their employment stated that they were engaged in gynecology and obstetrics.[2] Treatment of female disease by women physicians was a spur to the earlier detection of serious impairment and the greater possibility of cure because of, as John Steinbeck Wilson of Atlanta explained in 1854, "the almost insuperable objections of the fair sufferers, to the inevitable exposure of their sexual secrets to a male physician."[3]

In another instance, technology was used to block the careers of women seeking employment as midwives. Midwifery was merged into the specialty of obstetrics when special instruments became fashionable in the delivery room. Female midwives were discouraged from seeking advancement as obstetricians on the basis that they were unable to handle obstetrical forceps properly. The male physician who specialized in gynecology and obstetrics, in an effort to eliminate his midwife competitor, found reasons to belittle them for their purported lack of skills and strength in applying instruments. Physician obstetricians claimed that midwives could not effectively cope with difficult births because they could not adequately control unwieldy instruments, which were best manipulated by men who possessed greater muscular strength.[4]

PRECISION AND MEDICAL TECHNOLOGY:

The salient medical changes adopted by physicians during the nineteenth century that depended on the

use of instruments and medical technology were: (1) diagnosis and treatment of many diseases with the aid of instruments, (2) the definition of diseases based on the data supplied by instruments, and (3) the demarcation between health and disease according to the limits determined with instruments applied in the course of a physical examination given both to healthy and sick individuals.

These elements comprised a type of medical practice that S. Weir Mitchell characterized by the term *precision*. Precision began to influence industry and economics, as well as social activities, in this period. After 1880, physicians repeatedly commented on the introduction of precision into medicine. Norman Bridge of the Rush Medical College in Chicago in 1884 described the nature of medical practice: "If there is a single feature that, more than another, distinguishes the practice of the present from that of a former time, it is the use of numerous instruments of precision. Nearly all instruments are the product of the present period."[5] An editorialist of the *JAMA* commented in 1890 that "the paramount condition to successful medical practice must ever be that of precision in diagnosis."[6] He then explained that precision only could be achieved with medical instruments.

Instruments enabled physicians to gather vast quantities of data from patients and analyze these data according to the principles of statistics, the keystone of precision medicine. Statistics were employed to evaluate the safety, diagnostic value, and cure potential of new techniques. Hospital records were a prime source of the basic data needed for statistical analysis. Surveys of the profession concerning the diagnosis and treatment of disease, such as the Collective Investigation of Disease Committee project launched by the British Medical Association in 1882, demonstrated the importance of data collection and linked the provincial physician with the acknowledged medical leaders in medical schools and major urban hospitals. These surveys, which were supplemented by information gathered in other countries, and the whole process of quantification in medicine were facilitated by instrumentally derived information.

Instrumental diagnosis extended into surgery. Surgeons developed special surgical techniques that became routine diagnostic procedures. Diagnosis by the aid of instruments led T. Gaillard Thomas of New York to conclude in 1886 that "the modern development of the art of diagnosis has been accomplished by the subordination of theoretical methods of exploration and investigation to those which were purely physical.''[7] One dangerous procedure Thomas recommended, based on his own astounding success with it, was laparotomy or the exploration of the abdominal organs through surgical incision. He had performed 7,000 to 8,000 laparotomies successfully over the previous twenty-three years. Lawson Tait, the Birmingham gynecologist, argued forcefully in support of laparotomy as a replacement for ''the old-fashioned mechanical school of teaching of the speculum, the sound, the caustic stick and the pessary.''[8] Replacement of diagnosis by mechanical aids with surgical procedures soon was taken up by other medical specialists. When microscopic inspection of tissues became reliable, the demand for tissue specimens from all the organs increased. The location of the tissue determined the degree of skill and potential danger in obtaining a sample for analysis. But these procedures expanded despite the difficulties. Surgical exploration of the bodily tissues and organs became the standard method of analyzing tumors for malignancies.

What did numerically defined physiologic parameters demand of the medical practitioner? S. Weir Mitchell, who witnessed the transformation of medicine from an approximate to a precision-based enterprise, argued that instruments trained the physician to be more accurate and to devote more time to his diagnostic examinations.

The instrument trains the man; it exacts accuracy and teaches care. Certain interesting intellectual results have everywhere followed the generalization of precision by the use of instruments like the world-wide lesson in punctuality taught by the railway and made possible by the watch. We have so often timed the pulse that most of us can guess its rate, and constant use of the thermometer enables one to trust better one's own sense of heat, as the hand appreciates it. If, indeed, you use the sphygmograph much, you get to making visual images of the pulse curves whenever you, very carefully, feel a pulse. . . . instruments force us, by the time their uses exact, to learn to be rapid, and at the same time, accurate. Thinking over the number of instruments of precision, a single case may require, it is clearly to be seen that no matter how expert we may be, the diagnostic study of an obscure case must today exact an amount of time, far beyond that which Sydenham may have found need to employ. A *post mortem* section used to take an hour or two, and now, alas! it goes on for weeks in some shape until the last staining is complete, the last section studied, the last analysis made.[9]

And as Mitchell suggested, the first instrument to become a standard diagnostic tool revealed its labor-absorbing quality early. In 1824 John Forbes noted the time consumed and the difficulties encountered in applying the stethoscope.

Precision in diagnosis did not imply a fundamental change in the process of identifying diseases. Confirming a sign or symptom previously suspected was the purpose of much nineteenth-century instrumentation; searching for the sources of tuberculosis and heart diseases with the stethoscope, measuring expansion of the infected chest, and analyzing the urine for kidney disease were confirmatory methods for diagnosing signs suspected but not readily apparent. The instrument and the laboratory test made it possible for more physicians to confirm disease signs by comparing their instrumental results with established standards based on external observation.

APPLICATION OF MEDICAL TECHNOLOGY TO INDUSTRY:

The immediate social and economic consequences of instrumental diagnosis may be seen in the establishment of health standards for individuals seeking employment in various civil service occupations, especially the police and fire departments, as well as the military forces, and in hazardous jobs on the railroad and in the factory, as well as applicants for life insurance policies. Insurance companies and industries grew at an unprecedented rate in the United States after the Civil War. Procedures for staffing these industries and selecting those to whom insurance policies should be sold included evaluation of an individual's health with special emphasis on specific physical characteristics required for some jobs or those diseases known to shorten life. New criteria were developed through the use of instruments for distinguishing diseaes at an early stage.

Medical examiners were required to use selected instruments to complete the physical examination of life insurance and job-seeking applicants. Among the procedures for physically examining individuals, which provided a reliable index of future health, was measurement of the blood pressure with the sphygmomanometer. Placing a cuff around the upper arm, applying a stethoscope to the artery at the bend in the arm, and synchronizing the maximum and minimum pressure with the mercury column graduated in millimeters of mercury on the manometer linked to the cuff enabled the physician to find a correlation between a range of maximum and minimum readings and the onset of serious heart and vascular diseases. Determination of blood pressure was also the most direct and accurate indicator of a shortened life span. The level of the blood pressure became more decisive as the age of the individual increased. Blood pressure eventually became a prognostic sign used by specialists such as the ophthalmologist, who discovered refractive errors, which could manifest nephritis or retinal damage, that the blood pressure could confirm. The blood pressure measured in one part of the body became a sign of impending disease and length of life, as well as an indicator of the function of the circulation organs, chemistry of the blood, and one of a series of signs in acute and chronic diseases including apoplexy, kidney failure, stroke, and heart attack. Other tests including measurement of the vital capacity of the lungs with the spirometer, localization of the sounds of the heart and lungs with the stethoscope and plessimeter, chemical analysis of the urine, and microscopic analysis of the blood and body tissues contributed to the insights into human physiology and pathology attained through the use of instruments. Data gathered in medical examinations for industrial, civil service, and insurance purposes provided a wealth of figures to determine the statistical parameters of normality and abnormality for each instrument and test. The application of instruments to a wide spectrum of the healthy population was essential in establishing the normal limits for a variety of physiologic processes as indicated by different medical instruments.

Health standards were evaluated, along with skills and other talents, as part of the requirements for many jobs. Physical deficiencies that formerly were undetected and posed few problems were obstacles to the performance of certain jobs. Nearsightedness, which formerly was infrequently recognized or tested for, was a handicap for those engaged in office jobs, many of which did not exist until the nineteenth century. Color blindness presented serious hazards to the railroad engineer, the ship's pilot, and later, the automobile driver. For the diagnosis of both nearsightedness and color blindness, numerous tests were designed and produced. The constraints placed on the form of these tests included convenience in administering them, accuracy in the diagnosis the tests permitted, and availability to the physician. When numerous individuals needed to be tested quickly or when a physician could not be employed to administer the tests, there existed the optimal conditions for simplifying and organizing the information into tests that presented self-evident diagnoses.

Patients occasionally corroborated the diligence with which instruments and techniques were applied in the pursuit of a cure. While still in the midst of treatment for tuberculosis of the neck, one patient optimistically summarized the extensive measures employed to treat him over the previous three years:

Account of myself up to October 29, 1893.—Operated on May 10th, October 16th, 1890 and April 1, 1891. Have had 87 enlargements up to now and 66 suppurating openings. Have now 27 openings suppurating—6 in neck and throat, 6 in chest, 7 in back between waist and shoulder blade, 2 in thumb joint, 1 in right armpit, 3 in left armpit, 1 in left side five inches below armpit, 1 in right side five inches below armpit. No less than 160 quarts of pus has come from me. Have used no less than 6,000 yards of bandages, 15 yards of court plaster, 2 yards of oil-silk, 100 pounds of flaxseed, 20 pounds of absorbent cotton, 6 pounds of vaseline, 1 pound of salve, 1 pound of oakum, 2 pounds of licorice powder and salts, 1 ounce of aristol, 4 ounces of iodoform, 600 pills, mostly sulphite calcium, 10 plasters, 1 caustic pencil, 70 quarts inward medicine, 2 quarts peroxide hydrogen, 2 quarts carbolic acid, 12 quarts liquour, 1 pint iodine, half pint balsam Peru, 4 syringes. This does not reach the figure at all. Yet it is enough to convince the most morbid. I hope to get well yet.[10]

This record-keeping patient may not have been aware of the continuous attempts to improve and make more precise medical and surgical instruments, which undoubtedly encouraged their application. However, simplicity was sacrificed for the advantages to be gained in applying the instruments. Surgeons and physicians learned to balance the quality and style of the instrument with the goals they sought in uncovering and treating each patient's illness. Convenience of use was an important factor. Those instruments that were difficult to manage, such as the sphygmograph, and the pressure chamber, did not remain popular.

PUBLIC HEALTH AND THE PREVENTION OF DISEASE:

In a time when physicians were learning about the cause but not the cure of disease, prevention became of great importance, and, involving science, also included a great deal of technology. Preventive medicine in the nineteenth century primarily encompassed the control of the environment, and especially the sewerage, housing, streets, and factories so that poisonous emanations—later discovered to be primarily disease bacteria—could not contaminate the water, air, and articles used by the public. Removing the debris of the sick room and objects infected by victims of contagious disease was an obvious part of the campaign supported by physicians and laymen to prevent the spread of these diseases. Education and enforcing basic standards of good hygiene were tackled by medical, governmental, and lay groups.

In the United States, the American Medical Association from its inception investigated special areas of public health. In addition to groups with exclusive or heavy medical participation, such as the American Public Health Association, lay societies, such as the Ladies Health Protective Association of Allegheny County, New York, organized effective campaigns against public health nuisances. Originally formed to eliminate the odors pervading their community from a nearby slaughterhouse, the Allegheny group continued to tackle other health nuisances after their initial success in having these odors removed. Other women's groups, organized in New York City and Pittsburgh, campaigned successfully to have the streets cleaned and garbage removed regularly, and to protect food sold in shops from bacterial and other contaminants.[11] Persistant campaigns such as these, which focused on the physical environment of the community and depended on machines and devices to keep out bacteria, flies, rodents, and other pests in the processing, packaging, and delivery of food and personal articles, contributed to the community's awareness of the predisposing causes of diseases and their elimination. Devices provided a means to keep anything entering or used on the body sterile or less contaminated then by being directly transferred with the hands and passed between a number of people.

In England, public health reform was guided by strong medical leaders who practiced medicine and surgery. Two outstanding leaders were Thomas W. Smith and John Simon.[12] Simon combined medical knowledge, research experience, and public welfare consciousness in sound administration to shepherd into existence many types of sanitary improvements in London from the mid-nineteenth into the twentieth century. Technological refinements in devices and appliances enabled many of his and other reformers' objectives to be met. The reform in keeping surgical procedures free from bacterial contamination provides a significant example of the transfer of technology from a community practice into the hospital. In the 1860s, carbolic acid to keep surgical wounds antiseptic was suggested by Joseph Lister by its use to disinfect sewage in Carlisle, England.[13]

Urbanization accelerated the application of technology to preventive medicine. Apparatus was designed and manufactured in ever greater quantities to keep the home, street, and factory sanitary, as the concentrated populations of the cities demanded more stringent control of wastes, treatment of water, and cleansing of space and devices in common use. England, with the greatest population densities in the larger cities, contributed a great range of sanitary appliances, fixtures, and systems for house drainage, sewerage, heating units, ventilators, stoves, and radiators. In the United States, changes were made in some of these devices to make them adaptable to the climate and to local methods of construction. Flush toilets installed in homes and public buildings for the immediate removal of body wastes and elimination of odors were among the most effective sanitary appliances to improve public health. John Shaw Billings assessed the importance of the new sanitary devices in 1892. Although, he said, "the most important improvements in practical medicine made in the United States have been chiefly in surgery, in its various branches, the greatest progress in medical science during the next few years will be in the direction of prevention, and to this end mechanical and chemical invention and discovery must go hand in hand with increase in biological and medical knowledge."[14] Health exhibitions and museums of hygiene introduced sanitary appliances to large segments of the population, which resulted in increased understanding and use of the items. These patterns of sanitation control were introduced into other European countries and followed the pattern indicated for England and the United States.

Cremation of the dead provides an example of the extent to which technology became involved in preventive medicine and public hygiene. In this case, the campaign was inspired by a desire to protect health through the control of disease-causing bacteria, and special technology was required to carry it out. Burial grounds were studied during the last decades of the nineteenth century, and by the 1890s, most researchers concluded "that no serious epidemics have been attributed to graveyards, even during the period in which there was the best chance for such to have taken place, owing to the utter disregard of sanitary laws and to the great overcrowding of the burial grounds."[15] Numerous experiments demonstrated "that from a purely bacteriological standpoint there is no evidence that a buried body is a source of special danger to the living."[16] The bacteria of decomposition rapidly reduced the bodies of people dying of any diseases and converted them into the chemicals essential for vegetation.

Nevertheless, cremation appeared necessary to advocates of the bacterial origin of contagion. It was no longer safe, they said, to bury the infected corpse in the earth. To bury the diseased according to custom offered the possibility that water draining through the burial ground or eventual opening of the grave would release noxious gases and disease germs and could lead to a future epidemic. Waves of cholera, typhoid fever, diphtheria, and other epidemic diseases brought renewed activity on the part of medical cremation sponsors like Spencer Wells of Enggland, who in an important address at the annual meeting of the British Medical Association in Cambridge in 1880 argued for the cremation of cholera victims.[17] The Cremation Society of England was founded in 1874 in response to Sir Henry Thompson's articles in the *Contemporary Review*, but it was only in 1891 that the British Medical Association officially supported the society. The first English crematorium was erected by the society in Woking in 1880 and first used in 1885 after cremation was made legal by Parliament.[18] Although requested as early as 1891 through a resolution proposed at the annual meeting of the British Medical Society in 1891, the Cremation Act of 1902 first enabled local authorities in Britain to erect crematoria for public use.[19] In the meantime, two other crematoria sponsored by local societies had been built in Manchester and Liverpool.[20]

Response to cremation by the public was as cautious in the United States as it had been in England. Religious sanctions and the natural horror of fire were causes for opposing the practice.[21]

While "the day in which the idea that the whole function of medical men began and ended with the treatment and cure of disease"[22] was passing away, preventive medicine was not merely a consequence of good sanitation. Preventive medical care for the individual under the supervision of a doctor began with the selection of a family physician who could be expected to provide medical advice as well as treatment throughout a lifetime. Beginning with a complete medical history, the physician was expected to keep the health record up to date with information gained in the course of a thorough physical examination, which was repeated at intervals. The patient was encouraged to keep records of his or her own physical development with the aid of prepared forms such as those designed by Francis Galton. In the twentieth century, laymen were taught to use diagnostic instruments like the sphygmomanometer, thermometer, and stethoscope to monitor thier own functions, so that they only need to call upon the physician at a time when a crisis appeared and treatment seemed necessary.

Andrew H. Smith of St. George's Hospital in London reminded physicians that if they continuously followed the careers and health of their patients, they would be in the best position to help the patients avert major and unexpected illnesses. The physicians' intention to stave off all illness and injury led them to advise on the social and business situations to which their patients should expose themselves, warning of specific dangers and habits that a patient's particular constitution could not tolerate and yet remain healthy.[23] This aspect of preventive medicine is still being pursued in the United States. While social conditions were understood to be crucial to the rise of diseases, bacterial agents were the direct vectors that needed to be controlled to prevent disease. Knowledge of bacteria also had a formative influence on the design and manufacture of medical instruments after 1880.

STANDARDIZING INSTRUMENTS:

In addition to the standards developed for diagnosing disease, standards were required for calibrating each instrument so that it would provide comparable information for each patient to which it was applied and to determine the conditions under which it was accurate. Instruments of precision required constant evaluation to maintain their calibration and correctly interpret the data presented, although the procedures for doing so were tedious and difficult. Consequently, a number of medical instruments of this type were less popular among the medical profession. The sphygmograph presented physicians with some of the most complicated data to interpret. Differences in forms of this instrument, as well as differences in pulse graphs stemming from its mode of application, contributed to the variability of results and uncertainty of their meaning. An elaborate sphygmograph, the polygraph, which recorded the pulse from several bodily sources simultaneously, enabled the physician to designate a reference pulse to compare with the pulses recorded from other parts of the body. The designation of the blood pressure in precise figures obtained with the sphygmomanometer was challenged by those who noted different figures obtained with instruments manufactured by different companies. Methods of standardizing these instruments and of periodically testing those in use were devised to guard against inaccuracies and to correct faulty equipment.

Stethoscopes were not calibrated and remained the most personalized of medical instruments. Physicians learned to interpret specific sounds with their own stethoscopes, which they usually carried with them.

Sounds differed according to the type of material from which the stethoscope was constructed and the design of the instrument. Charts for recording data, combined with stylized diagrams, assisted the physician in organizing the information gathered with stethoscopes and other instruments that did not provide clear-cut numerically based data. Tables of standards were constructed for consultation as a guide to the interpretation of the data obtained with an instrument.

The three forms of standardization that grew out of the use of medical instruments—health, disease, and instrument standards—introduced a degree of precision into medical practice that changed the economic, social, and personal aspects of medicine. Health and disease were described in greater detail with ramifications for everyone. However, the comparative element introduced into an instrument-standardized medicine led to a decreased emphasis on the uniqueness of the individual treated for disease. The special procedures required time and careful application, which could distract the physician from listening to and observing his patient for other reasons.

SPECIALISM AND SPECIALIZATION:

Medicine in a technological era adopted technical aids in various guises for various purposes. These long- and short- terms uses included diagnosis, therapy, experimentation, and via publications, films, and museums, education of laymen concerning health and disease. The physician's attitude toward disease and patients was altered by the use of technology in both expected and less obvious ways. Directly related changes included the use of instruments on the body in the physician's office, in the clinic, and in the hospital to measure functions and structures for diagnostic and prognostic purposes. This change in technique of coping with disease led to the segregation of a minimal body part to be elected for study and possible treatment. Fortified with special tools, the physician met this intellectual challenge by centering all of his or her attention on one organ or system and turning over the study and care of other organs and systems to other physicians. The view that treating detailed structures of the body provided the optimal chances of success in helping a patient prevent or resist disease eventually prevailed in medical circles. Medical specialists practicing medical specialties followed upon the introduction of instruments that made possible this type of medical practice. Without particular instruments, it is unlikely that specialism

would have appealed to the physician or even have been feasible.

The types of specialties regular physicians learned to practice grew directly out of the instruments invented to diagnose and treat disease invading different parts of the body. The ophthalmologist, endoscopist, cardiologist, otolaryngologist, and internist were all educated to use special instruments and techniques that distinguished their practices from those of the general practitioner. With instruments to define normal and abnormal bodily functions and to measure and record organic changes, the medical specialist created a type of medical practice that expanded the opportunities, as well as the constraints, stemming from medical technology.

Physicians aspired to adopt the veneer, as well as the more substantial role, of the scientist, which provided them with compelling incentives to become specialists even when their sensibilities and social consciences made them oppose this separation within their own ranks. The assumption that disease was discrete and more scrutable than the sick individual followed from the medical specialist's technological methods of diagnosing and treating disease.

The transformation of medical diagnosis from a technique based on a personal interview and visual inspection of the body into a process centered on direct observation with the aid of instruments, machines, devices, and so on was accompanied by some doubt on the part of the medical profession. Physicians criticized the process, the instruments, and the achievements through lectures to medical students, addresses at professional meetings, articles in medical journals, and their textbooks. Organized opposition was limited and consisted mainly of the activities carried out by the various medical sectarians who emphasized minimal treatment consisting of drugs or a single cure-all therapy. These irregular practitioners offered unorthodox alternatives frequently based on little understanding of human physiology, which made them unacceptable to regular physicians even when they were in agreement about the problems created by medical specialism and the use of medical technology.

Although physicians developed a special technology, they did not adopt all of the customs and practices associated with other technologies. One practice physicians condemned was applying for a patent on an instrument invented by a doctor. The medical profession almost unanimously frowned on physicians and surgeons who sought patents for instruments and devices they had invented. The American Code of

Medical Ethics included a provision against owning a medical patent. Holding a monopoly on medical instruments became controversial as early as the seventeenth century when the Chamberlens invented and applied the obstetrical forceps, but would not allow others to use them, with few exceptions.[24] An occasional inventor would try to raise the conscience of the profession by pointing out how unfair it was to the physician-inventor if he could not patent his invention, especially in a society where all other inventors were given this privilege. One correspondent to a medical journal who had witnessed the "skill and ingenuity" that produced the splendid medical instruments on display in Philadelphia to celebrate the American Centennial in 1876, wondered if it would be possible to make

some arrangement with the trade, to allow the profession a *royalty* on all designs and inventions accepted, manufactured and sold, leaving to the former the sole right and privilege of *patenting* and selling? This plan would save the dignity of the profession, and though not so renumerative as the holding of a patent, it would nevertheless give a physician some pecuniary recompense for the outlay of his time and means, and for the labor of his brain.[25]

He noted that "scarcely a day elapses without a new design being furnished to an instrument maker, for the making of which he takes good care to charge a round sum to the designer, and then he manufactures and sells the article at an immense profit to himself."[26] It seemed equitable that some of the profit made by the manufacturer be shared with the medical profession. Manufacturers found it convenient to appease inventors and increase sales by applying the name of the medical inventor to an instrument or the modification a physician proposed for an existing instrument. This practice seemed to be recompense enough, but a study of business records might reveal that royalties on some instruments sold were, in fact, paid to the physicians whose names were applied to specific instruments.[27]

The possibility of patenting medical instruments is suggested by the practice of dentists. Largely because of the mechanical nature of their practice and their dependence on tools, dentists remained close to mechanical artists in their attitude toward and use of patents. Dentists frequently obtained patents for their inventions, a practice that helped to maintain the philosophical gulf between the medical profession and dentistry. Leading dental instrument manufacturers bought patents from the dentist-inventor and mechanician, in some cases to keep other firms

from producing competitive types of equipment. Occasionally, patent controversies arose out of the sale of licenses to dentists who wished to use a patented item. The fees were not exorbitant, but the sense of exploitation this practice engendered aroused opposition until it became unfashionable for respectable dentists to sell licenses for devices they had invented. The attitude of dentists toward the morality of advertising their skills and patenting their inventions has its roots in the evolution of dentistry as a medical specialty in which the devices employed, whether they were for operating on the teeth or the prosthesis itself, had a much larger role in the perception of the specialty by all concerned.

The need for dentists to introduce themselves and their techniques to the public and make their presence known was more urgent than for the physician to do the same. From the Renaissance until the end of the nineteenth century, dentists advertised their skills and techniques. Most people did not understand the value of having someone with special training remove or repair decayed teeth. They understood even less about the need for prosthetic replacements and often could not afford the specially carved teeth made from ivory and attached to metallic plates. To encourage people to care for their teeth and patronize reputable dentists, who had learned their techniques from respected practitioners, the pamphlet and single sheet flyer, extolling the skills of a dentist, was distributed by mail, printed in newspapers, and later, in magazines and trade journals. These notices frequently announced the arrival of a dentist into a town or city, since seldom could the practitioner make a living in dentistry by remaining in one locale. This tradition continued for several centuries. Dental advertisements provide a rich source for the history of dental pioneers and their techniques and technologies in various parts of the United States and Europe.[28]

MEDICAL TECHNOLOGY EXHIBITIONS AND COLLECTIONS:

The discovery of disease-causing bacteria and the measures taken to prevent these diseases—antisepsis, sterilization, and the design and manufacture of numerous forms of cleansing devices—combined with medical instruments to alter the type of medicine practiced in Western society. Bacterial control and mechanization were essential components of the period, which few educated people could ignore or fail to incorporate into their techniques. Mechanization and elimination of bacteria were brought together in community-wide campaigns and projects at the time that physicians were refining their own instruments and methods to lessen bacterial contamination. These included the application of many technological devices and systems (sewerage, drainage, garbage disposal, pasteurization) to maintain germ-free conditions where human exposure was common. Hygiene technology was demonstrated and discussed in many forums including international fairs, hygiene exhibitions, and museums.

The success of temporary, traveling, and permanent health-centered exhibitions in spreading antibacterial ideas and information concerning the types of technology that would help maintain a bacteria-free environment in a variety of settings led physicians to understand the teaching value of technological museums. Medical groups turned to the museum as a vehicle for explaining the fundamental tenets of health and disease control. Since the eighteenth century, physicians regularly had learned anatomy and pathology through the study of specimens displayed in medical and hospital museums.

The instruments, devices, and machines used by physicians in the course of examining and treating patients were first shown at medical society meetings. The earliest and most technological of these displays were sponsored by the British Medical Association and American Medical Association at their annual meetings. The BMA began in 1867 to mount medical instrument displays. In small stages, surgical and medical instruments were introduced to the public through national and international expositions beginning with the archetype Industrial Fair of 1851 in London.

Medical instruments entered the ranks of major collector's objects in the nineteenth century. Private individuals, such as the French physician Pierre Hamonic, gathered implements employed in antiquity and others in later periods up through the nineteenth century. His collection contained many representative surgical instruments, including scarificators, scalpels, obstetrical forceps, and surgical sets, as well as contemporary diagnostic instruments. Hamonic's collection was purchased by Henry Wellcome in 1928 and became the nucleus of the most comprehensive medical instrument collection in existence.

With the exception of the Smithsonian Institution, the Armed Forces Institute of Pathology, the Wellcome Historical Museum, and a few individuals including Pierre Hamonic, medical collections were developed by hospitals, medical societies, and medical libraries. These institutions became the custodians of medical instruments since they were the most accessible and suitable locations known to the inventors, users, and their families and friends who wished to preserve these medical objects for posterity. Other medical items were given to local, state, and regional museums and historical societies as separate items or as a part of the papers and artifacts of a locally respected physician. (See figures 10.3, 10.4, and 10.5) With relatively little space and almost no trained staff in these institutions, coping with the preservation, documentation, and cataloguing of these items has been difficult. The most enterprising keepers displayed some of the more interesting pieces based on appearance, association, application and relationship to the history of the field.

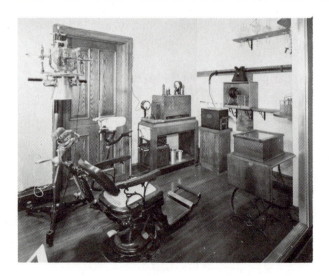

Figure 10.3. Dr. Charles Kell's office on exhibit in the National Museum of American History, Smithsonian Institution. *SI Photo No. x4325.*

Medical museum collections testify to the technological skills developed by physicians primarily in the nineteenth and twentieth centuries. These instruments and objects also symbolize the conceptual and institutional changes within medicine. The cost of medical treatment grew in proportion as the number of technological devices and the number of people to manufacture, sell, service, and apply them increased. By the twentieth century, the reputation of the physician depended, in large part, on his skill in applying medical instruments and on his possessing a full array of medical equipment.

The foregoing discussion of resources, narrative, and analysis in the history of medical technology, centering on the initial stages in the nineteenth century, should serve not to close, but to open up discussion of the subject. Knowledge about instruments and techniques and where the remnants of them can be found and studied is essential. The discussion of the clinical and social events that give technology its significance can expand appropriately—whether on the model of the stethoscope and pulse or the prevailing standardization that penetrated even into medicine. It is hoped that a number of volumes, essays, and papers discussing the history of the myriad aspects of medical technology will appear in the next decades.

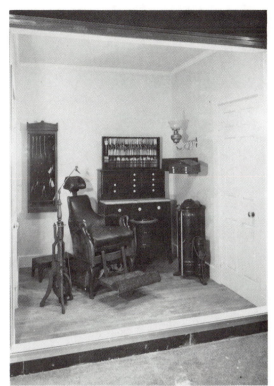

Figure 10.4. Dr. Green Vardiman Black's office on exhibit in the National Museum of American History, Smithsonian Institution. *SI Photo No. x3796.*

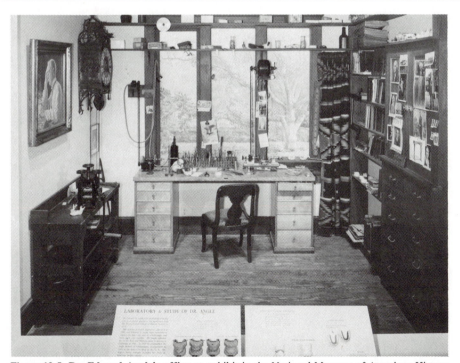

Figure 10.5. Dr. Edward Angle's office on exhibit in the National Museum of American History, Smithsonian Institution. *SI Photo No. x4315.*

NOTES

Journals which are cited infrequently are given with their full titles or containing standard abbreviations. The most frequently cited journals are abbreviated in the following manner:

AJC American Journal of Cardiology
AJMS American Journal of Medical Sciences
AJPH American Journal of Public Health
AS Annals of Science
BMSJ Boston Medical and Surgical Journal
BMJ British Medical Journal
BHM Bulletin of the History of Medicine
BMLA Bulletin of the Medical Library Association
BNYAM Bulletin of the New York Academy of Medicine
DSB Dictionary of Scientific Biography
GHR Guy's Hospital Reports
JAMA Journal of the American Medical Association
JEH Journal of Economic History
JHMAS Journal of the History of Medicine and Allied Sciences
JNMA Journal of the National Medical Association
MH Medical History
MR The Medical Record
M-CT Medico-Chirurgical Transactions
MTG Medical Times and Gazette
NEJM New England Journal of Medicine
NYMJ New York Medical Journal
NYSJM New York State Journal of Medicine
PMJ Pennsylvania Medical Journal
PT Philosophical Transactions
SMJ Southern Medical Journal
USNMB United States National Museum Bulletin

Trade catalogues are listed by manufacturer followed by the word Catalogue and relevant pages. The most frequently cited Trade Catalogues include:

1. Kny-Scheerer, 1923
2. A. S. Aloe, circa 1893
3. George Tiemann, 1889
4. Charles Lentz and Son, 1882

CHAPTER 1

1. Henry Taylor Bovey, *International University Lecture at the Congress of Arts and Sciences, University Exposition St. Louis* (New York: Alliance Inc., 1912), vol. 7, pp. 200, 212. The applied nature of medicine is further emphasized in the fact that the physician's instruments were not given the same status by the Customs Office. Imported scientific instruments were not taxed in this period as were surgical and diagnostic instruments. The Board of U.S. Customs General Appraisers at New York decided on 30 December 1893 that "instruments used by the physicians and surgeons of a hospital, for the purpose of carrying on their professions, are mechanical implements . . . and cannot be classed as either philosophical or scientific instruments, or apparatus, for the assessment of duties, when imported and can't be admitted free." Notice, *MR* (1894) 45:466.

2. The only specific bibliography on surgical instruments was prepared by Anne Honor Clulow, "A Bibliography of the Literature on Surgical Instruments, 1875-1900," London: Diploma in Librarianship Thesis, May 1961, in the University Library.

3. Stanley J. Reiser, *Medicine and the Reign of Technology* (Cambridge: Cambridge University Press, 1978). See also Sandra Harding's review of Reiser's book, "Knowledge, Technology and Social Relations," in *Journal of Medicine and Philosophy* (1978) 3:346-58. Harding believes that "the prevailing social relations in a society limit the development and adoption of technological alternatives" to a far greater extent than Reiser has shown in his text. Technology, she claims, is a means of organizing labor, a concept overlooked by Reiser and one which Harding believes contributes some of the most meaningful interpretations of the social dimensions of technology as applied in medicine. I develop some of the implications of this relationship in my chapter on the social implications of medical standards.

4. Quoted by Bruno Zambia, "The Restoration of Pavia Version of Giovanni Alessandro Brambilla's Surgical Armamentarium," in *Wien und die Welt Medizin*, Erna Lesky, (Koln, Graz: Hermann Bochlaus, 1974), p. 54.

5. Among the various definitions provided in the *Oxford English Dictionary* is the one, which may be applied to surgical and medical instruments that is "applied technically to small steel articles, as hammers, pincers, buckles, button-hooks, nails, etc.," vol. 11 (Oxford: At the Clarendon Press, 1933) p. 208.

6. Ed. "The Bicycle Doctor," *MR* (1896) 49:138; A. C. Getchell, "Bicycling in its Relation to Heart Disease," *Med News* (1899) 75:36, 37; Grahme M. Hammond, "The Influence of the Bicycle in Health and in Disease," *MR* (1895) 47:129-33 from *J Nervous and Mental Disease* (1892).

7. Richard Asher, "Clinical Sense, the Use of the Five Senses," *BMJ* (1960) I:992.

8. Paul Starr, "Medicine, Economy and Society in Nineteenth Century America," *J Social Hist* (1977) 10:595, 596, 599.

9. Ibid., p. 598.

10. In 1913 A. Dale Covey described a well-equipped physician's office, which cost about one thousand dollars to furnish. It consisted of modern appliances, chairs, carpets, furniture, a reception room, consultation room, operating room, electric room, and bathroom, each of which contained the appropriate equipment. Covey claimed a population of 5,000 citizens was needed to support the well-outfitted physician's office. *The Secrets of Specialists* (Detroit, Mich.: Physicians Supply Co., 1903), pp. 23-25. The manufacturer Charles Lentz and Sons claimed circa 1882 that "it having been fully demonstrated that those (physicians and surgeons) supplied with the best and most elaborate office outfits (other things being equal) are the most successful in building up a lucrative practice." *Illustrated Catalogue and Price List of Surgical Instruments*, 3d ed. (Philadelphia, ca. 1882, pref. Division of Medical Sciences, The National Museum of American History Collections).

11. Abstract from *Archives d'Ophthalmologie* "Instrument Cases," *JAMA* (1883) I:214.

12. E. B. Meyrowitz, *Bulletin* No. 18, 1896. Film, Box 8, in the Division of Medical Sciences, The National Museum of American History.

13. S. Weir Mitchell, *The Early History of Instrumental Precision in Medicine* (New Haven: Tuttles, Morehouse and Taylor, 1892), pp. 8, 9.

14. H. E. Fish, "The Development and Growth of the American Sterilizer Company," typescript, 1961, pp. 6, 9, 13, 14.

15. Audrey B. Davis, "The Emergence of American Dental Medicine: The Relationship of the Maxillary Antrum to Focal Infection," *Texas Rep. on Biol. and Med.* (1974) 32:144, 145.

16. Editorial, "The Defect in the Dentist," *MR* (1894) 45:114.

17. Roswell O. Stebbins, "Painless Dentistry," *MR* (1893) 44:524.

18. Ibid.

19. Ilza Veith, *Huang Ti Nei Ching Su Wen The Yellow Emperor's Classic of Internal Medicine* (Berkeley: University of California, 1960), p. 167.

20. James J. Gregory, "Some Facts Regarding Chinese Medical Practice with a Brief History of their Method," *MR* (1893) 44:167.

21. I. E. Cohn, "The Chinese and their Peculiar Medical Ideas," *MR* (1892) 42:477.

22. H. A. Huntington, "The Post-Mortem Pulse," *MR* (1899) 56:383.

23. Ibid.

24. Richard Selzer, *Mortal Lessons: Notes on the Art of Surgery* (New York: Simon and Schuster, 1974).

25. L. T. C. Rolt, *Tools for the Job: A Short History of Machine Tools* (London: B. J. Batsford, Ltd., 1965), pp. 187, 192, 226; Aubrey F. Burstall, *A History of Mechanical Engineering* (Cambridge, Mass.: MIT Press, 1965), p. 359. The critical nature of precision medical instruments was brought out by complaints such as that of Warren Sneden in 1885, who found that urethral instruments were not always the exact sizes that they were marked. "Inaccurate Urethral Instruments," *MR* (1885) 27:670, 671.

Chapter 2

1. S. Weir Mitchell, *The Early History of Instrumental Precision in Medicine* (New Haven: Tuttles, Morehouse and Taylor, 1892), p. 10.

2. Girindranath Mukhopadhyoya, *The Surgical Instruments of the Hindus with a Comparative Study of the Surgical Instruments of the Greek, Roman and the Modern Europeans* (Calcutta: Calcutta University, 1913, 1914); John Stewart Milne, *Surgical Instruments in Greek and Roman Times* (London, 1902; reprint New York: Augustus M. Kelly, 1970).

3. Ernst Julius Guerlt, *Geschichte der Chirurgie und ihrer Ausuebung*, 3 vols. (Berlin, 1898; reprint Hildesheim: Georg Ulm, 1964).

4. Henry Sigerist, *A History of Medicine: Primitive and Archaic Medicine.* (New York: Oxford University Press, 1951), p. 19. Sigerist called attention to a method of studying medical technology that also applied to technology in general. Edwin T. Layton, Jr., recently summarized the major studies in the history of technology and concluded: ". . . the idea of technologists cannot be understood in isolation; they must be seen in the context of a community of technologists and of the relations of this community to other social agencies." "Technology as Knowledge," *Technology and Culture* (1974) 15:41.

5. C. J. S. Thompson, *The History and Evolution of Surgical Instruments* (New York: Schuman's, 1942).

6. V. Moeller-Christensen, *The History of the Forceps*, trans. W. E. Calvert (Oxford: Oxford University Press, 1938).

7. Ruth and Edward Brecher, *The Rays: A History of Radiology in the United States and Canada* (Baltimore: The Williams and Wilkins Co., 1969).

8. Guido Majno, *The Healing Hand: Man and Wound in the Ancient World* (Cambridge, Mass.: Harvard University Press, 1975).

9. See for review Audrey B. Davis, *Am Sci* (1975) 63: 720-21.

10. Eugene Ferguson, *Bibliography of Sources for the Study of the History of Technology* (Cambridge, Mass.: MIT Press and the Society for the History of Technology, 1968).

11. Fielding H. Garrison and L. T. Morton, *A Medical Bibliography*, 3d ed. (New York: J. B. Lippincott Co., 1970).

12. Kedarnath Das, *Obstetric Forceps, its History and Evolution* (St Louis: The C. V. Mosby Co., 1929).

13. Leonard J. T. Murphy, *The History of Urology* (Springfield, Ill.: Charles C. Thomas, 1972).

14. George E. Burch and N. P. Pasquale, *A History of Electrocardiography* (Chicago: Yearbook Medical Publs. Inc., 1964).

15. Arthur Master, Charles I. Garfield, Max B. Walters, *Normal Blood Pressure and Hypertension* (Philadelphia: Lea and Febiger, 1952).

16. Gustav Gaujot, *Arsenal de la Chirurgie Contemporaine*, (Paris, 1867).

17. Albucasis, *On Surgery and Instruments*, trans. M. S. Spink and G. L. Lewis (London: The Wellcome Institute of the History of Medicine, 1973). See Emily Savage-Smith, *Hist Sci* (1976) 14:245-64 on the merits of this translation. Savage-Smith recommends that "someone should be persuaded to undertake a comprehensive study of Greco-Roman, Byzantine and Islamic surgical instruments on the basis of manuscript illustrations and museum artifacts," p. 254. See also Sami Hamarneh, "Drawings and Pharmacy in al-Zahrawi's Tenth Century Surgical Treatises," *USNM Bulletin* 228 (Washington, D.C.: Smithsonian Institution, 1961).

18. Albucasis, *On Surgery and Instruments*, p. 2.

19. Hermann Schoene, *Apollonius von Kitium illustrieter Kommentar zu der Hippokrateischer Schrift.* (Leipzig: B. C. Teubner, 1896), pl. 25.

20. Albucasis, *On Surgery and Instruments*, p. 346.

21. Robert Herrlinger, *History of Medical Illustration from Antiquity to 1600*, trans. Graham Fulton Smith (Munich: Heinz Moos, 1970), p. 44.

22. Eugene Ferguson, "The Mind's Eye: Nonverbal Thought in Technology." *Science* (1977) 197:831. See also: Ellen B. Wells, "Medical Illustration and Book Decoration in the Eighteenth Century," *Medical and Biological Illustration* (1970) 20:78-84; Ellen B. Wells, "Graphic Techniques of Medical Illustration in the Eighteenth Century," *J Biocommunications* (1976) 3:24-27.

23. Hans von Gersdorff, *Feldbuch der Wundartzney* (Strasbourg: Joannes Schott, 1517); Hieronymus Brunschwig, *Buch der Chirurgia* (Strasbourg: Johannes Gruninger, 1497). This was the first illustrated surgical textbook to be printed. It is mainly a compilation.

24. R. Herrlinger, *History of Medical Illustration*, p. 140.

25. Jacques Guilleneau, *The French Chirurgerye . . .*, trans. A. M. (Paris 1594). To the reader, unnumbered.

26. R. Herrlinger, *History of Medical Illustration*, p. 143.

27. Johannes Scultetus, *Armamentarium Chirurgicum* (Ulm: Balthasar, 1655), Table 41, Fig. V.

28. Albucasis, *On Surgery and Instruments*, pp. 490-93, Fig. 147.

29. J. Scultetus, *Armamentarium Chirurgicum*. The book contains 43 plates.

30. Audrey B. Davis and Toby Appel, *Bloodletting Instruments in the National Museum of History and Technology* (Washington, D.C.: Smithsonian Institution Press No. 41, 1979), pp. 6, 7, 64, 65.

31. Réné Jacques Croissant de Garengeot, *Nouveau Traité des Instrumens de Chirurgie les plus utiles*, 2d ed. (Paris, 1727), p. 2.

32. Laurence Heister, *A General System of Surgery in Three Parts*, 7th ed. trans. (London, 1759) p. 12. John Savigny also produced an excellent illustrated surgical instrument text with illustrations in actual size. *A Collection of Engravings Representing the Most Modern and Approved Instruments Used in the Practice of Surgery with Appropriate Explanations* (London, 1798). Savigny explained in the preface: "It will be readily admitted that there is no species of manufacture whatever that requires such minute attention in its progress, such precise perfection in its completion, and that on these are dependent in all cases the proportion of pain they necessarily inflict, and in many even life itself. Hence I am persuaded, that there will not be found one considerate mind that will not reward it accordingly, especially when it is accompanied by the reflection, that the operator's sensibility in the use of a good or a bad instrument, must, in a great degree, be affected by the consequent increase or diminution of his patient's sufferings; and, independent of these natural effects upon him mental feelings . . . and that the trifling differences of expense between a well finished and high conditioned instrument, and its inferior, will never fail of being amply repaid, both in profit and in fame." One example of a text prepared by a cutler, which gives manufacturing details for a great variety of surgical instruments, is Jean J. Perret, *L'Art du Coutelier expert en Instruments de Chirurgie*. (Paris, 1772), 2 vols. His goal, stated on page iv, was to "d'établir les règles et d'ensiegner les moyens sous de le fabriquet dans les formes les plus convenables pour chacun d'opérations."

33. R. Herrlinger, *History of Medical Illustration*, p. 146.

34. Anon., Review of *Chirurgische Kupfertafeln, eine answerlesene sammlung der noethigsten Abbildungen von Ausserlich sichtbaren Krankheitsformen: u.s.f. zur gebrauch für Praktische Chirurgen*. *AJMS* (1927) I: 188. Ambroise Paré explained in 1564 that there were limitations to the printed and illustrated text for learning manual surgery. He wrote: ". . . . but you must consider that it is a very difficult thing to put manual surgery clearly and entirely in writing, for it is rather to be learned by imagination and by seeing good and experienced masters perform, if you have the

means or, indeed, to try it on dead bodies as I have done many times." *Ten Books of Surgery with the Magazine of the Instruments Necessary for it*, trans. Robert White Linker and Nathan Womak, (Athens, Ga.: University of Georgia Press, 1969). Paré also published *An Explanation of the Fashion and Use of Three Hundred and Fifty Instruments of Chirurgery*, trans. (London, 1631).

35. Joseph Pancoast, *A Treatise on Operative Surgery Comprising a Description of the Various processes of the Art including all the New Operations . . .* (Philadelphia: Carey and Hart, 1844).

36. Anon., Review of P. S. Wade, *Mechanical Therapeutics* in *MR* (1868) 3:60.

37. W. P. Northrup, "Memorial Address on Joseph O'Dwyer," *MR* (1898) 53:361-64.

38. A. L. Ranney, "Practical Hints Regarding the Methods of Examination employed as Aids in the Diagnosis of Nervous Disease," *MR* (1884) 25:309.

39. J. W. H. review *AJMS* (1886) 91:567; review of John Draper's book in *JAMA* (1886) 7:83-84. John Draper's book was called the first book to be published on medical physics in the United States. Charles J. B. Williams produced one of the earliest texts to explain the physical laws of acoustics and their relevance to auscultation with a stethoscope. He wrote, "physical signs stand on the broad and intelligible basis of physical laws, and are as readily explained as other simple phenomena, illustrated by natural philosophy. It has been my endeavour to exhibit them, as far as possible, in this intelligible view; to show the mechanism by which the signs are produced, and the manner in which, according to fixed laws, they result as phenomena; to make a knowledge of the pathology predicate the signs, and a knowledge of the pathology indicate the pathology; and by thus familiarising the mind with their principles, to enable it to understand the multifarious forms which, by combination, these signs may assume, and to judge of the corresponding physical changes that modify or produce them."

40. Arndt VonHippel, *Chest Tubes and Chest Bottles* (Springfield, Ill.: Charles C. Thomas, 1970), p. vii.

41. George Tiemann, *The American Armamentarium Chirurgicum* (New York, 1889), pref. p. iii.

42. Ibid.

43. Charles Truax, *The Mechanics of Surgery* (Chicago, 1899), p. 7.

44. The catalogues of these manufacturers are in the collection of the National Museum of American History of the Smithsonian Institution, and The Wellcome Institute of the History of Medicine.

45. John Frederic Charrière, *Exposition Nationale de l' Industrie de 1839: Extrait du Catalogue de la Maison Charrière* (Paris, 1843), p. vi.

46. Ibid., p. iii.

47. Anon., To the Medical Profession, *Modern Surgical Instruments Chiefly of France and Germany Illustrated* (London, 1844), p. 2.

48. E. B. Meyrowitz, *Bulletin* No. 54, 1931. In the collection of the New York Academy of Medicine Library. Film No. 8 in The National Museum of American History, Smithsonian Institution.

49. Medical texts and articles often assumed that the medical reader would be familiar with the instruments discussed through medical school or apprenticeship training.

50. Charles A. King, *Catalogue* (London, 1933). In the Wellcome Institute of the History of Medicine Collection.

51. See, for succinct historical account of the development of physical medicine and its evolution into rehabilitation medicine, Audrey B. Davis, *Triumph Over Disability: The Development of Rehabilitation Medicine in the U.S.A.* (Washington, D.C.: Smithsonian Institution, 1973).

52. Reinhold Wappler and Thomas H. Holgate, To the Editor, "Inaccuracy of Glass Graduates," *MR* (1877) 12:47.

53. E. B. Meyrowitz, *Bulletin* No. 17, 1895. Film No. 8 in The National Museum of American History, Smithsonian Institution. Making instruments and supplies for hospitals forced the medical instrument producer to adopt the competitive marketing practices of other large industries. As medical suppliers competed for the same hospital accounts, they began to offer sales and discounts. The sales inducement method of advertising was not always acceptable to the physician or the manufacturer. E. B. Meyrowitz in 1892 condemned the practice of offering discounts on surgical instruments since he believed that physicians and hospitals were captive buyers. Meyrowitz believed that these buyers should be in a position to know the real value of their implements and would want to purchase the best equipment at all times. Sales and discounts continued to be offered on medical equipment, especially by large companies, such as Charles Betz and Company of Chicago.

54. George Shrady, Editorial, "The Reason Why," *MR* (1882) 32:21-22.

55. Editorial, "Public Surgical Operations," *MR* (1891) 39:144.

56. "News of Medicine," *MR* (1866-67) 1:238.

57. Ibid.

58. G. L. E. Turner, "The Use of Scientific Collections for Research," *Museums J* (1967) 66:275.

59. Correspondence with Dr. Robert Hudson and my visit to the library center.

60. George Bowditch, "Cataloguing Photographs," *Am. Assoc. for State and Local Hist. Technical Leaflet* (1971) 57:2.

61. Robert G. Chenhall, "Museum Cataloguing in the Computer Age," *Am. Assoc. for State and Local Hist. Leaflet* (1975) 61: 9, 11. This article contains a bibliography of articles on using the computer to catalogue museum collections.

62. Geoffrey Lewis, "Information Retrieval in Museums," *Museums J* (1967) 66:283.

63. R. G. Chenhall, "Museum Cataloguing in the Computer Age," pp. 242, 243.

64. Division of Medical Sciences, USNMAH Records.

One of the most comprehensive computer-formated systems has evolved over the past decade from staff discussions and special cataloguing projects undertaken at the National Museum of American History of the Smithsonian Institution. The present system was theoretically structured by 1973 and tested initially in the same year. Information on objects is stored on magnetic tapes for running through the computer, to be printed on paper or cards as desired. Microscopes were among the first items in the museum to be entered into the system as a group. A sample computer printout of several microscopes reveals the types of categories most easily supplied by study of the accession records and those properties of the instrument revealed by inspection and measurement. Since the cataloguing system was designed to include the characteristics of the widest variety of objects, it may be used by historical museums of all types. As in all computer programs, information may be added and corrections made as desired, which is an essential requirement in documenting and making accessible a museum collection.

The system is used routinely by the registrar's office of the museum and is being adopted by divisions and curators as time and funds permit the scheduling of delineated cataloguing projects, including bibliographies related to documentation such as the instruments, the listing of instrument makers, and patents.

65. For example, the excellent conservatory laboratory directed by Dr. Robert Organ, Smithsonian Institution located in USNMAH.

66. D. S. Lamb, "The Army Medical Museum—A History," *Wash. Med. Annals* (1916) 15:26; *The Billings Microscope Collection of the Medical Museum Armed Forces Institute of Pathology* 2d ed. (Washington, D.C.: AFIP, 1974).

67. Division of Medical Sciences, USNMAH Records.

68. P. H. van Cittert, *Descriptive Catalogue . . . in Charge of the Utrecht University Museum* (Utrecht, 1923); G. L. 'E. Turner, *Descriptive Catalogue of van Marum's Scientific Instruments in Teyler's Museum* (Leiden, 1974); Ellis Kellert and Leonard B. Clark, *The Microscope Collection at Union College* (Schenectady, New York, 1967); *A Catalogue of the Collection of Antique Microscopes formed by the Late Sir Frank Crisp* (London, 1925).

69. Edwin Clarke, ed., *Modern Methods in the History of Medicine* (London: The Athlone Press of the University of London, 1971), pp. 358-75; Brian Bracegirdle, "The Performance of Seventeenth and Eighteenth Century Microscopes," *MH* (1978) 22:187-95.

70. Brian Bracegirdle, *A History of Microtechnique* (Ithaca: Cornell University Press, 1978).

71. Brian Bracegirdle, "The History of Histology," *Hist Sci* (1977) 15: 79-101.

72. C. J. S. Thompson, *Guide to Surgical Instruments and Objects in the Historical Series with Their History and Development* (London: Taylor and Francis, 1929).

73. Some of these instruments were part of the Loan Collection of the Royal Society of Medicine. *Catalogue of and Report of Obstetrical and Other Instruments Exhibited at Conversazione of Obstetrical Society of London.* 28 March 1866.

74. Alban Doran, *Descriptive Catalogue of the Surgical Instruments . . . Lord Lister* part I, 1925 and C. J. S. Thompson, *Lord Lister the Discoverer of Antiseptic Surgery* (London: John Bale, Sons and Danielsson, Ltd., 1934), appendix.

75. K. Bryn Thomas, *The Development of Anesthetic Apparatus* (Oxford and London: Blackwell Scientific Publs., 1975).

76. Ibid.

77. The title continues: *With Special Reference to the Years 1846-1900* (London: The Wellcome Historical Medical Museum by Geoffrey Cumberlege, Oxford University Press, 1947).

78. John Crellin, *Medical Ceramics: A Catalogue of the English and Dutch Collections in the Museum of the Wellcome Institute of the History of Medicine* (London: Wellcome Institute of the History of Medicine, 1969); John Crellin and J. R. Scott, *Glass and British Pharmacy, 1600-1900: A Survey and Guide to the Wellcome Collection of British Glass* (London: Wellcome Institute of the History of Medicine, 1972); Philip Reichert, *The Reichert Collection Illustrative of the Evolution and Development of Diagnostic Instruments and Techniques in Medicine,* Loan Exhibit Catalogue (New York: Burroughs Wellcome and Co., 1942); Kenneth W. Berger, *The Hearing Aid: Its Operation and Development* (Detroit, Mich.: The National Hearing Aid Society, 1970). This book contains a sixty-one page listing of manufacturers and indicates the specific models of instruments each company produced. Audrey B. Davis and Toby Appel, *Bloodletting Instruments in the National Museum of History and Technology*; Samuel Joseph Platt and Mary Louise Ogden, *The Medical Museum at the Knoxville Academy of Medicine* (Knoxville, Tenn., 1971); J. Menzies Campbell, *Catalogue of the Menzies Campbell Collection of Dental Instruments, Pictures, Appliances, Ornaments, Etc.* (Edinburgh: Royal College of Surgeons of Edinburgh, 1966); Sami Hamarneh, "Dental Exhibition and Reference Collection at the Smithsonian Institution," *Health Service Reports* (1972) 87:291-303.

Among the current catalogues in which the prices of antique and collectible medical instruments are listed are: *An Exhibition of Antique Medical Instruments* (London: Simon Kaye, 1976); Crystal Payton, *Scientific Collectibles Identification and Price Guide.* (Sedalia, Missouri: Flat Creek Press, 1978). An auction catalogue of excellent medical and surgical instruments is *Instruments et Livres de Chirurgie et de Divers Arts provenent des anciennes collections des Maisons Charrière, Collin et Gentile* compiled by M. Alain Brieux (Paris, 1978).

Brochures and pamphlets on historical medical, pharmaceutical, and dental instruments include: Michael Harris, "Drugs and their Dispensers," (Washington, D.C.: Smithsonian Institution, 1977), 12 pp.; Audrey B. Davis, "The Dentist and His Tools," (Washington, D.C.: American

College of Dentists and Smithsonian Institution, 1975), 12 pp.; "The Apothecary in Eighteenth Century Williamsburg," (Williamsburg, Va., Williamsburg Craft Series, 1973).

79. See my review of Elisabeth Bennion, *Antique Medical Instruments* (Berkeley: Sotheby Parke Bernet and University of California Press, 1979) in *BHM* (1979) 53:626-28.

80. M. L. review of Isambard Owen, *A Supplementary Catalogue of the Pathological Museum of St. George's Hospital: A Description of the Specimens added during the Years 1866-81* in *AJMS* (1882) 85:557-58.

81. W. O. review of Morris Longstreth, *Supplement to the Descriptive Catalogue of the Pathological Museum of the Pennsylvania Hospital (1882)* in *AJMS* (1882) 84:229.

82. Anon. Review of Catalogue of the U.S. Army Medical Museum prepared under the Direction of the Surgeon-General U.S. Army, *MR* (1867) 1:494-95.

83. For a series of articles on the development of wax models see: *La Ceroplastica Nella Scienza e Nell'Arte*. Atti del i Congresso Internazionale, 2 vols. (Firenze: Leo S. Olschki, 1977).

84. E. J. Pyke, *A Biographical Dictionary of Wax Modellers* (Oxford: At the Clarendon Press, 1973).

85. Ibid., p. 49.

86. Maria Luisa Azzaroli, "La Specola, the Zoological Museum of Florence University," *La Ceroplastica Nella Scienza*, pp. 14, 15, 16.

87. Paolo Buffa, "On the Accuracy of the Wax Models of Biological Microscopical Preparations of Giovan Battista Amici (1786-1863)," *La Ceroplastica Nella Scienza*, pp. 217-41.

88. Konrad Allmer, Marlene Jantsch, *Katalog der Josephinische Sammlung Anatomischer und Geburtshilf-lisher Wachspraparate im Institut fur Geschichte der Medizin an der Universitat Wien* (Graz-Koln: Hermann Bohlaus, 1965).

89. E. J. Pyke, *A Biographical Dictionary*, p. 89.

90. Thomas Bryant, "Joseph Towne Modeller to Guy's Hospital for Fifty-Three Years," *GHR* (1882) 26:1-12.

91. Ed. Note, *BMJ* (1891) I:234. Louis Baretta is not identified by E. J. Pyke.

92. Linda Deer, "Italian Anatomical Waxes in the Wellcome Collection, The Missing Link," *La Ceroplastica Nella Scienza*, pp. 281-97.

93. Thomas C. Haviland and Laurence C. Parrish, "A Brief Account of the Use of Wax Models in the Study of Medicine," *JHMAS* (1970) 25:66.

94. Jacqueline Sonolet, "A Propos d'un Mannequin Anatomique en Bois; Napoleon Bonaparte et Felice Fontana," *La Ceroplastica Nella Scienza*, pp. 443-57.

95. Audrey B. Davis, "Louis Thomas Jerome Auzoux and the Papier Maché Anatomical Model," *La Ceroplastica Nella Scienza*, pp. 257-79.

96. The French were leading supporters of plans to introduce the teaching of physiology into the lower school levels. Articles in medical journals of the last quarter of the nineteenth century testify to this special interest, which was becoming of equal interest to American physicians. A study of the origin, methods, and appeal of science teaching in the secondary and grammar schools, with an emphasis on human and comparative anatomy and physiology, is highly desirable. Factors that encouraged the widespread teaching of anatomy and physiology included the increasing need to practice approved habits of sanitation and other good health habits, to maintain government-sponsored institutions such as the military forces, and to teach farmers how to safeguard their livestock and plants from epidemic diseases.

97. J. Clifton Edgar, "Aids in Obstetric Teaching," *MR* (1896) 50:810.

98. Ibid., p. 809.

99. Wellcome Exhibit catalogues include: (1) The Curator, *Handbook to the Wellcome Historical Medical Museum* (London, 1920); (2) *Medicine in 1815, An Exhibition to Commemorate the 150th Anniversary of the End of the Napoleonic Wars* (London: The Wellcome Historical Medical Museum and Library, 1965); (3) *Chinese Medicine, an Exhibition Illustrating the Traditional Medicine of the Chinese People* (London: Wellcome Historical Medical Museum and Library, 1966); (4) *Medicine and Surgery in the Great War 1914-1918* (London: Wellcome Institute of the History of Medicine, 1968); (5) *The History of Cardiology* Exhibition Catalogue No. 6 (London: Unwin Bros. Ltd., 1970); (6) *Psychiatry and Mental Health in Britain* (London: Wellcome Institute of the History of Medicine); (7) *Dickens and Medicine* (London: Wellcome Institute of the History of Medicine).

100. *Kobenhavns Universitets Medicinsk-Historiske Museum* (Copenhagen: Kirurgisk Akademi, 1969); *Istituto de Storia della Medicina dell'universita di Roma* (Roma: Il Museo, 1958); Josep Antell, ed., *Pictures From the Past of the Healing Arts* (Budapest: Semmelweis Medical Historical Museum, 1972). See my review of this catalogue in *Isis* (1977) 68:123-24. Sami Hamarneh, "History of the Division of Medical Sciences," *Contributions from the Museum of History and Technology* (Washington, D.C.: Smithsonian Institution Press, 1964).

101. Audrey B. Davis, *Triumph Over Disability*.

102. Victor Seidel, "New Technologies and the Practice of Medicine," in E. Mendelsohn et al., eds., *Human Aspects of Biomedical Innovation*, (Cambridge, Mass.: Harvard University Press, 1971) pp. 131, 135.

103. S. Putnam, "Fatal Use of the Aspirator," *BMSJ* (1880) 102:404-05. Putnam calls attention to Hall C. Wyman of Detroit.

104. Editorial, "Laparotomy as a Diagnostic Resource," *JAMA* (1886) 7:603-605. See also: To editor from A. D. Bundrey, "Death from Introduction of Stomach Tube," *MR* (1884) 25:504; F. Huber, "Drainage Tubes Accidentally Left in the Pleural Cavity in Cases of Empyema," *MR* (1885) 127:3-8; Key Aberg, "Rupture of the Stomach from the Use of the Stomach Pump," *MR* (1891) 40:458; Jacob Frank, "The Breaking of a Lithotrite in the Bladder," *MR* (1887) 32:17-18; Dillon Brown, "Dangers and Accidents of Intubation," *MR* (1887) 31:705.

105. Abstract of Negebauer of Warsaw "Count Sponges

and Instruments,'' *BMJ* (1900) I:1047-48. Taken from *Monats. f.Geburts. u. Gynaek.* (1900) 40. See also Editorial, "The History of an Abdominal Compress," *MR* (1892) 41:518.

CHAPTER 3

1. Réné Jacques Croissant de Garengeot, *Nouveau Traité des Instrumens de Chirurgie les plus utiles* 2d ed. (Paris, 1727), p. 2.

2. Ivor Nöel-Hume, *A Guide to Artifacts of Colonial America* (New York: Alfred A. Knopf, 1972), p. 5.

3. Henry Sigerist, *A History of Medicine, Early Greek, Hindu and Persian Medicine*, vol. II (London: Oxford University Press, 1961), p. 70. See also J. N. Svoronos, *Das Athener National Museum* (Athens, 1908-1911).

4. George Griffenhagen, "Tools of the Apothecary," *J Am Phar Assoc* (1956) 156:7, and Alma Wittlin, *The Museum, Its History and Its Tasks in Education* (London: Routledge and Kegan Paul, 1949).

5. Silvio Bedini, "The Evolution of Science Museums," *Technology and Culture* (1965) 6:1.

6. Ibid., p. 7. See also for a listing of some significant medical collections: Henry Sigerist, *A History of Medicine: Primitive and Archaic Medicine.* (New York: Oxford University Press, 1951), pp. 525-31.

7. S. Bedini, "Evolution of Science Museums," p. 7.

8. Ibid., p. 8.

9. Ibid., p. 9.

10. George Griffenhagen "Tools of the Apothecary," p. 8.

11. Ibid.

12. S. Bedini, "Evolution of Science Museums," pp. 2-6.

13. E. Andrews, "Fossil Trusses, A Clinical Lecture," *JAMA* (1885) 4:197.

14. W. B. McDaniel, "Medical Museum as an Adjunct to Medical Library," *BMLA* (1934) 23:91.

15. Ed., "The International Health Exposition," *MTG* (1883) 2:657.

16. *Official Catalogue of the Great Exhibition* (London: W. Clowes and Sons, 1851), pp. 60-74; Bruno Gebhard, "The Changing Ideology of Health Museums and Health Fairs since 1850," *BHM* (1959) 33:160-67.

17. Bruno Gebhard, "Sights and Thoughts on the Brussels's World's Fair" presented to Adult Education Council of Greater Cleveland 23 October 1958, typescript, Gebhard Papers, Allen Memorial Library, Cleveland, Ohio.

18. Bruno Gebhard, "The Changing Ideology of Health Museums," p. 162.

19. Bruno Gebhard, "History of World Fairs," 4 January 1939, typescript, Gebhard Papers, Allen Memorial Library, Cleveland, Ohio; Kenneth W. Luckhurst, *The Story of Exhibitions* (London and New York: The Studio Publs., 1951), pp. 63, 70.

20. I. M. H., Review of *International Exhibition, 1876 Official Catalogue*, 4 vols. *AJMS* (1876) 72:238.

21. A collection of photographs is on file in Philadelphia in the American Philosophical Society Library.

22. "Bureau of Hygiene and Sanitation of the World's Columbian Exposition," *MR* (1892) 42:745.

23. G.-E. Mergier avec la collaboration de Dr. Mosay, L. Audaine, F. de Grandmaison, *Technique Instrumentale* (Paris, 1891), p. viii.

24. Editorial, "The Educational Value of Museums," *Lancet* (1880) II:386.

25. Alice R. Kruse, "Bruno Gebhard: Father of the American Health Museum Movement," M.A. thesis, 1976, University of Toledo, Gebhard Collection, Allen Memorial Library, Cleveland, Ohio; Bruno Gebhard, "The Development of the Health Museum," *Museum News* (1964) 43.

26. "The Pathological Society of London 1848-1896," *MR* (1896) 49:728.

27. Jonathan Hutchinson, "Scheme for an Annual Museum," *BMJ* (1868) II:44.

28. Ibid.

29. Ibid.

30. Anon., "The Annual Museum at the Oxford Meeting," *BMJ* (1868) II:196.

31. Ibid., p. 197.

32. Anon., "The Annual Museum and Library," *BMJ* (1869) II:197.

33. Anon., "The Association Annual Museum," *BMJ* (1870) II:13.

34. Anon., "The Annual Museum, Newcastle," *BMJ* (1870) II:19, 190.

35. "The Collections of Instruments in the Annual Museum," *BMJ* (1874) II:320.

36. "Edinburgh Annual Museum," *BMJ* (1875) II:146.

37. "Annual Exhibition," *BMJ* (1902) II:139.

38. Anon., "The Annual Museum of Foods, Drugs, Instruments, Books and Sanitary Appliances," *BMJ* (1901) II:270. The selection of the medical instruments for major exhibitions such as the International Exhibition of 1861-62 occasionally presented difficulties to the jury that made the selection. James Syme reported in 1862, "If you only saw the outrageous increase in the way of surgical instruments that have been submitted for our approval. I sometimes think of taking down a bagful to laugh at." Robert Paterson, *Memorials of the Life of James Syme* (Edinburgh: Edmonston and Douglas, 1878), p. 143.

39. *BMJ* (1901), p. 270.

40. Note "Annual Exhibition," *BMJ* (1902) II:139; *"Annual Museum,"* *BMJ* (1886) II:41–42, 31, 427; "The Annual Museum," *BMJ* (1886) II:453; "The Annual Museum," *BMJ* (1888) II:426-40.

41. Editorial, "The Sanitary Exhibition in New Jersey," *MR* (1881) 20:437.

42. "An AMA Museum," *JAMA* (1892) 18:721.

43. Ibid.

44. "Notice to Exhibitors," from D. C. Patterson, *JAMA* (1884) 2:241.

45. Thomas G. Hull, "Bureau of Exhibits," in Morris Fishbein, *A History of the American Medical Association, 1847 to 1947* (Philadelphia and London: W. B. Saunders Co., 1943).

46. News of the Week, "Medical Exhibition in Berlin," *MR* (1886) 29:733.

47. Reported in *JAMA* (1900) 35:43, 44 and quoted in M. Fishbein, *A History of the American Medical Association*, p. 1043.

48. M. Fishbein, *A History of the American Medical Association*, p. 1044.

49. Ibid., p. 1046.

50. Ibid., pp. 1057-65.

51. Ibid., p. 1055.

52. Ibid., p. 1053.

53. "Black Historical Exhibit prepared by Dr. William Babb, Auditorium Hotel, Chicago 5-9 August 1918; C. Alvin Small, "The Black Historical Exhibit," *Oral Health* (1918) 8:334, 335.

54. "Medical Museums in St. Petersburg," *MR* (1898) 53:633.

55. "Trained Nurses' Educational Exhibit," *MR* (1898) 53:416.

56. Colin A. Sizer, "The Museum of the Wellcome Institute of the History of Medicine," *The Museums J* (1970) 80:13. Not all the medical treasures in Great Britain are preserved in the Wellcome Collection. For instance, a surgical chest containing over one hundred instruments, which was presented to the College of Physicians of London by Thomas Prujean in 1653, remains in the RCP possession and is on exhibit in the Museum of London. See C. J. S. Thompson, "An Historical Case of Surgical Instruments in the Possession of the Royal College of Physicians of London," *Medical Proceedings* (1927) 3 unnumbered pages.

57. See note 82 Chap. 2.

58. C. A. Sizer, "The Museum of the Wellcome Institute," p. 13.

59. Pierre Hamonic, *La Chirurgie et la Médecine d'autrefois d'après une premiére série d'instruments anciens renfermes dans mes Collections* (Paris: A Maloine, 1900) and typed list "Hamonic Collection 1928" in Wellcome Institute of the History of Medicine.

60. S. H. Daukes, "The Historical Medical Museum: its Future and Possibilities," *Museums J* (1944) 44:17-21.

61. C. A. Sizer, "The Museum of the Wellcome Institute," p. 13.

62. Ibid., p. 13.

63. Ibid., pp. 16, 20.

64. Ibid., p. 18.

65. Ibid., p. 19.

66. Sami Hamarneh, "History of the Division of Medical Sciences," *Contributions from the Museum of History and Technology* (Washington, D.C.: Smithsonian Institution Press, 1964), pp. 272, 273.

67. Ibid.

68. James M. Flint, "Directions for Collecting Information and Objects Illustrating the History of Medicine," *Bulletin USNM* (1905) 39:3-5.

69. Audrey B. Davis and Toby Appel, *Bloodletting Instruments in the National Museum of History and Technology* (Washington, D.C.: Smithsonian Institution Press, 1979).

70. Sami Hamarneh, "Dental Exhibition and Reference Collection at the Smithsonian Institution," *Health Service Reports* (1972) 87:291-303.

71. Ella N. Wade, "A Curator's Story of the Muetter Museum and College Collections," *Trans. and Studies of the College of Physicians* (1974) 42:122. Some notable physicians presented medical instruments to the museum. For example, J. M. DaCosta donated in 1892 a stethoscope that belonged to S. Weir Mitchell. Judson gave in 1927 a wooden stethoscope made from the timber of the Edinburgh Infirmary. DaCosta also presented a thermometer that had belonged to William Cullen, then had been passed on to a Virginian, then to Prof. J. T. Metcalfe, and finally to DaCosta.

72. Ibid., pp. 123, 125.
Whether the museum is worth the labor, care and money necessarily expended to maintain and increase it continuously, without end, is a question not easily answered. While the usefulness of such collections to help teachers of medical science in their demonstrations may not be doubted, their value in possession of a medical society chiefly composed of busily employed practitioners of medicine and surgery is not quite certain. Many visit the museum merely to gratify curiosity. How many resort to it only for study, or consult it for information alone, has not been ascertained. Possibly, the founder did not underestimate the general benefit which would flow from his munificent gift; but up to this time, conclusive evidence that medical science has gained anything from it is wanting.

73. Ibid., pp. 141, 142.

74. Ibid., pp. 150, 157, 166.

75. John Shaw Billings, *Medical Museums with Special Reference to the Army Medical Museum at Washington* (New Haven, 1888).

76. Ibid., p. 373.

77. D. L. Huntington, "The Army Medical Museum and Library," reprint of address before the Union Meeting of the Maryland State and Washington City Dental Societies, 8 May 1896, pp. 5, 6.

78. Helen R. Purtle, "Notes on the Medical Museum of the Armed Forces Institute of Pathology," *BMLA* (1956) 44:302.

79. Charles H. Mayo, "Educational Possibilities of the National Medical Museum," *JAMA* (1919) 73:411-13.

80. Howard Dittrick, "Medical History Collection in the U.S. and Canada." II. "A Description of Medical History Collections in Cleveland, Ohio," *BHM* (1940) 8:1214.

81. Barbara Smith Cooper, "Doctor's Office," *Bull. Acad. Med. Cleveland* (1966) reprint, 2 pp.

82. Howard Dittrick, "Medical History Collections," pp. 1214-32.

83. Ibid., p. 1216.

84. Ibid., p. 1226.

85. Samuel Joseph Platt, Mary Louise Ogden, *The Medical Museum at the Knoxville Academy of Medicine* (Knoxville, Tenn., 1971).

86. Erna Lesky, "Professor Jellinek's Electropathological Museum," *Ciba Symposium* (1961) 9:248-52.

87. Josep Antell, ed., *Pictures From the Past of the Healing Arts* (Budapest: Semmelweis Medical Historical Museum, 1972).

88. Leonard F. Menczer, Michael Mittelmann, *The Historical Museum of Medicine and Dentistry*. A Catalogue of Selected Objects, Hartford Medical Society and Hartford Dental Society, 1979.

CHAPTER 4

1. G. Sims Woodhead and P. C. Varrier-Jones, "Investigations on Clinical Thermometry: Continuous and Quasicontinuous Temperature Records in Man and Animals in Health and Disease," *Lancet* (1916) 1:176. Gibson wrote "On the Use of the Thermometer as a Guide in the Diagnosis of Pyrexial Diseases," *BMJ* (1866) I:249, 278.

2. C. A. Wunderlich *On the Temperature in Diseases: A Manual of Medical Thermometry* 2d German ed. 1870 trans. W. Bathurst Woodman (London: The New Sydenham Society, 1871), p. 20.

3. W. Ainslie Hollis, "On the Value of the Thermometer as an Aid to the Physician," *St. Bartholomeu's Hospital Reports* (1867) 3:287.

4. Review of Wunderlich's 1868 text *Das verhalten der Eigenwarme in krankheiten* (Leipzig, 1868), *AJMS* (1869) 57:431. This review was signed by J. C. R. and is twenty-two pages long.

5. J. F. Goodhart, "Thermometric Observations in Clinical Medicine," *GHR* (1869) 15:365.

6. J. W. Stickler, "Temporary Febrile Rise after Simple Fractures" *MR* (1882) 21:153-54.

7. Review of Wunderlich's text, p. 428.

8. C. A. Wunderlich, *On the Temperature in Diseases*, pp. 100, 120; A. S. Aloe, *Aloe's Illustrated and Priced Catalogue of Superior Surgical Instruments*, 6th ed., (St. Louis, ca. 1895), p. 575. Garrison described Wunderlich as the individual "who found fever a disease and left it a symptom." *An Introduction to the History of Medicine* 3d ed. (Philadelphia and London: W. B. Saunders Co., 1922), p. 453.

9. William Carter, "Observations on the normal temperature of the human body," *JAMA* (1884) 2:376, article abstracted from the *Liverpool Medico-Chirurgical Journal*.

10. Pierre Adolph Piorry, *Traité de la diagnostic* vol. III, 1838; cited in C. A. Wunderlich, *On the Temperature in Diseases*, pp. 28, 29. Piorry, of course, used the example of the magnetic compass in his statement.

11. John B. Bradbury, "Reports of Societies: Modern Scientific Medicine," *MR* (1880) 18:353. See also A. T. H. Waters, "The Present and Future Prospects of Medicine," *MR* (1883) 24:142.

12. C. A. Wunderlich, *On the Temperature in Diseases*, p. 19.

13. Review of Wunderlich's text and C. A. Wunderlich *On the Temperature in Diseases*, p. 19.

14. C. A. Wunderlich, *On the Temperature in Diseases*, p. 19.

15. T. Clifford Allbutt, "Medical Thermometry," Review of Wunderlich's book, *British and Foreign Medico-Chirurgical Review* (1870) 47:431, 432.

16. *Opera medica* (1676) pp. 11, Audrey B. Davis, *The Circulation of the Blood and Medical Chemistry in England, 1650-1680.* (Lawrence, Kans.: Coronado Press, 1973), p. 155.

17. Gerard van Swieten, *The Commentaries upon the Aphorisms of Dr. Hermann Boerhaave* vol. VI, (London, 1759) p. 182; G. A. Lindeboom, *Hermann Boerhaave: The Man and His Work* (London: Metheun and Co., Ltd., 1968), p. 294.

18. Everett Mendelsohn, *Heat and Life: The Development of the Theory of Animal Heat* (Cambridge, Mass.: Harvard University Press, 1964), pp. 123-139.

19. H. F. A. Goodridge, "Address in Medicine: The Pathology of Fever," *BMJ* (1878) II:200.

20. *Lancet* (1855) I:228 and see Editorial "A Theory of Fever," *MR* (1882) 22:375.

21. H. F. A. Goodridge, "Address in Medicine," p. 203.

22. Ibid., p. 200.

23. Editorial, "The Thermotaxic Heat Centres," *MR* (1887) 32:739; Horatio C. Wood, "A Study of the Nature and Mechanism of Fever," The Toner Lectures, *Smithsonian Miscellaneous Collections* No. 282, 1875, 45 pp.

24. John Burdon Sanderson, "Address in Physiology," *BMJ* (1873) II:154 ". . . in fever the elevation of the bodily temperature is characteristic of the whole process."

25. T. Clifford Allbutt, "The Clinical Thermopile," *BMJ* (1873) II:309; G. S. Woodhead and P. C. Varrier-Jones, "Investigations on Clinical Thermometry," p. 176.

26. "A New Thermograph," *MR* (1879) 20: 629. Marey's account appears in *Annales et Bulletin de la Société de Médecine de Gand* July 1881. W. B. Bowkett of the Leeds Fever Hospital engaged Salt and Son of Birmingham to construct a continuous curve recording thermograph. "The Clinical Thermograph," *BMJ* (1881) II:903.

27. H. F. A. Goodridge, "Address in Medicine," p. 200.

28. Ibid.

29. Ibid., p. 202.

30. Ibid., pp. 200, 202.

31. Ibid., p. 202.

32. Ibid., p. 203.

33. Richard Quain, "On the History and Progress of Medicine," *BMJ* (1885) II:779.

34. T. Lauder Brunton, "Address in Medicine. Twenty-Five Years of Medical Progress," *BMJ* (1891) II:231.

35. Editorial, "Antipyresis," *MR* (1885) 28:205.

36. S. Sambursky, *The Physical World of the Greeks* (London: Routledge, 1956).

37. W. E. Knowles Middleton, *A History of the Thermometer and Its Uses in Meteorology* (Baltimore: The Johns Hopkins Press, 1966), p. 3.

38. Michael McVaugh, "Quantified Medical Theory and Practice at Fourteenth Century Montpellier," *BHM* (1969) 43:413. See also Edith Sylla, "Medieval Quantifications of Qualities: The 'Merton School'," *Archives for the History of the Exact Sciences* (1971), pp. 9-39.

39. W. E. K. Middleton, *A History of the Thermometer*, p. 4.

40. M. McVaugh, "Quantified Medical Theory," for discussions of their ideas, p. 399.

41. Eric Ebstein, "Die Entwicklung der Klinischen Thermometrie," *Ergebnisse der Innerin Medizin und Kinderheilkunde* (1928) 33:438.

42. W. E. K. Middleton, *A History of the Thermometer*, p. 13.

43. Ibid., pp. 10, 11.

44. Ibid., p. 20.

45. J. A. Chaldecott, "Bartholomeo Telioux and the Early History of the Thermometer," *Annals of Science* (1952) 8:195-201.

46. W. E. K. Middleton, *A History of Thermometry*, p. 22.

47. Ibid., p. 9.

48. Ibid., p. 13.

49. Ibid., p. 39.

50. Ibid., p. 52.

51. Ibid., p. 50.

52. Ibid., pp. 78, 79.

53. S. Weir Mitchell, *The Early History of Instrumental Precision in Medicine* (New Haven: Tuttles, Morehouse and Taylor, 1892), p. 10.

54. W. E. K. Middleton, *A History of the Thermometer*, p. 9.

55. "Scala gradum caloris," *PT* (1701) 22. Samuel Wilks, physician, studied the history of the Fahrenheit scale, since it was the first thermometer scale to use body temperature as an endpoint. He traced it to Newton's paper.

56. W. E. K. Middleton, *A History of the Thermometer*, pp. 57, 58; "'Nova et vera', The Scale of Fahrenheit's thermometer," *BMJ* (1900) II:1212, 1213.

57. R. T. Gunther, *Early Science in Oxford* (Oxford: Oxford University Press, 1923-25) vol. III p. 69 and vol. IV p. 66.

58. C. A. Wunderlich, *On the Temperature in Diseases*, chap. 2.

59. E. Ebstein, "Die Entwicklung," pp. 407-503 and note one.

60. *Report on Italian Instruments South Kensington Special Collections* (1876) p. 941 illus. p. 94.

61. S. Weir Mitchell, "The History of Instruments of Precision in Medicine," *MR* (1878) 14:286.

62. G. A. Lindeboom, *Hermann Boerhaave*, p. 295.

63. Ibid.

64. Ibid.

65. Ibid., p. 295.

66. G. Van Swieten, *Commentaries*, p. 182.

67. J. Boersma, "Antonius de Haen 1704-1776: Life and Work," *Janus* (1963) 50:285, 286.

68. Cornelius Fox, "The thermometer in Disease," *MTG* (1869) II:459.

69. Eduoard Seguin, trans. *Medical Thermometry and Human Temperature*, by C. A. Wunderlich (New York: William Wood and Co., 1871, 2d ed., 1876).

70. Ibid., (1871), p. 208.

71. W. E. K. Middleton, *A History of the Thermometer*, p. 74.

72. Robert Fludd, *Integrum morborum mysterium*, "Pulsus seu nova et arcana pulsuum historia e sacro fonte radicaliter extracta, nec non medicorum ethnicorum dis tis . . ." (1631).

73. E. Seguin, *Medical Thermometry* (1871) p. 242 and (1876) p. 264.

74. Ibid., (1876) p. 261.

75. "A New Thermometer," *MR* (1896) 50:502.

76. W. E. K. Middleton, *A History of the Thermometer*, p. 109.

77. Ibid., p. 143.

78. Ibid., p. 155.

79. Bradford Noyes, Jr., "The History of the Thermometer and Sphygmomanometer," *Bulletin Medical Library Association*, 24 (1936), p. 160.

80. *Report on Italian Instruments*, p. 942.

81. Louis P. Casella, "Letter on Clinical Thermometers," *MTG* (1869) II:611.

82. Ibid.

83. "An Improved Clinical Thermometer," *BMJ* (1900) I:647.

84. "The New Phoenix Thermometer," *BMJ* (1885) II:768.

85. B. Noyes, "The History of the Thermometer," p. 161.

86. *Lancet* (1895) I:39.

87. "Broken Thermometers," *MR* (1882) 22:699.

88. A. T. H. Waters, "The Present and Future Prospects of Medicine," *MR* (1883) 24:141; W. R. Fisher of Hoboken, "Letter to Editor," *MR* (1883) 23:15; T. F. Houston, Charles C. F. Gay, William R. Leonard, and F. H. Darby of Morrow, Ohio, *MR* (1883) 24:111.

89. James Finlayson, "On the Use of the Clinical Thermometer," *BMJ* (1874) I:261.

90. Andrew Shrewsbury, *BMJ* (1868) p. 447.

91. T. Clifford Allbutt, "Medical Thermometry" Review of Wunderlich's book, pp. 437, 438.

92. F. C. Curtis, "Thermometry in Health and Medicine," *NYMJ* (1872) 16:619.

93. J. Finlayson, "On the Use of the Clinical Thermometer," p. 261.

94. W. E. K. Middleton, *A History of the Thermometer*, p. 135.

95. W. B. Kesteven, "Clinical Thermometers and Their Derivatives," *Lancet* (1873) I:824.

96. W. E. K. Middleton, *A History of the Thermometer*, p. 146.

97. Ibid., p. 145.

98. Ibid., p. 147.

99. B. Noyes, "The History of the Thermometer," p. 160.

100. T. Clifford Allbutt, Review of Wunderlich's book, p. 438. For a commentary by an American see "Clinical Thermometers," *MR* (1882) 21:164.

101. C. Fox, "The Thermometer," p. 459. Hawksley patented and advertised his thermometer in the *MTG* 1870

to 1872 and the *Lancet* 1869 and mentioned Fox's endorsement.

102. Anon., "A New Clinical Thermometer," *Lancet* (1869) II:12.

103. Other scales for the medical thermometer are mentioned by Allbutt J. Finlayson, "On the Use of the Clinical Thermometer," p. 262; C. A. Wunderlich, *On the Temperature in Diseases*, p. 62; James Flint, "Remarks on the Use of the Thermometer in Diagnosis and Prognosis," *NYMJ* (1866) 4:83.

104. W. E. K. Middleton, *A History of the Thermometer*, p. 163.

105. "The Clinical Thermoscope," *MR* (1875) 10:204, 205. The Truax Company of Chicago produced a thermometer that formed a new index each time it was used. *Price List of Physicians' Supplies*, Charles Truax and Co. (Chicago, 1893), p. 963.

106. Leonard Waldo, "The Thermometric Bureau of Yale College," *NYMJ* (1882) 36:222, 223.

107. W. R. Leonard, "An Improvement in Clinical Thermometers," *MR* (1883) 24:305.

108. Leonard Waldo, "Thermometric Bureau," *BMSJ* (1880) 103:185.

109. Anon., "The Accuracy of Clinical Thermometers," *BMSJ* (1881) 104:187.

110. L. Waldo, "The Thermometric Bureau of Yale College," p. 222.

111. *Med. Ann.* (1897) p. 828. B. Noyes of the Taylor Instrument Company claimed in 1936 "A so-called half-minute thermometer has a smaller bulb than the one-minute or two-minute, but I should point out at this time that this half-minute registration, so called, is nonsense and is put out by certain manufacturers for sales reasons only." "The History of the Thermometer," p. 162.

112. L. Waldo, "The Thermometric Bureau of Yale College," p. 221.

113. Leonard Waldo, "Note on the Errors of Clinical Thermometers," *MR* (1880) 18:179.

114. E. Seguin, *Medical Thermometry*, (1876), p. 262.

115. Orran T. Sherman, "An Improvement in Clinical Thermometers," *MR* (1883) 24:305.

116. Herbert T. Wade, "How Clinical Thermometers are Standardized and Tested," *Scientific American* (1905) 93:296.

117. Rexmond C. Cochrane, *A History of the National Bureau of Standards* (Washington, D.C.: National Bureau of Standards, U.S. Department of Commerce, 1966), p. 78.

118. H. Wade, "How Clinical Thermometers," p. 296.

119. B. Noyes, "A History of the Thermometer," p. 162.

120. E. Seguin, *Medical Thermometry*, (1876), p. 262 and W. B. Kesteven, "Clinical Thermometers and Their Derivatives."

121. R. T. Gunther, *Early Science in Oxford*, p. 69.

122. G. S. Woodhead and P. C. Varrier-Jones, "Investigations on Clinical Thermometry," p. 175.

123. L. P. Casella, "Letter," p. 611.

124. *Official Exhibition Catalogue*, p. 943.

125. C. Fahrney, "A Shorter Scale for the Thermometer," *MR* (1895) 48:322.

126. Anon., "Arnold's Patent Clinical Thermometer," *BMJ* (1875) I:649.

127. Review of Wunderlich's text, p. 430. Wunderlich described the characteristics of a good instrument: "The reservoir or bulb should not be too large or too small; when it is too large it suffers in sensibility, when too small it does not come closely in contact with the parts. A diameter of about one-half or three-fourths of a centimeter (.18 to .28 of an inch) is best. The spherical form is to be preferred for measurements in the axilla to the cylindrical; at least a cylindrical reservoir should not be very long, but approach the spherical form. . . . The tube of the instrument must be everywhere of the same calibre, and of such a bore that a distance of two-fifths of a degree can be divided by the eye without difficulty into halves and quarters. The length of the tube must be such that the scale reaches at least twelve centimetres (4.5 inches) from the bulb, so that when the instrument is applied, the height of the mercury can be easily seen. On account of portability, however, the length should not be too great. . . . The scale need only extend from 32.5 degrees Centigrade to 45 degrees Centigrade (90.3 degrees Fahrenheit to 113 degrees Fahrenheit), and if the thirty-fifth degree is twelve centimetres from the bulb the length will be satisfactory."

128. *MTG Advertiser* 5 (5 February 1872).

129. G. S. Woodhead and P. C. Varrier-Jones, "Investigations on Clinical Thermometry," p. 178; *MTG Advertiser* 5 (9 March 1872), p. 302.

130. Austin Flint, "Remarks on the Use of the Thermometer in Diagnosis and Prognosis," *NYMJ* (1866-67)4:83.

131. G. S. Woodhead and P. C. Varrier-Jones, "Investigations on Clinical Thermometry," p. 179.

132. Byron Bramwell, *Practical Medicine and Medical Diagnosis* (Edinburgh: Pentland, 1887), p. 61.

133. "The Annual Museum," *BMJ* (1888) II:433 and (1891) II:429.

134. Primavesi Bros. *BMJ* (1891) II:430.

135. "The Annual Museum," *BMJ* (1887) II:468.

136. William Aitkin, *The Science and Practice of Medicine* (1886), p. 34.

137. Advertisement, Codman & Shurtleff, *JAMA* (1884) 2, p. ii.

138. "English-made Thermometers," *Lancet* (1897) I:898 and *JAMA* (1889) 13:21 *The Journal General Advertiser*; A. S. Aloe, *Aloe's Illustrated and Priced Catalogue of Superior Surgical Instruments*, 6th ed. (St. Louis, ca. 1895), p. 577. The cheaper and less accurate German-made thermometers were compared unfavorably with English instruments by Drs. Johnson and Garrod, who attempted to encourage use of the thermometer in 1865. "The Thermometer in Specific Fevers; Three Cases of Typhus Fever," *Lancet* (1865) II:647.

139. "Weinhagen's Magnifying Normal Index Fever Thermometers," *BMSJ* (1893) 129, p. 5.

140. *JAMA* (1887) 9:16.

141. *Official Exhibition Catalogue*, pp. 943, 944.

142. *Lancet* (1865) II:647.

143. James J. Hicks, "Climax Clinical Thermometer," *Lancet* (1895) I:995.

144. Aloe, *Catalogue*, p. 574; Moritz Immisch, "Comparison between Mercurial and Avitreous Thermometers," *NYMJ* (1889) 50:313.

145. *JAMA* (1887) 9:16.

146. Maurice Perkins, "How to Restore the Scale of Thermometers," to the editor, *MR* (1877) 12:767.

147. J. Gall, "Improved Fever Thermometer," *MR* (1880) 17:273.

148. The Kny-Scheerer Co., *Illustrated Catalogue of Surgical Instruments*, 16th ed. (New York, 1917), p. 1042.

149. Arnold and Son, *BMJ* (1896) I:853.

150. "The Autosterilizing Thermometer Case," *MR* (1896) 48:497.

151. "Duplex Instanter Clinical Thermometer," *BMJ* (1890) II:347.

152. *Lancet* (1897) I:898.

153. Editorial, *BMSJ* (1893) 129:46-47.

154. Aloe, *Catalogue*, p. 575.

155. E. Ebstein, "Die Entwicklung," p. 23. "Seit dieser zeit sind Gebeite der Medizin, nicht zür der praktischen sondern auch der theoretischen von der anwendung der thermometris der methoden stark beeinflusst worden."

156. "On Cerebral Thermometry," *MR* (1878) 14:37, 157; "Cerebral Thermometry," *MR* (1879) 16:490.

158. "Facts and Figures on Cerebral Thermometry," *MR* (1880) 17:706.

159. "Instruments of Precision," *MR* (1879) 16:470.

160. C. K. M., *Experimental Researches on the Temperature of the Head* by J. S. Lombard, reviewed in the *AJMS* (1881) 82:221-24. See also J. S. Lombard, "Description of a New Portable Thermoelectric Apparatus for Medical and Physiological Investigations," *BMJ* (1875) I:98-102.

161. "The Value of Cerebral Thermometry on Diseases of the Brain," *MR* (1883) 23:625, 626.

162. *MR* (1883) 24:94, 95.

163. Bogdan Flitner, *Thermometry of Ear in Physiologic and Pathologic Aspects*, in Russian (St. Petersburg, 1882).

164. Abstracted from *MR* (1 November 1884), "Aural Thermometry," *JAMA* (1884) 2:549.

165. G. Sterling Ryerson, "Thermometry in Diagnostic Relation to Ear Disease," *MR* (1891) 40:211.

166. Abstract, "A Urine Thermometer for Gynecological Practice," *MR* (1879) 15:466.

167. Ibid., p. 466. This account is abstracted from the *Centralblatt fur gynakologie* (15 February 1879).

168. E. Ebstein, "Die Entwicklung," p. 498.

169. E. Seguin, *Medical Thermometry* (1871).

170. Ibid., (1876), introd.

171. *Idiocy and its Treatment by the Physiological Method with a Bibliographical Note by* Harold Runn and Francesco Cordasco (New York: Augustus M. Kelly, 1971); Mabel Talbot, "Edouard Seguin: A Study of an Educational Approach to the Treatment of Mentally Defective Children," (New York: Columbia University Teachers College, 1964).

172. "Obituary," *MR* (1880) 18:531-32.

173. E. Seguin, *Medical Thermometry* (1871), p. 199.

174. See the section on thermometry instruments above for details.

175. E. Seguin, *Medical Thermometry* (1871) p. 203. Seguin added: ". . . that its use could become general, and could be extended to the solution of social and economical problems far more important than those of individual disease and recovery."

176. Ibid., p. 251.

177. Ibid., p. 233.

178. Ibid.

179. Ibid., p. 240.

180. Ibid., p. 243.

181. Ibid., p. 245.

182. Ibid., p. 265.

183. Ibid., p. 256.

184. Ibid., p. 266. "Thus rendered *human* thermometry protects the life of children and invalids, as well as the sick; guides and justifies the physician; enfranchises the mother from the imposition of the bonzes; reconstitutes the antique unity of diagnosis around the phenomenon of ustion; and connects the laws of animal heat—as far as they are discovered with the known laws of the universe. Thermometry begat thermography, and thermography is pregnant with medical mathematism," p. 384.

185. "Patients Notions of the Clinical Thermometer," *MR* (1876) 11:43.

186. Charles Wilson Ingraham, "Spreading Disease by the Clinical Thermometer," *MR* (1895) 40:25; "Dirty Thermometers," *MR* (1896) 49:142. Excerpt from *Charlotte M J*.

187. "The First Symptoms of Pulmonary Tuberculosis," *MR* (1895) 47:557.

188. Ibid.

189. Joseph G. Richardson, "Cases Illustrative of the Assistance Afforded in Diagnoses by Thermometric Observation in Private Practice," *MR* (1868) 6:79. "When any new scientific instrument is introduced among the implements of our profession, it often happens that many practitioners, after a partial test of its capacities, become dissatisfied with its failure to aid them in solving all the problems which disease, modified by the infinitely diverse idiosyncracies of patients, present and in the disappointment which they feel over its shortcomings, renounce even the benefits which it is able to confer."

Chapter 5

1. Henry E. Sigerist, *A History of Medicine* (Oxford: Oxford University Press, 1951), pp. 310-15; L. Stern, *Papyros Ebers* II (Leipzig, 1875); Robert W. Buck, "Physical Diagnosis Prior to Auenbrugger," *NEJM* (1933) 211:240.

2. Joseph Sailor, "Auscultation in the Physical Examination of the Abdomen," *JAMA* (1923) 81:728; Book 2, Chap. 9 of Soranus. See also *Gynecology*, trans. with an introduction by Owsei Temkin. (Baltimore: Johns Hopkins Press, 1956).

3. I. E. Drabkin, *Caelius Aurelianus on Acute Diseases and on Chronic Diseases* (Chicago: University of Chicago, 1950), p. 695.

4. *Exercitatio anatomica de motu cordis et sanguinis* (Frankfurt, 1628), p. 30.

5. Alfred Hudson, "Laennec: His Labours and Their Influence in Medicine," *BMJ* (1879) II:204.

6. D. M. Cammann, "An Historical Sketch of the Stethoscope," *NYMJ* (1886) 46:465. Cammann, originator of the most popular flexible binaural stethoscope, reviewed the claims that Hippocrates, Bayle, Hooke, and Laennec had each invented the instrument.

7. H. A. McCallum, Discussion of "Paracentesis of the Pericardium: Its Induction and Methods by George Dock," *Lancet* (1906) II:802.

8. A. Hudson, "Laennec," p. 206.

9. D. C. Abrahams-Auriel, *Laennec His Life and Times*, trans. Roger Kevram (New York: Pergamon Press, 1960), p. 149.

10. James T. Whittaker, "The History of Auscultation," *MR* (1879) 16:413; P. J. Bishop, "Evolution of the Stethoscope," *JRSM* (1980) 73:449.

11. Robert W. Buck, "Physical Diagnosis Prior to Auenbrugger," *NEJM* (1933) 209:240; Émile Littré, *Oeuvres complètes d'Hippocrate*, vol. 7 (Paris: J. B. Baillière, 1851), p. 70.

12. D. C. Abrahams-Auriel, *Laennec*, p. 148. Paré, *Table méthodique pour cognoistre les maladies par les cinq sens* (A Systematic Table for the Recognition of Diseases by the Five Senses) (1560).

13. D. C. Abrahams-Auriel, *Laennec*, p. 133.

14. Ibid.; Fielding H. Garrison, *An Introduction to the History of Medicine* 2d ed. (Philadelphia: W. B. Saunders Co., 1917), p. 167 reference to Sudhoff. See also for surgical instruments depicted in other paintings Romulus Popescu, "Instruments Médico-chirurgicaux dans la peinture Féodale de Roumania," 23d Congrès International d'Histoire de la Médecine Bucharest 1970, pp. 461, 462.

15. *The Posthumous Works of Robert Hooke* (1705), pp. 39, 40. Quoted in K. D. Keele, *The Evolution of Clinical Medicine* (Springfield, Ill.: Charles C. Thomas, 1963), p. 46.

16. John Forbes, trans., *A Treatise on the Diseases of the Chest and on Mediate Auscultation* by R. T. H. Laennec, 4th ed. (London, 1834), p. 4.

17. James Clark, *Medical Notes on the Climate, Diseases, Hospitals and Medical Schools of France and Italy and Switzerland . . . in Cases of Pulmonary Consumption* (London, 1820). Clark met Jean-Bruno Cayol, a colleague of Laennec's, at the Hospital Necker who showed him Laennec's stethoscope, which was thirteen inches long and perforated by an opening four or five lines in diameter.

18. Henry Bennett, "Remarks on the Comparative Value of Auscultation Practiced with and without the Stethoscope," *Lancet* (1844) I:462.

19. Richard Quain, "History and Progress of Medicine," *BMJ* (1885) II:779. Quain was a consulting physician to the Hospital for Consumption and Diseases of the Chest at Brompton.

20. William Stokes, *An Introduction to the Use of the Stethoscope* (Edinburgh: Maclachlan and Stewart, 1825); Charles J. B. Williams, *A Rational Exposition of the Physical Signs of the Diseases of the Lungs and Pleura* (London: T. and G. Underwood, 1830).

21. J. Forbes, *A Treatise*, p. xxvi.

22. Ibid., pp. ix, x.

23. Ibid., p. xiii.

24. Ibid., pp. xxv, xxvii.

25. John Forbes, trans., *Original Cases with Dissection and Observations Illustrating the Use of the Stethoscope and Percussion in the Diagnosis of Diseases of the Chest* (London, 1824). Thirty-six pages and second, third and fourth editions of Laennec's book in 1830, 1834, 1838.

26. A. Hudson, "Laennec," p. 206.

27. "A Note on the Reception of the Stethoscope in England," *BHM* (1939) 7:93.

28. "Physical Signs in the London Hospital," *MH* (1958) 2:198.

29. Edmond I. Bluth, "James Hope and the Acceptance of Auscultation," *JHMAS* (1970) 25:202-10; Lester S. King, "Auscultation in England, 1821-1837," *BHM* (1959) 33:446-53.

30. Iago Galdston, "Diagnosis in Historical Perspective," *BHM* (1941) 9:369, 370.

31. Saul Jarcho, "John Eberle's Lectures on Medicine," 1827 *AJC* (1969) 8:508-12.

32. Joseph H. Pratt, "The Development of Physical Diagnosis," *NEJM* (1935) 213:641, 642 and see Saul Jarcho, "The Young Stethoscopist," *AJC* (1964) 13:808-19.

33. Austin Flint, *Physical Exploration and Diagnosis Affecting the Respiratory Organs* (Philadelphia: Blanchard and Lea, 1856). See also Francis J. Heringhaus, "Austin Flint," *J. Mich. State Med. Soc.* (1932) 31:133. "As a diagnostician in diseases of the chest he has few equals. . . . I know of no one who is so well entitled as Austin Flint, Sr., to be regarded as the American Laennec."

34. Review of *A Treatise of Auscultation* by Robert Spittal, *Lancet* (1831) II:618.

35. R. T. H. Laennec, *A Treatise on the Diseases of the Chest*, trans. John Forbes (New York: Hafner Publishing Co., 1962), p. 284. Charles J. B. Williams, who had studied with Laennec, claimed that Laennec's "knowledge of acoustics was by no means profound; and clever as he had been in tracing the signs empirically he was not equally successful in explaining them rationally." *Memoirs of Life and Work* (London: Smith, Elder and Co., 1884), p. 49. Williams attempted to remedy this defect and the difficulty created by Laennec's omission by publishing his book, which appeared in several editions, *Rational Exposition of the Physical Signs of Diseases of the Chest* (1828).

36. Fielding Garrison, *A History of Medicine*, 3d ed. (Philadelphia: W. B. Saunders Co., 1922), p. 430.

37. J. Forbes, *A Treatise* (1834), pp. 132, 133.

38. *MR* (1885) 27:499.

39. Ibid.

40. Ibid.

41. Ibid., p. 500.

42. *An attempt at Medical and Surgical Diagnosis, in Tables; or Recognition and Discrimination of Internal and External Disease, by Comparison of Their Resembling Forms*, which originally was published in German in 1812 and in later editions in 1816, 1825 and 1830. *AJMS* (1828-29) 3:153.

43. J. Lisfranc, *A Memoir on the Diagnostic Signs afforded by the Use of the Stethoscope in Fractures and in some other Surgical Diseases* trans. J. R. Alcock, with notes and additions by Alcock (London, 1827), pp. 186, 187. Lisfranc published in 1823.

44. Charles Scudamore, *Observations on M. Laennec's Method of Forming a Diagnosis of the Diseases of the Chest by Means of the Stethoscope and of Percussion* (London: Longman, Rees, Orme, Brown, and Green, 1826), p. 9.

45. Review of *Physical Diagnosis including Diseases of the Thoracic and Abdominal Organs: A Manual for Students and Physicians* by Egbert Le Fevre, (Philadelphia and New York: Lea Bros. and Co.), *AJMS* (1906) 125:128.

46. C. Scudamore, *Observations*, p. 42.

47. Laennec, *Diseases of the Chest*, p. 366.

48. Arthur Leared, "On the Mechanism of the Acoustic Phenomena of the Circulation of the Blood, with an Exposition of a new Element in the Causation of the First Sound of the Heart," *AJMS* (1852) 58:340.

49. Ibid., p. 346.

50. Ibid., p. 349.

51. Austin Flint, "The Mitral Cardiac Murmurs," *AJMS* (1886) 91:29.

52. Review of *A Treatise of Auscultation* by Robert Spittal, *Lancet* (1831) II:618.

53. Aldo A. Luisada, *From Ausculation to Phonocardiography* vol. 4 (St. Louis: C. V. Mosby Co., 1965), p. 1.

54. H. A. Frederick and H. F. Dodge, "The Stethophone, An Electrical Stethoscope," *The Bell System Technical Journal* (1924) 3:531, note one.

55. D. C. Hawley, "Heart Sounds and Cardiac Murmurs," *JAMA* (1892) 18:666.

56. See for review and detailed description of a variety of chest measuring methods and devices: Arthur Ransome, *On Stethometry* (London: Macmillan and Co., 1876).

57. Albert Abrams, "Stethophonometry," *NYJM* (1901) 75:265. Abrams became the inventor of a popular radiographic medical device, which eventually was condemned as a quack device. I am indebted for this information to Prof. Thomas Creed, who is working on a history of alternative medical methods and devices. He has consulted the papers of Abrams in the collection of the Bakken Museum of Electricity and Life Archives in Minnesota. The quack device is on display in the medical museum in St. Louis. See also Nancy Roth, "Albert Abrams and his 'Electronic Reactions'," *Medical Instrumentation* (1977) 11:351.

58. Ibid.

59. Howard Kelly, "Every Patient His Own Case-Book," *JAMA* (1883) 1:535.

60. Editorial, "A New Departure in Physical Diagnosis," *MR* (1892) 42:625-26.

61. James M. DaCosta, "Respiratory Percussion," *AJMS* (1875) 139:17-26.

62. C. Dennison, "The Essentials of a Good Stethoscope," *MR* (1892) 42:494.

63. Henry Sewall, "The Role of the Stethoscope in Physical Diagnosis," *AJMS* (1913) 145:234.

64. J. B. Dawson, "Auscultation and the Stethoscope," *The Practitioner* (1964) 193:317.

65. Ibid., p. 318.

66. David Littmann, "An Approach to the Ideal Stethoscope," *JAMA* (1961) 178:504.

67. Bowles Pat. Nos. 700,728 (27 May 1902); 693,487 (18 February 1902); 677,172 (25 June 1901); 526,802 (2 October 1894). Bowles designed a pear- or flat-iron-shaped diaphragm to combine the maximum vibration obtained in a larger stethoscope with the adaptability of a smaller instrument. It was manufactured by George P. Pilling and Son of Philadelphia. "A New Pattern of Bowles Stethoscope," *MR* (1904) 66:719.

68. Littmann, "An Approach," p. 504.

69. Ibid. See also Maurice B. Rappaport and Howard B. Sprague, "The Effects of Tubing Bore on Stethoscope Efficiency," *AMJ* (1951) 42:605-09. These authors report on tests they conducted to show that the most efficient stethoscope was composed of a rubber tube having a bore reduced from 3/16 to 1/8 inch and its length made no longer than ten inches.

70. J. B. Dawson, "Auscultation," pp. 320, 322.

71. Edward MacCurdy, *The Notebooks of Leonardo da Vinci* (New York: Reynal and Hitchcock, 1938), p. 277; Wilhelm Ebstein, "Einige Bermerkungen zu der Geschichte des Stethoskops," *Deutsch Archiv. fur Klin. Med.* (1900-1901), pp. 488-502.

72. A. Wolf, *A History of Science, Technology and Philosophy in the 16th and 17th Centuries*, 2d ed., vol. I (New York: Harper Torchbooks, 1959), pp. 285-89.

73. Laennec, *Diseases of the Chest*, p. 285.

74. Ibid., p. 284.

75. Ibid., p. 286.

76. Kenneth D. Keele, *The Evolution of Clinical Methods in Medicine* (Springfield, Ill.: Charles C. Thomas, 1963), p. 47.

77. H. Landouzy, *Mémoire sur les procédés acoustiques de l'auscultation et sur un nouveau mode de stéthoscopie applicable aux études cliniques* (Paris and London: J.-B. Baillière, 1841), p. 29.

78. C. J. B. Williams, "Stethoscope," in *The Cyclopedia of Practical Medicine*, vol. IV, (Philadelphia: Lea and Blanchard, 1845), p. 237.

79. Ibid., p. 238.

80. H. Landouzy, *Mémoire*, p. 14.

81. C. J. B. Williams, "Stethoscope," p. 237.

82. Charles Moore Jessop, "Reports and Analyses and Descriptions of New Instruments—The Finger-Ended Stethoscope," *BMJ* (1879) I:514. The stethoscope was manufactured by Ferris and Co. of Bristol, England. See for a succinct discussion and illustrations of a variety of stethoscopes P. J. Bishop, "Evolution of the Stethoscope," pp. 448-56.

83. C. J. B. Williams, "Stethoscope," p. 237.

84. Laennec, *Diseases of the Chest*, p. 286; Williams, "Stethoscope," pp. 237-38.

85. Victor A. McKusick, William D. Sharpe, and Allen O. Warner, "An Exhibition on the History of Cardiovascular Sound Including the Evolution of the Stethoscope," *BHM* (1957) 31:471. Some basic types of stethoscopes are illustrated in Morris Leikind, "The Stethoscope, Some Notes on Its History," *JNMA* (1955) 47:177-80.

86. George Tiemann, *The American Armamentarium Chirurgicum* (New York, 1899), pp. 5-7. Hereafter *Catalogue.*

87. Charles Truax Co., *Price List of Physicians Supplies* (circa 1895) pp. 644-47.

88. The Kny-Scheerer Co., *Illustrations of Surgical Instruments*, Section I (New York, 1899), pp. 1029-31.

89. C. J. B. Williams, "Stethoscope," p. 238.

90. C. Theodore Williams, "A Lecture on Laennec and the Evolution of the Stethoscope," *BMJ* (1907) II:7; John Shaw Billings, *Principles of Medicine* (1842), p. 15.

91. Ibid., p. 7. One of the earliest stethoscopes was brought to London by Charles Scudamore, who introduced a Laennec stethoscope in 1826 after having studied in Paris with Laennec. Scudamore employed Mr. Garden of Oxford St. to copy Laennec's model and make up instruments for physicians seeking them. C. Scudamore, *Observations*, pp. 117-18.

92. Noel Adler, "A New Form of Straight Monaural Stethoscope," *Lancet* (1920) II:856. This was manufactured by Allen and Hanbury of London.

93. "Reports and Analyses and Descriptions of New Instruments, A New Portable Stethoscope," *BMJ* (1882) II:950, illus. p. 1024, No. 2989.

94. Anon., "The Flexible Clinical Stethoscope," *BMJ* (1875) II:302.

95. Conversation tubes continued to be sold in the twentieth century. See, for example, John Bell and Croyden in association with Savory and Moore Ltd. and Arnold and Sons, *Illustrated List of Acoustic Instruments* (London, circa 1920), pp. 29-31.

96. *Porte-caustique* is a case for carrying caustic drugs. Charles Frederick Power, "Reports and Analyses and Descriptions of New Instruments, A Combination Stethoscope," *BMJ* (1882) II:900; W. H. Taylor, "Combination Stethoscope," *BMJ* (1882) II:1159. This stethoscope was first announced in *BMJ* (18 September 1880).

97. Adolphe Piorry, *De la Percussion Médiate* (Paris, 1828), p. 16.

98. Ibid., p. 18. See Tiemann, *Catalogue*, p. 5 for Elliotson's model and Martin's model of combination stethoscope and pleximeter. Piorry's double-purpose instrument was adapted to the binaural stethoscope and reintroduced by several inventors in a slightly different form. For instance, F. W. Koehler, "An Improved Stethoscope for Use in Auscultatory Percussion," *MR* (1892) 42:170. See also Editorial, "Auscultatory Percussion and American Priority," *MR* (1885) 27:600. Cammann is given credit for the method and Dr. McBride is mentioned as introducing a solid binaural stethoscope circa 1880.

99. D. M. Cammann, "An Historical Sketch of the Stethoscope," *NYMJ* (1886) 46:466.

100. V. Huter, "The Somatoscope, *MR* (1877) 12:311; see for another combination stethoscope, thermometer, nasal or anal speculum, ophthalmometer, and reflector: Charles Frederick Power, "A Combination Stethoscope," *BMJ* (1882) II:900. It was made by Arnold and Sons.

101. Felix von Niemeyer combination percussor, stethoscope, 1868.

102. Erna Lesky, "Zur Geschichte diagnostischer Methoden perkussion und Auskultation," I Documenta Geigy (1970), p. 13.

103. *Official Catalogue of the Great Exhibition* (London: W. Clowes and Sons, 1851), Class 10.

104. V. Poulain, "Finger-Ended Stethoscope," *BMJ* (1879) I:612. This instrument was suggested to Poulain by the "Finger-ended stethoscope" designed by Charles Moore Jessop of Bristol and manufactured by Ferris and Co. and Matthews. It could be applied to any small area. Other temporary substitutes included: two cotton reels to be used on either side of a lead pencil or penholder. Letter of G. R. Moore, *BMJ* (1882) II:604. A wineglass was suggested by David A. Alexander of Clifton, Bristol in 1907. Comment on C. Theodore Williams, "Laennec and the Evolution of the Stethoscope," *BMJ* (1907) II:184.

105. C. Theodore Williams, "A Lecture on Laennec and the Evolution of the Stethoscope," *BMJ* (1907) II:7.

106. Samuel Wilks, "Correspondence—The Evolution of the Stethoscope," *BMJ* (1907) II:113; Nicholas P. Comins, "New Stethoscope," to the editor, *London Medical Gazette* (1829) 4:427-30.

107. H. Landouzy, *Mémoire*, p. 25.

108. Samuel Wilks, "Abstract of Lecture on the Evolution of the Stethoscope," *Lancet* (1882) II:883 and Sam Wilks, "Correspondence," p. 113.

109. *Official Catalogue of the Great Exhibition*, Class 10.

110. George L. Carrick, "On the Differential Stethoscope and Its Value in the Diagnosis of Diseases of the Lungs and Heart," *Aberdeen Medical and Chirurgical Tracts* 12, Tract 9 (1873), p. 895.

111. George P. Cammann, *NYMT* (1855) 4:140. An editorial in *JAMA* (17 June 1885), claimed "that Cammann's binaural stethoscope just as he left it, is really the best instrument . . . for auscultatory purposes that we have." 4:75. Arthur Leared made a claim for priority for the binaural stethoscope after he had noticed an American claim in the *British and Foreign Med. and Chir. Review*, "Progress of Medicine," in "A Hint About the Stethoscope," *MTG* (1855) 32:521. He made one of gutta percha with two earpieces, which he sent to the Great Exhibition in 1851.

112. G. L. Carrick, "On the Differential Stethoscope," p. 896.

113. *The Reichert Collection Illustrative of the Evolution and Development of Diagnostic Instruments and Techniques in Medicine*, Loan Exhibit Handbook, (New York: Burroughs Wellcome and Co., 1942), p. 53.

114. D. M. Cammann, "Historical Sketch," p. 465.

115. Kny-Scheerer, *Catalogue* p. 1025; Charles Dennison,

"An Improved Binaural Stethoscope," *MR* (1885) 27:391.

116. Letter of Ferris and Co., "Spencer's Compound Stethoscope," *BMJ* (1875) II:661.

117. R. Harvey Hilliard "On a New Double Stethoscope: The Headspring Stethoscope," *BMJ* (1875) II:610.

118. Charles Dennison, "The Essentials of a Good Stethoscope," *MR* (1892) 42:494.

119. "An Improved Binaural Stethoscope," *MR* (1885) 27:391.

120. *The Reichert Collection*, p. 54. A stethoscope with an enlarged opening in the tube free of any material proved to be a better sound conductor. Therefore, C. B. Longenecker suggested in 1892 that "the possessors of stethoscopes take them to a mechanic and have their internals curetted, and some of the strictures enlarged, and they will find themselves possessing a decidedly more efficient instrument." "The Essentials of a Good Stethoscope," *MR* (1892) 42:575.

121. See for example: R. K. Valentine, "An Improved Binaural Stethoscope and Improved Soft Rubber Bell," *MR* (1895) 47:30-31; R. Harvey Hilliard, "On a New Double Stethoscope: the Head Spring Stethoscope," *BMJ* (1875) II:610; R. K. Valentine, "An Improved Stethoscope," *MR* (1892) 42:82; Mark L. Knapp, "An Improved Stethoscope," *MR* (1895) 48:43-44; Dickson L. Moore, "An Articulated Knapp's stethoscope," *MR* (1896) 49:824; John R. Philpots, "A New Stethoscope," *BMJ* (1892) I:562; W. J. Burroughs, "A Portable Binaural Stethoscope," *BMJ* (1892) I:721; J. Inman Langley, "Improved Stethoscope," *BMJ* (1907) II:1720; George Herschell, "An Improved Binaural Stethoscope," *BMJ* (1891) I:706; William Rollins, "A Smaller Seehear," *BMSJ* (1901) 154:112; Aubrey Leatham, "An Improved Stethoscope," *Lancet* (1958) I:463.

122. T. C. Blackwell, "An Improved Stethoscope," *Lancet* (1911) I:1361; J. Birney Guthrie, "Modification of the Bowles Stethoscope," *JAMA* (1923) 81:1013-14.

123. G. L. Carrick, "Differential Stethoscope," p. 897.

124. Ibid., p. 898.

125. Ibid., p. 902.

126. Samuel Wilks, "Correspondence," p. 113.

127. G. L. Carrick, "Differential Stethoscope," p. 896.

128. William Ewart, "Analysis in Auscultation," *BMJ* (1888) I:1086. See also Constantin Paul, *Diseases of the Heart* (Philadelphia: William Wood and Co., 1884).

129. O. Leyton, "Differential Stethoscopes," *Lancet* (1916) II:24.

130. Ibid.

131. Ibid.

132. Dr. Bock, designer, "Differential Stethoscope for the Examination of the Heart and Lungs," *Mod. Hosp.* (1915) 4:449.

133. William J. Kerr, "Stethoscope and Symballophone," in *Medical Physics*, ed. Otto Glaser (Chicago: The Year Book Publishers, 1944).

134. Ibid., p. 1474.

135. Ibid.

136. Anon., "Salt's Portable Stethoscope," *BMJ* (1881) II:821.

137. F. W. Koehler, "An Improved Stethoscope for Use in Auscultatory Percussion," *MR* (1892) 42:170. For illustrations and brief descriptions of a personal collection of binaural stethoscopes, see Stephen Morris, "The Advent and Development of the Binaural Stethoscope," *The Practitioner* (1967) 199:674-80.

138. J. T. Whittaker, "History of Auscultation," p. 413.

139. Ibid., p. 412.

140. C. Dennison, "The Essentials," p. 494.

141. C. C. Henry, "The Heartphone," *NYMJ* (1918) 107:162.

142. Albert Abrams, "Measuring the Intensity of the Heart Tones," *Medical News* (1899) 75:40-42.

143. Ibid., p. 40; A. Abrams, "Studies in Stethophonometry," *NYMJ* (1902) 76:679.

144. Ibid.

145. Ibid., p. 678.

146. H. Landouzy, "Mémoire," pp. 25-28.

147. C. T. Williams, "A Lecture on Laennec," p. 7. This stethoscope was much used in the Polyclinic lectures. Another multiple stethoscope was devised in Europe and copied in the United States by George Pilling and Son of Philadelphia. Called a phonendoscope, it was reported by A. S. Walsh of New York. "New Attachments for the Phonendoscope," *MR* (1898) 53:755.

149. Jenner Hoskin, "A Multiple Electrical Stethoscope," *Lancet* (1925) II:1164.

148. Charles H. Larned quote, 1900.

150. R. C. Cabot, "A Multiple Electrical Stethoscope for Teaching Purposes," *JAMA* (1923) 81:298; C. J. Gamble, "Multiple Electrical Stethoscope and Electrical Filters as Aids to Diagnosis," *JAMA* (1924) 83:1230-32.

151. H. A. Frederick and H. F. Dodge, "The Stethophone," p. 547.

152. Aldo A. Luisada, *From Auscultation to Phonocardiography* (St. Louis: C. V. Mosby Co., 1965), p. 52.

153. S. Weir Mitchell, "The History of Instruments of Precision in Medicine," *MR* (1878) 14:287.

154. V. Collin, *Des Diverses Méthodes D'Exploration de la Poitrine et de leur Application au Diagnostic de ses Maladies* (Paris: J.-B. Baillière, 1831), p. vi and xiii. Trans. mine.

155. William Stokes, "The Cavendish Lecture on the Altered Relations of Surgery to Medicine," *BMJ* (1888) I:1197.

156. C. T. Williams, "A Lecture on Laennec," p. 7.

157. The experimentalist was not always the earliest to appreciate the stethoscope and other diagnostic instruments. For instance, Hermann Von Helmholtz and some of his colleagues believed that auscultation, percussion, temperature recording, and ophthalmoscopic investigation of the eye were coarsely mechanical and disparaging to the dignity of the patient and unnecessary for a physician with a clear mental insight. G. S. Hull, *Founders of Modern Psychology* (New York and London: D. Appleton and Co., 1912), p. 274.

CHAPTER 6

1. L. Emmett Holt, "Medical Tendencies and Medical Ideals," *JAMA* (1907) 48:845.

2. Eduoard Seguin, "Sphygmometry," *MR* (1867) 2:248.

3. Ibid., p. 248.

4. *The Seven Books of Paulus Aeginata* "On the pulse, from the Works of Galen" I Section XII, trans. from Greek with a commentary by Francis Adams (London, 1844), p. 219.

5. Charles Daremberg and Charles Émile Ruelle, eds. *Oeuvres de Rufus d'Ephese* (Paris: J. B. Baillière et fils, 1879), p. 614.

6. R. B. Amber, A. M. Babey-Brooke, *The Pulse in Occident and Orient: Its Philosophy and Practice* (New York: Santa Barbara Press, 1966), p. i.

7. V. Bugiel, *Un célèbre médecin Polonais au XVIe siècle: Joseph Struthius (1510-1568)* (Paris: G. Steinheil, Editeur, 1901), p. 51.

8. Ilza Veith, *Huang Ti Nei Ching Su Wen The Yellow Emperor's Classic of Internal Medicine*, trans. with an introductory essay (Berkeley and Los Angeles: University of California Press, 1966), pp. 4-9. See also for other aspects of Chinese physical diagnosis: Ronald Chen, *The History and Methods of Physical Diagnosis in Classical Chinese Medicine* (New York: Vantage Press, 1969). It is believed that the text of the *Nei Ching* was not written earlier than the third century A.D. K. C. Wong, "The Pulse Lore of Cathay," *The Chinese Medical Journal* (1928).

9. K. Chimin Wong and Lien-Teh Wu, *History of Chinese Medicine*, 2d ed. (Shanghai, China, 1936), p. 42.

10. Francis Adams, *Paulus Aeginata*, p. 221; Boleslaw Szczesniak, "John Floyer and Chinese Medicine," *Osiris* (1954) 2:127-56.

11. John Floyer, *The Physician's Pulse Watch: or an Essay to Discover the Causes of Diseases, and a Rational Method of Them by Feeling of the Pulse*, vol. I (London: S. Smith and B. Walford, 1707), p. 345; vol. II (London: J. Nicholson, 1710).

12. K. C. Wong and L. T. Wu, *History of Chinese Medicine*, pp. 57, 58.

13. R. B. Amber and A. M. Babey-Brooke, *The Pulse*, p. 1.

14. G. M. Ebers, ed., *Papyrus Ebers*, trans. H. Joachim, 2 vols. (Berlin, 1880); J. H. Breasted, *The Edwin Smith Surgical Papyrus* II, 2 vols. (Chicago: Chicago University Press, 1930).

15. Charles R. S. Harris, *The Heart and the Vascular System in Ancient Greek Medicine from Alcmaon to Galen* (Oxford: Clarendon Press, 1973), p. 182.

16. D. Evan Bedford, "The Ancient Art of Feeling the Pulse," *BHJ* (1951) 13:424, 426; C. R. S. Harris, *The Heart and the Vascular System*, pp. 184, 185.

17. D. E. Bedford, "The Ancient Art," p. 426.

18. C. R. S. Harris, *The Heart and the Vascular System*, pp. 187, 194.

19. D. E. Bedford, "The Ancient Art," p. 426.

20. C. R. S. Harris, *The Heart and the Vascular System*, p. 184; W. H. Broadbent, *The Pulse* (Philadelphia: Lea Bros. and Co., 1887), p. 3.

21. C. R. S. Harris, *The Heart and the Vascular System*, pp. 182, 183, 185, 186.

22. Ibid., pp. 257, 261, 262, 263.

23. V. Bugiel, *Un Célèbre Médecin*, p. 50.

24. Francis Adams, *Paulus Aeginata*, p. 202.

25. C. R. S. Harris, *The Heart and the Vascular System*, p. 397.

26. Robert Willis, trans. *The Works of William Harvey, M.D.* (London: The Sydenham Society, 1847), p. 22.

27. C. R. S. Harris, *The Heart and the Vascular System*, p. 401.

28. Ibid., p. 401.

29. Ibid., p. 405. Galen claimed that "just as sculptors, painters, wine-tasters, cooks, scent-makers, or musicians need many years to acquire their skills, in spite of the opportunity of unlimited practice on their materials in unlimited quantity, so the physician needs even more time to acquire his."

30. D. E. Bedford, "The Ancient Art," pp. 428, 429.

31. Sir Thomas Clifford Allbutt, *Greek Medicine in Rome* (New York: Benjamin Blom, Inc., 1970), pp. 135, 139.

32. Henry Viets, "De Staticis Experimentis of Nicolaus Cusanus," *Ann. Med. Hist.* (1922) 4:123.

33. Ibid., p. 127.

34. Ibid., p. 128.

35. Silvio Bedini, "The Seventeenth Century Table Clepysdra," *Physis* (1968) 10:27.

36. Ibid.

37. Ibid., p. 30.

38. Piero E. Ariotti, "Aspects of the Conception and Development of the Pendulum in the Seventeenth Century," *Archives of the History for the Exact Sciences* (1972) 8:329.

39. Silvio Bedini, "The Instrument of Galileo Galilei," in *Galileo, Man of Science*, ed. Ernan Mc Mullin (New York: Basic Books, 1967), p. 257.

40. *Commentaria in primum fen primi libri canon is Avicennae* (Venice, 1625).

41. Piero Ariotti, "Aspects of the Conception" p. 376.

42. Ibid., p. 377.

43. Ibid.

44. Ibid.

45. R. Willis, *The Works of William Harvey*, p. 49.

46. Ibid., p. 92. William Salmon provides the pulses counted by several seventeenth-century physicians. These include James Primerose (700/hour); Jean Cardan (4,000/hour); Waleous and Regius (3,000/hour; Thomas Bartholin (4,400/hour); Plempius (4,450/hour) Harvey and Riolan (2,000/hour) and Salmon (3,600/hour or 60/min.) *Synopsis medicinae A Compendium of Physick, Chirurgery and Anatomy in IV Books*, 2d ed. (London, 1681), p. 1119. Hermann von Helmholtz and other German physicians in the 1840s thought it was not in good taste to time the pulse with a watch. Richard Shyrock, "Quantity in Medical Science," *Isis* (1961) 52:223. Methods of counting the pulse

with a watch or clock varied. A. W. Abbott of Minneapolis suggested in 1882 that the physician should make dots on a piece of paper in synchronization with the pulse and count the dots. Letter "How to Count a Rapid Pulse," *MR* (1882) 22:194.

47. R. Willis, *The Works of William Harvey*, p. 51.

48. Ibid., p. 125.

49. Gary Townsend, "Sir John Floyer (1649-1734) and His Study of Pulse and Respiration," *JHMAS* (1967) 22:298. See also F. J. Britten, *Old Clocks and Watches and their Makers*, 3d ed. (London: B. J. Batsford, 1911), p. 225.

50. J. Floyer, *The Pulse Watch*, p. iv.

51. B. Szczesniak, "John Floyer," p. 137; D. E. Bedford, "The Ancient Art," p. 426.

52. G. Townsend, "Sir John Floyer," p. 315.

53. J. Floyer, *The Pulse Watch*, p. 14, i, vol. II.

54. Ibid., pp. ix, x, vol. I.

55. Ibid., p. 346, vol. II.

56. Ibid., p. 368; V. Bugiel, *Un Célèbre Médecin*, p. 50.

57. J. Floyer, *The Pulse Watch*, p. 433, 436, vol. I.

58. Ibid., p. i, vol. I.

59. Ibid., pp. 327, 328, vol. II.

60. R. T. H. Laennec, *A Treatise on Diseases of the Chest*, p. 368. Laennec added: "It may seem surprising that the practice of feeling the pulse has been so generally in all ages. It is of easy performance and gives little inconvenience either to the physician or patient; the cleverest, it is true, can derive from it but a few indications and uncertain conjectures; but the most ignorant can, without exposing themselves, reduce from it all sorts of indications. Its very uncertainty gives it a preference with persons of inferior qualifications, over means quite certain in their nature."

61. William Hall Lewis, "The Evolution of Clinical Sphygmomanometry," *BNYAM* (1941) 17:871-81.

62. Irving S. Wright, Ralph F. Schneider, and Harry E. Ungerleider, "Factors of Error in Blood Pressure Readings," *AHJ* (1938) 16:469. See also N. S. Korotkoff, "Experiments for Determining the Efficiency of Arterial Collaterals," Harold N. Segall, Ed. of Russian translation, 1980. Montreal, privately printed. Distributed by Mansfield Book Mart Ltd. 2065 Mansfield St., Montreal Quebec 174 A IY7, Canada.

63. E. Seguin, "Sphygmometry," p. 248.

64. Ibid., p. 251.

65. Ibid., p. 244.

66. Hebbel E. Hoff and L. A. Geddes, "Graphic Recording Before Carl Ludwig, an Historical Summary," *AId'HS* (1959) 12:3.

67. Julius Herrison, *The Sphygmometer, an Instrument which records the Action of the Arteries Apparent to the Eye* (London: Longmans, 1835).

68. L. Waldenburg, *Die Messung des Pulses und des Blutdrucks* (Berlin, 1880).

69. Etienne Jules Marey, *La Méthode Graphique dan les Sciences Expérimentale* (Paris, 1878).

70. Robert E. Dudgeon, *The Sphygmograph* (London: Baillière, 1882). See also Arnold and Sons, *Catalogue* (London, 1895), p. 314; Christopher Lawrence, "Physiological Apparatus in the Wellcome Museum. 2. The Dudgeon Sphygmograph and its Descendents," *Med Hist* (1979) 23: 96-101.

71. B. W. Richardson modified sphygmograph in Arnold and Sons, *Catalogue* (London, 1895), p. 314 and A. S. Aloe (circa 1893), p. 354.

72. "Standard Pulse Readings," *Asclepiad* (July 1885).

73. J. M. Poiseuille, *Récherches sur la Force du Coeur Aortique* (Paris: thèse 1828).

74. Octavius A. White, "The Haemarumascope," *AJMS* (1877) 74:136.

75. William Ewart, *Heart Studies Chiefly Clinical: A Study in Tactile Sphygmology* (London: Baillière, 1894), pp. viii, 1; James Mackenzie, *The Study of the Pulse, Arterial, Venous and Hepatic and the Movement of the Heart* (Edinburgh and London: Young J. Pentland, 1902), p. 95.

76. Alex Mair, *Sir James Mackenzie, M.D. 1853-1925: General Practitioner* (Edinburgh and London: Churchill Livingstone, 1973), p. 243.

77. Ibid., p. 148.

78. Ibid., p. 149.

79. Ibid., p. 90.

80. Ibid.

81. Ibid., p. 91.

82. A. E. Wales and J. Shafer, "Sir James Mackenzie: The Burnley Years," *MH* (1967) II:298. Mackenzie used the polygraph extensively between 1883 and 1890.

83. A. Mair, *Sir James Mackenzie*, p. 182.

84. Ibid.

85. J. Mackenzie, *The Study of the Pulse*, p. 95.

86. Ibid., p. 165.

87. James Mackenzie, *The Future of Medicine* (London: Henry Frowde, Hodden and Stoughton, 1919), pp. 35-37.

88. Ibid.

89. Ibid., p. 7.

90. William Sydney Thayer, "On the Importance of Fundamental Methods of Physical Examination in the Practice of Medicine," *SMJ* (1914) 7:933-42.

91. J. Mackenzie, *The Future of Medicine*, p. 6.

92. Ibid., p. 7.

93. Ibid., p. 33.

94. Ibid., p. 41.

95. Ibid., p. 44. Mackenzie wrote in 1922, "Moreover, in any case, knowledge, revealed by mechanical devices, however, valuable it may be, is not of the kind required for prognosis or treatment." "The Position of Medicine at the Beginning of the Twentieth Century illustrated by the State of Cardiology," *NYMJ* (1922) 115:61.

96. George E. Burch and N. De Pasquale, *A History of Electrocardiography* (Chicago: Yearbook Medical Publishers Inc., 1964). There also exists a fine monograph on the development of the ekg published by the Cambridge Instrument company. S. L. Barron, *The Development of the Ekg*, Cambridge Monograph No. 5 (London: Cambridge Instrument Co., Ltd., 1952).

CHAPTER 7

1. A. D. Farr, "Some Problems in the History of Haemoglobinometry (1878-1931)," *MH* (1978) 22:151-53.

2. "Function," *Encyclopédie des sciences médicales* (Paris, 1878) cited in Joseph Schiller, "Physiology's Struggles for Independence in the First Half of the Nineteenth Century." *Hist Sci* (1968) 7: 74.

3. Joseph Schiller, "Physiology's Struggles for Independence," p. 65.

4. A. D. Farr, "Some Problems in the History of Haemoglobinometry," pp. 151-53.

5. Editorial, "The Influence of Medical Journals on the March of Science," *JAMA* (1889) 13:339.

6. Ilza Veith, ed., *Perspectives in Physiology: An International Symposium* (Washington, D.C.: American Physiological Society, 1953), p. ix.

7. Rufus Cole, "Progress of Medicine During the Last Twenty-Five Years as Exemplified by the Harvey Society Lectures," *Science* (1930) 71:624.

8. Dietmar Rapp, *Die Entwicklung der physiologischen Methodik von 1784 bis 1911: Eine quantitative Untersuchung* (Muenster, 1970).

9. Frederick L. Holmes, ed., *Animal Chemistry or Organic Chemistry in its Application to Physiology and Pathology* by Justus Liebig, reprint (New York: Johnson Reprint Co., 1964), p. xvi.

10. Karl Rothschuh, *History of Physiology*, trans. and ed. Guenter B. Risse Huntington, (New York: Robert E. Kruger Publ. Co., 1973), pp. 269, 270, 271.

11. Claude Bernard, *An Introduction to the Study of Experimental Medicine*, trans. Henry Copley Greene (New York: Collier Books, 1961). "Our instruments for vivisections are indeed so coarse and our senses so imperfect that we can reach only the coarse and complex parts of an organism," p. 133.

12. Frederic L. Holmes, Book Review. *BHM* (1965) 39:490; C. Bernard, *An Introduction to the Study of Experimental Medicine*, p. 128.

13. Gerald Geison, *Michael Foster and the Cambridge School of Physiology* (Princeton, N.J.: Princeton University Press, 1978).

14. "The Beginnings of Physiological Research in America," *Science* (1923) 58:185-95; Henry Sewall, "Henry Newell Martin," *Johns Hopkins Hosp Bull* (1911) 22:327-33; Walter B. Cannon, "The First American Laboratory of Physiology," *Science* (1933) 78:365-66; C. S. Breathurch, "Henry Newell Martin (1848-1893) A Pioneer Physiologist," *Med Hist* (1969) 13:27-29. For the names and locations of early physiology laboratories and related bibliography, see K. E. Rothschuh, *History of Physiology*. H. P. Bowditch described the "universally acknowledged . . . most complete establishment of the kind in Europe" in his article "The Physiological Laboratory at Leipzig," *Nature* (1870) 3:142-43. J. Burdon Sanderson places the "Physiological Laboratories in Great Britain" in perspective in *Nature* (1871) 4:189.

15. Paul Klemperer, "The Pathology of Morgagni and Virchow," *BHM* (1958) 32:25, 26.

16. Saul Jarcho, "Giovanni Battista Morgagni: His Interests, Ideas and Achievements," *BHM* (1948) 22:505.

17. Ibid., p. 505. See also W. T. Gairdner, "On the Progress of Pathology," *BMJ* (1874) II:515, 517. Gairdner wrote: "Without him [Morgagni] we should almost certainly have been without those means and appliances in all our hospitals, which produced for use in this country Baillie, the Hunters, Richard Bright, Astley Cooper and a host of others both at home and abroad, who have contributed their stores of experience to an investigation of disease at once clinical and pathological," p. 517.

18. Saul Jarcho, "Morgagni and Auenbrugger in the Retrospect of Two Hundred Years," *BHM* (1961) 35:489-96.

19. Jean-Nicolas Corvisart, *An Essay on the Organic Diseases and Lesions of the Heart and Great Vessels*, reprint (New York: New York Academy of Medicine, Hafner Publ. Co., 1962).

20. Paul Klemperer, "Morbid Anatomy before and after Morgagni," *NYAM* (1961) 37:749.

21. Stephen Hales, *Statical Essays: containing Haemastaticks* (1733), introd. Andre Cournand, reprint (New York: Hafner Publ. Co., 1964), p. xii.

22. P. Klemperer, "Morbid Anatomy," p. 750.

23. Ibid., p. 755.

24. Ibid., pp. 755, 756.

25. W. S. Greenfield, "An Inaugural Address on Pathology, Past and Present," *BMJ* (1881) II:731.

26. Lionel Beale, *The Microscope and its Application to Clinical Medicine* (London, 1854), p. 10; William Rutherford, *Outlines of Practical Histology*, 2d ed. (London: J. and A. Churchill, Philadelphia: Linsay and Blakiston, 1876), p. 33. See also Brian Bracegirdle, *A History of Microtechnique* (Ithaca, N.Y.: Cornell University Press, 1978).

27. E. B. Krumbhaar, *History of Pathology* (1937) reprint (New York: Hafner Publ. Co., 1962), p. 107.

28. Ibid., p. 150.

29. A. W. Mayo Robson, "Position of Pathology with Respect to Clinical Diagnosis," *BMJ* (1906) I:603, 604.

30. Ibid., p. 605.

31. John Ritchie, *History of the Laboratory of the Royal College of Physicians of Edinburgh* (Edinburgh: The Royal College of Physicians, 1953).

32. Ibid., p. 15.

33. Charles Newman, *The Evolution of Medical Education in the Nineteenth Century* (London: Oxford University Press, 1957).

34. James Cassedy, *Demography in Early America: Beginnings of the Statistical Mind* (Cambridge, Mass.: Harvard University Press, 1969), p. 283.

35. Ibid., p. 280.

36. Lester King, "What Is a Diagnosis?" *JAMA* (1967) 202:716.

37. Robley Dunglison, *Medical Lexicon: A Dictionary of Medical Science* (Philadelphia: Lea and Blanchard, 1848), p. 586. See also Knud Faber, *Nosography in Modern Internal Medicine* (New York, 1923).

38. Ibid.

39. James Currie, *Medical Reports on the Effects of Water, Cold and Warm* vol. I (Philadelphia, 1808), p. 48.

40. N. S. Davis, "The American Medical Association and Its Relation to Public Health," *JAMA* (1889) 13:122.

41. Editorial, "The Classification of Disease," *BMJ* (1891) I:186, 187.

42. John Adam, "Medical Diagnosis and Modern Discoveries," *BMJ* (1902) I:500; Book Review, *AJMS* (1879) 77:499.

43. Jacob M. DaCosta, *Medical Diagnosis; with Special Reference to Practical Medicine* (Philadelphia: J. B. Lippincott and Co., 1864).

44. James C. Wilson, *A Handbook of Medical Diagnosis* (Philadelphia and London: J. B. Lippincott Co., 1909), p. v.

45. Lester King, "Signs and Symptoms," *JAMA* (1968) 206:1064. King does not consider the cause to be related to the use of medical instruments.

46. James Cuming, "The Control of Pathological Research by Clinical Observation," *BMJ* (1884) II:202.

47. Ibid., p. 203.

48. Lester King, "The Meaning of Medical Diagnosis," *Etc.* (1951) 8:202.

49. Walter Hayle Walshe, *A Practical Treatise on the Diseases of the Lungs and Heart including the Principles of Physical Diagnosis* (London: Taylor, Walton, and Maberly, 1851), pp. 1-2.

50. H. Power, reviewer of Clifford Allbutt, *On the Use of the Ophthalmoscope in Diseases of the Nervous System and of the Kidneys. Nature* (1871), p. 3. See also Henry Juler, "A Lecture on the Use of the Ophthalmoscope in Medical Diagnosis," *MR* (1885) 27:673-76.

51. Francis Delafield, "On the Diseases of the Kidneys Popularly called Bright's Disease," *AJMS* (1891) 102:319, 320.

52. Royston Lambert, *Sir John Simon (1816-1904) and English Social Administration* (London: Macgibbon and Kee, 1963), p. 45; John Simon, "On Sub-Acute Inflammation of the Kidney," Medico-Chirurgical Transactions (1847) 30:141. See also Editorial, "The Bradshore Lecture," presented by Dr. Goodhart for Dr. Mahomed, who studied arterial tension and kidney disease. Other contributions to the study of kidney disease are also mentioned. *BMJ* (1885) II:401.

53. Austin Flint, *Manual of Chemical Examination of the Urine in Disease* (New York: D. Appleton and Co., 1870).

54. Henry G. Piffard, *A Guide to Urinary Analysis for the Use of Physicians and Students* (New York: W. Wood and Co., 1873); Alfred Loomis, *Lessons in Physical Diagnosis* (New York: W. Wood and Co., 1868).

55. George Tiemann, *The American Armamentarium Chirurgicum* (New York, 1889), pp. 1-3 for illustrations of typical equipment.

56. A. Von Koranyi, *Die Wissenschaftlichen Grundlagen der Kryoskopie in ihrer klinischen Anwendung* (Berlin, 1904).

57. Ottomar Rosenbach, "Die Mechanismus und die Diagnose der Mageninsufficienz." *Samml Klin Vortr* (1878) pp. 1315-46; *Grundlagen Aufgaben und Grenzen der Therapie nebst einem Anhange: Kritik des Koch'schen Verfahrens'* (Vienna and Leipzig: Urban and Schwarzenberg, 1891).

58. Thomas Clifford Allbutt, *A System of Medicine*, vol. I (New York and London, 1896-98), p. xxxii.

59. Michel Foucault, *The Birth of the Clinic*, trans. A. M. Sheridan Smith (New York: Pantheon Books, 1973), p. 164.

60. Ibid., pp. 3, 4.

61. J. B. Bouillard, *Traité des fièvres dites essentielles* (Paris, 1826) p. 13, cited in M. Foucault, p. 192.

62. M. Foucault, *The Birth of the Clinic*, p. 164.

63. Austin Flint, "A Uniform Nomenclature of Auscultatory Sounds in the Diagnois of Diseases of the Chest," *Cong. Period Internat. d. Sc. Med. Compt. Rendu* (1884), p. 1881.

64. Austin Flint, "On the Clinical Study of the Heart Sounds," *JAMA* (1884) 3:88.

65. First Official *The Nomenclature of Diseases drawn up by a joint committee* appointed by the Royal College of Physicians of London. 1869. In the United States: "A Nomenclature of Diseases, with the Reports of the Majority and of the Minority of the Committee thereon," *Trans Am Med Assoc* (1872) 23:1-94.

66. Alex R. Simpson, "Uniformity in Obstetrical Nomenclature," *MR* (1887) 32:332. A Committee on the Nomenclature of Mental Disorders was founded at the Antwerp Medical Congress in 1885, *BMJ* (1885) II:1175.

67. H. R. M. Landis, "Austin Flint: His Contribution to the Art of Physical Diagnosis and the Study of Tuberculosis," *John Hopkins Hosp Bull* (1912) 23:183.

68. Austin Flint, *Clinical Medicine: A Systematic Treatise on the Diagnosis and Treatment of Disease* (Philadelphia: Henry C. Lea, 1879), p. 22.

69. Ibid.

70. Sir Henry Thompson, "Leiter's Endoscope in the Treatment of Vesical Disease," *BMJ* (1888) I:775.

71. E. Hurry Fenwick, "The Value of Electric Illumination of the Urinary Bladder (The Nitze Method) in the Diagnosis of Obscure Vesical Disease," *BMJ* (1888) I:786.

72. T. S. K. M. review of *The Electric Illumination of the Bladder as a Means of Diagnosis of Obscure Vesico-Urethral Disease* (London, 1888). *AJMS* (1888) 96:611; Josef Leiter, *Elektro-Endoscopische Instrumente Beschreibung und Instruction zur Handhabung der von Dr. M. Nitze und J. Leiter Construirten Instrumente und Apparate* (Vienna: W. Braumueller und Sohn, 1880). Dr. Antel first used the instrument on a patient, p. vi. The use of the electric cautery first siggested the use of electric light to see into the body cavities, p. 1.

73. See for example: D. S. Adam, "The Differential Diagnosis of Mammary Tumours," *MR* (1876) 16:13.

74. Morell Mackenzie, "On the Differential Diagnosis of Treatment of Bronchocele," *Lancet* (1872) I:606-08, 642-45.

75. Editorial, "Studying Phthisis," *MR* (1880) 18:98.

See also E. Darwin Hudson "The Physical Examination of Weak Chests," *Lancet* (1872) I:645; "Differential Diagnosis of the Several Forms of Early Phthisis," *MR* (1885) 27:505.

76. "On the Importance of Recognizing the Conditions known as Sthenic and Asthenic in Differentiating the Caucasian and African Races; and in Disease Generally," *MR* (1883) 23:538, 539.

77. R. C. Cabot, *Differential Diagnosis Presented Through an Analysis of 383 Cases*, 2 vols. (Philadelphia: W. B. Saunders Co., 1911), p. 19.

78. Frank Dennette Adams, ed., *Physical Diagnosis* by R. C. Cabot, 14th ed. (Baltimore: William and Wilkins Co., 1958), p. 2.

79. Richard C. Cabot, "Diagnostic Pitfalls Identified during a Study of Three Thousand Autopsies," *JAMA* (1912) 59:2295.

80. L. King, "The Meaning of Medical Diagnosis," p. 204.

81. A. H. Douthwaite, *Index of Differential Diagnosis*, (Baltimore: Williams and Wilkins 9th ed., 1967), p. vii. Operations for diagnosis also were used successfully. See for example: Editorial, "Laparotomy as A Diagnostic Resource," *JAMA* (1886) 7:603-05.

82. Robert S. Ledley and Lee B. Lusted, "Reasoning Foundations of Medical Diagnosis," *Science* (1959) 130: 9, 10.

83. W. R. Houston, "Diagnosis: Purpose and Scope," *Inter. Med. Classics* (1937) 1:232, 233.

84. John Burdon Sanderson, "Note of his Address, Remarks Before His Address," *BMJ* (1873) II:196.

85. John Burdon Sanderson, "Address in Medicine," *BMJ* (1873) II:153.

86. L. King, "Signs and Symptoms," p. 1065.

87. J. B. Sanderson, "Address in Medicine," p. 153.

88. Ibid., p. 154.

89. Ibid., p. 155.

90. Editorial, "The Nature of Fever," *MR* (1887) 31: 497, 498.

91. J. B. Sanderson, "Address in Medicine," p. 198.

92. Samuel Wilks, "The Use and Abuse of the Term 'Fever'," *Lancet* (1871) I:10.

93. Richard Quain, "The Harveian Oration on the History and Progress of Medicine," *BMJ* (1885) II:779. The American physician William Wood Gerhard distinguished typhoid and typhus fevers for American physicians in 1837. See *AJMS* (1837) 20:289-322.

94. Public Health Notice, "The Removal to Fever Hospitals of Patients who Have Not Fever," *Lancet* (1872) I: 661, 702.

95. W. H. Thomson, *MR* (1876) 11:45.

96. Nelson E. Jones, "Pyrexia, A Conservative Force in Fever," *MR* (1882) 21:537.

97. N. S. Davis, "The Basis of Scientific Medicine and the Proper Methods of Investigation," *JAMA* (1891) 16: 116; see also Henry Mitchell Hunter, "Therapeutic Uses of the Coal Tar Derivatives," *Trans. of the Medical Association of the State of Alabama*, (1894):358-69.

98. J. B. Sanderson, "Address in Medicine," p. 156.

99. Ibid., p. 198.

100. William Seller, "On the Signification of Fact in Medicine, and on the Hurtful Effects of the Incautious Use of Such Modern Sources of Fact as the Microscope, Stethoscope, Chemical Analysis and Statistics, etc.," *Edin Med Surg J* (1848) 70:343.

101. Ibid., p. 344.

102. Anon., "On Functional Diseases," *MTG* (1883) 2:659.

103. W. Seller, "On the Signification of Fact in Medicine," pp. 344, 345.

104. Ibid., pp. 347, 348.

105. E. A. Parkes, "Address in Medicine," *Lancet* (1873) II:177.

106. Anon., "On Functional Diseases," p. 659.

107. Ibid.

108. W. S. Greenfield, "An Inaugural Address on Pathology," p. 731.

109. "Report on Lecture to BMA Meeting," *MR* (1880) 18:355.

110. Thomas C. Allbutt, *On the Use of the Ophthalmoscope in Diseases of the Nervous System and of the Kidneys* (London and New York: Macmillan Co., 1871), p. 10.

111. Ibid., pp. 3, 4.

112. Ibid., p. 5.

113. Henry Juler, "A Lecture on the Use of the Ophthalmoscope in Medical Diagnosis," *MR* (1885) 27:674.

114. "BMA Meeting Report by Dr. Humphrys," *MR* (1880) 18:354.

115. William A. Fisher, *Ophthalmoscopy, Retinoscopy and Refraction*, 2d rev. ed. (Philadelphia: F. A. Davis, 1927), pp. 16, 17.

116. James Cuming, "The Control of Pathological Research," *BMJ* (1884) II:202.

117. Ibid.

118. Thomas Huxley, *Science, Culture and Other Essays* (London: E. Arnold, 1881), pp. 326-45.

119. Charles Creighton, *A History of Epidemics in Britain*, vol. II (Cambridge: Cambridge University Press, 1891-94), p. 145.

120. Isaac Hays and R. Eglesfeld Griffith, trans., *Principles of Physiological Medicine . . .* (Philadelphia: Carey and Lea, 1832), p. 27.

121. Claude Bernard, *Leçons de physiologie expérimentale appliquée à la médecine*, vol. I (Paris, 1855), p. 29.

122. "du principe de pathologie, si souvent encore invoque, selon lequel l'état morbide n'est, chez l'être vivant, qu'une simple variation quantitatives des phénomènes physiologiques qui définissent l'état normal de la fonction correspondante." Georges Canguilhem, *Le Normal et le Pathologique*, 2d rev. (Paris: Presses Universitaires de France, 1972).

123. Sir William Gull, "Presidential Address to the Clinical Society," *MTG* (1872) I:131.

124. Ibid.

125. George Murray Humphry, "An Address at the Opening of the Section of Physiology," *BMJ* (1873) II:161.

126. M. A. Quetelet, *A Treatise on Man and the Develop-*

ment of His Faculties, introd. by Richard Well (Edinburgh: Gregg International Publs., Ltd., 1842), p. 99.

127. Ibid., pp. 67, 68.

128. Ibid., p. 73.

129. Ibid., p. 99.

130. F. J. Gant, "What has Pathological Anatomy Done for Medicine and Surgery?", *Lancet* (1857) II:240.

131. M. A. Quetelet, *A Treatise*, p. 49.

132. "The Life History Album," *BMJ* (1884) II:1166.

133. C. Bernard, *An Introduction to the Study of Experimental Medicine*, pp. 158, 159.

134. Pierre C. A. Louis, *Researches on the Effect of Bloodletting in Some Inflammatory Diseases*, (Boston: Hilliard, Gray and Co.) trans. C. G. Putnam, 1836), p. 63.

135. Ibid., p. 58.

136. Ibid., p. 60.

137. Ibid., p. 63. Erwin Ackerknecht sums up the opposition to Pierre Louis and the Sociètè Médicale d'Observation. *Medicine at the Paris Hospital 1794-1848* (Baltimore: Johns Hopkins University Press, 1967), p. 104.

138. P. C. A. Louis, *Researches On the Effects of Bloodletting*, p. 69.

139. William A. Guy, "On the Value of the Numerical Method as Applied to Science, but especially to Physiology and Medicine," *J Stat Soc* (1839) 2:27, 32.

140. Ibid., pp. 38, 39, 40.

141. Ibid., p. 42.

142. Ibid., p. 45.

143. Norman T. Gridgeman, "Francis Galton," in *Dictionary of Scientific Biography* (New York: Charles Scribner's Son, 1972) vol. 5, p. 266.

144. Ibid.

145. Ruth Schwartz Cowan, "Nature and Nurture: The Interplay of Biology and Politics in the Work of Francis Galton," *Studies in Hist Bio* (1977), pp. 133-208.

146. Ernest Hart, "Abstract of a Lecture on the International Health Exhibition of 1884: Its Influence and Possible Sequels," *BMJ* (1884) II:1120, 1121.

147. "Charles Roberts," in section entitled "Bibliographical Notices, Discussion of Charles Roberts' 'The Physical Development and the Proportions of the Human Body'," *AJMS* (1877) 74:492.

148. Charles Roberts, "Practical Anthropometry," *BMJ* (1888) I:740.

149. Ibid. Charles Roberts assembled a fourteen-page bibliography on anthropometry, which included books published as early as the sixteenth century. *A Manual of Anthropometry* (London, J. and A. Churchill, 1878). Hawksley's of London advertised several dozen instruments in this text.

150. Ibid., pp. 26-36.

151. Kny-Scheerer, *Catalogue*, p. 1029; A. S. Aloe (circa 1893), pp. 636-37, 40, 41 for models by Collin, Hammond and Mathieu.

152. Ibid., p. 617.

153. C. Roberts, "Practical Anthropometry," p. 741.

154. Kny-Scheerer, *Catalogue*, p. 1034.

155. A. S. Aloe, *Catalogue*, p. 636.

156. E. C. Seguin, "Methods of Diagnosis in Diseases of the Nervous System," *MR* (1881) 22:617.

157. A. L. Ranney, "Practical Hints Regarding the Methods of Examination Employed as Aids in Diagnosis of Nervous Diseases," *MR* (1884) 25:687.

158. Ancienne Maison Chez Verdin G. Boulitte, rue Linné, Paris (n.d.) New York Academy of Medicine Collection, pp. 280, 350-53.

159. Allan McLane Hamilton, *Railway and Other Accidents with Relation to Injury and Diseases* (New York: William Wood and Co., 1905), pp. 63, 68.

160. Eduoard Seguin, "The Aesthesiometer and Aesthesiometry," *MR* (1866-67) 1:510.

161. A. L. Ranney, "Practical Hints Regarding the Methods of Examination employed as Aids in the Diagnosis of Nervous Diseases," *MR* (1884) 25:713, 714.

162. Ibid. Vierordt, Kottenkamp, Ullrich, Paulus, Riecher, and Hartmann confirmed Weber's tables. Sieveking and Valentin provided other scales. The distances able to be distinguished between points were found to be considerably shorter for Weber. Grace Peckham, "Aesthesiometry," *MR* (1885) 26:232. Tables appeared in John C. Dalton, *Human Physiology*. (Philadelphia: Blanchard, 1864), p. 463. and volume 4 of Robert B. Todd, ed., *The Cyclopedia of Anatomy and Physiology*. (London: Sherwood, Gilbert and Piper, 1836-1847), pp. 1169.

163. A. L. Ranney, "Practical Hints," p. 714.

164. Brown-Sequard, "Recherches sur nos moyens de mesurer l'Anaesthésie et l'hyperaesthésie," *Comptes Rendus des Séances de la Sociètè de Biologie* (1866), p. 162; *MR* (1866-67) 1:501.

165. "The Annual Museum at the Oxford Meeting," *BMJ* (1868) II:196.

166. Lewellys F. Barker, "A New Aesthesiometer," *Johns Hopkins Hosp Bull* (1897) 8:125.

167. Ibid.

168. Alfred Gordon, "A New Precision Esthesiometer," *JAMA* (1909) 52:1257. See also S. Auerbach, "A New Aesthesiometer," *J Nervous and Mental Disease* (1913) 40:106-08.

169. Ibid., p. 126.

170. Ibid.

171. Audrey B. Davis and Uta C. Merzbach, *Early Auditory Studies. Activities in the Psychology Laboratories*, Studies in History and Technology No. 31 (Washington, D.C.: Smithsonian Institution Press, 1975).

172. Review of J. A. Myers, *Vital Capacity of the Lungs*, *Lancet* (1925) II:1073.

173. Bruno Gebhard, "Sights and Thoughts of a Scandinavian Museum's Tour from 30 June to 5 August 1959," Trip Report in Gebhard Papers, Allen Memorial Medical Library, Cleveland, Ohio, p. 4.

174. Frederick, L. Hoffman, "Research Work in Life Insurance Medicine," *MR* (1912) 82:418.

175. Ibid., p. 422.

176. Lester King, "What is Disease?" *Phil Sci* (1954), p. 46.

177. Cited in Georges Canguilhem, *Le normal et le Pathologique*, p. 111. Translation of the French: "These states are at the limit of physiology and pathology. From the

point of view of the European, these states are pathologic, from the point of view of the native, they are so closely linked to the usual state of the black person that if one did not have comparable information for the white person one could consider it almost as physiologically normal.''

178. Ibid., p. 138.

179. Wilfred Trotter, "Observation and Experiment and Their Use in the Medical Sciences," *BMJ* (1930) II:130.

180. Thomas Lewis, "Research in Medicine: Its Position and its Needs," *BMJ* (1930) I:479.

181. G. Canguilhem, *Le Normal et le Pathologique*, p. 93.

182. Ibid.

183. Ibid., p. 156.

184. Ibid., p. 215.

185. Ibid., p. 110.

186. Ibid., p. 155.

187. J. Mitchell Bruce, "The Dominance of Etiology in Modern Medicine," *BMJ* (1910) II:246, 251.

188. J. Ritchie, *History of the Laboratory of the Royal College*, p. 3.

189. William A. Womer, "One Hundred Cases Treated with Autogenous Vaccines," *PMJ* (1918) 22:137-39; H. G. Adamson, "On Disappointments of Vaccine Therapy," *Lancet* (1918) II:172.

190. Theodore L. Sourkes, *Nobel Prize Winners in Medicine and Physiology*, revision of work by Lloyd Stevenson (London and New York: Abelard-Schuman, 1967), pp. 15-19.

191. J. M. Bruce, "The Dominance of Etiology," p. 247.

192. W. Stokes, "Altered Relation of Surgery to Medicine," cited in William Aitkin "On the Progress of Science and Pathology," *BMJ* (1888) II:350.

193. Ibid.

194. William Gull, "Presidential Address delivered before the Clinical Society of London," *Lancet* (1871) II:146.

195. J. M. Bruce, "The Dominance of Etiology," p. 250.

196. For instance, editorials appeared regularly in the Medical Record of the 1870s and 1880s.

197. Note "Nomenclature of Diseases of the Mouth and of the Gastroenteric Tract," *MR* (1894) 46:85. Appeared in *Archives of Pediatrics*.

198. W. T. Gairdner, "On the Progress of Pathology," *BMJ* (1874) II:515.

199. Ibid.

200. Ibid., p. 516.

201. Ibid., p. 517.

202. C. F. Hoover, "The Reputed Conflict between the Laboratories and Clinical Medicine," *Science* (1930) 71:492, 494.

203. Albert Sterne, "Interpretations of Negative Laboratory Findings in Syphilis," *JAMA* (1918) 71:87.

204. Thomas Lewis, "The Relation of Physiology to Medicine," *BMJ* (1920) II:460.

205. C. F. Hoover, "The Reputed Conflict between the Laboratories and Clinical Medicine," p. 496.

206. Ibid., p. 493.

207. T. Lewis, "The Relation of Physiology," p. 483; C. F. Hoover, "The Reputed Conflict," p. 491.

208. R. Cole, "Progress of Medicine," p. 620.

209. Ibid., p. 621.

210. Ibid., p. 624.

211. Ralph J. Stillman, "The Significance of Laboratory Tests and Methods," *NYSJM* (1935) 35:761.

212. Andrew F. Downing, "The Physical Examination as a Civil Service Instrument," *BMSJ* (1918) 179:181-92.

213. Brandreth Symonds, "Blood Pressure in Health," *Am Med* (1923) 29:412.

214. R. Max Goepp, "Blood Pressure as a Prognostic Factor," *PMJ* (1919) 22:300.

215. Maurice Fremont-Smith, "Periodic Examination of Supposedly Well Persons," *NEJM* (1953) 248:170.

216. Kendall Emerson, "Responsibility of Organized Medicine," *AJPH* (1940) 30:117.

CHAPTER 8

1. Frederick L. Hoffmann, "Research Work in Life Insurance Medicine," *MR* (1912) 82:417, 419.

2. Ibid., p. 418. See Karl Pearson, *The Chance of Death and Other Studies in Evolution* (London: E. Arnold, 1897).

3. E. D. Hudson, *MR* (1885) 27:505. "The physician has come to regard physical diagnosis, in the hands of experts, as affording exact knowledge of the conditions of the intrathoracic organs."

4. James Paget, "Imperfect Symmetry," *AJMS* (1886) 91:41-44. See also Milton Josiah Roberts, "Anatomical Geometry and Toponymy," *MR* (1885) 27:197-201. Roberts discusses and provides illustrations to indicate the movements of the body and limbs, as well as some of the instruments for measuring the various angles of motion. He explained that with these "instruments the orthopedic surgeon will find himself as thoroughly equipped for the accurate measurement of angular deformities of the body as the oculist is with his ophthalmoscope and set of trial glasses for the measurement of errors of refraction," p. 201.

5. Simon Baruch, "Precision in the Technique of Hydrotherapy," *MR* (1896) 49:284.

6. Rexmond C. Cochrane, *Measures for Progress: A History of the National Bureau of Standards* (Washington, D.C.: U.S. Dept. of Commerce, 1966), pp. 38, 39, 60.

7. Harold W. Dingman, *Insurability Prognosis and Selection: Life, Health Accident* (Chicago: The Spectator Co., 1927), p. 6.

8. Solomon S. Huebner, *Life Insurance: A Textbook* (New York: D. Appleton and Co., 1923), p. 3.

9. Ibid., p. 5.

10. H. W. Dingman, *Insurability Prognosis and Selection*, p. 23. Thomas Roe Edwards developed life tables in the 1830s based on age-specific mortality. His articles appear in *The Lancet* for the years 1835-1837. John Eyler has shown that Edwards was a strong influence on William Farr. See *Victorian Social Medicine, The Ideas and Methods of William Farr* (Baltimore: The Johns Hopkins University Press, 1979). One of the earliest tables based on the experience of an insurance company was computed by Charles Beard in 1778. H. W. Dingman, p. 30.

11. Thomas Laycock, *The Principles and Methods of Medical Observation and Research for the Use of Advanced Students and Junior Practitioners*, 2d ed. (Edinburgh and London, 1864), pp. 162, 163.

12. H. W. Dingman, *Insurability Prognosis and Selection*, p. 16.

13. Ibid., p. 80.

14. Terence O'Donnell, *History of Life Insurance: Its Formative Years* (New York: American Conservation Co., 1936), p. 348.

15. H. W. Dingman, *Insurability Prognosis and Selection*, p. 12.

16. Louis I. Dublin, *A Family of Thirty Million* (New York: Metropolitan Life Insurance Co., 1943), pp. 401, 402.

17. William Detmold, "Examination for Life Insurance," *MR* (1877) 12:81.

18. Nathan Allen, "The Law of Longevity," *MR* (1874) 9:111.

19. John Stockton Hough, "Longevity and Other Biostatic Peculiarities of the Jewish Race," *MR* (1873) 8:241-44. This was the first article to appear in the new life insurance section of the *Medical Record*. The same author compared the lives of men and women and concluded that women lived longer and contracted fewer hereditary diseases. See *MR* (1873) 8:297, 353.

20. Medical Director, "On Method in the Examination of Applicants," *MR* (1873) 8:304.

21. Edward H. Sieveking, "The Duties of the Medical Officer," *MR* (1874) 9:276.

22. E. G. Marsh, "Value of Family History and Personal Condition in Estimating a Liability to Consumption," *Report to the President of the Mutual Life Insurance Company, MR* (1896) 49:267.

23. A series of articles on the environmental factors conducive to disease appeared in the life insurance sections of the *Medical Record*.

24. H. W. Dingman, *Insurability Prognosis and Selection*, p. 73.

25. C. A. Wunderlich, *Medical Thermometry and Human Temperature*, trans. Edouard Seguin (New York: William Wood and Co., 1871). Part II. Suggestions on Thermometry and Human Temperature by E. Seguin, p. 247.

26. H. W. Dingman, *Insurability Prognosis and Selection*, p. 73.

27. The low opinion of the medical examination "does not result so much from a want of confidence in the professional skill of the examiners, as from the absences, too frequently observable, of a certain *moral* qualification, not less essential in the exercise of his responsible duties," Secretary of a Life Insurance Co., "On the Relation of the Medical Examiner to the Business of Life Insurance," *MR* (1873) 8:245.

28. Oliver Pillsbury, compiler, "On the Selection of Medical Examiners by a Medical Director from Report of the Proceedings of the National Insurance Convention of the U.S.," *MR* (1873) 8:636.

29. George M. Cox, "Let the Good Work Go On," to the editor, *MR* (1874) 9:277; Walter B. Chase, "Annoyances of Medical Life Insurance Examiners," *MR* (1873) 8:415.

30. Editorial, "Frauds in Life Insurance," *MR* (1877) 12:57, 58.

31. Editorial, "Physicians and Insurance Certificates," *MR* (1886) 30:294.

32. Anon., "Wholesale Graveyard Insurance," *MR* (1892) 41:408.

33. A Medical Director, "Medical Experts in the Selection of Lives," *MR* (1874) 9:222, 223.

34. Editorial, "Medical Officers of Insurance Offices," *BMJ* (1878) II:332.

35. L. I. Dublin, *A Family of Thirty Million*, p. 403.

36. Editorial, "Medical Examinations for Life Insurance," Letter from W. F. McNutt to the Editor from H. S. Purdon, *MR* (1873) 8:229, 230, 528. This national distribution of journals helped the *Medical Record* to grow into a medical journal of importance to physicians throughout the United States. *MR* (1886) 30:13, 14.

37. Editorial, "The Mutual Relations of Life Insurance and the Medical Press," *MR* (1910) 78:68. Frederick L. Hoffman, statistician of the Prudential Insurance Co. of America, complimented the medical press for these articles.

38. George W. Wells, Editorial, "The Purpose of this Paper," *Medical Examiner* (1891) 1:1.

39. S. S. Huebner, *Life Insurance*, p. 4.

40. N. Allen, "The Law of Longevity," p. 111. Almost half a century later in 1921, there were 288 American companies selling life insurance. S. S. Huebner, *Life Insurance*, p. 5.

41. Douglas C. North, "Life Insurance and Investment Banking at the Time of the Armstrong Investigation of 1905-1906," *JEH* (1954) 14:210.

42. Henry A. Riley, "Some New Factors in Life Insurance," *MR* (1891) 40:477.

43. Mary Dublin, "The Extent and Adequacy of Life Insurance Protection in the U.S.," *Misc. Contrib. on the Costs of Medical Care*, No. 11 (Committee on the Costs of Medical Care, 1932). See also "Periodic Examinations of Supposedly Well Persons," *NEJM* (1973) 248:170-73; Ralph G. Stillman, "The Significance of Laboratory Tests and Methods," *NYSJM* (1935) 35:757-66.

44. Edward Henry Sieveking, *The Medical Advisor in Life Insurance*, 2d ed. (Hartford, Conn.: N.P. Fletcher and Co., 1886), p. 51.

45. John M. Keating, *How to Examine for Life Insurance* (Philadelphia: William F. Fell and Co., 1890), p. 175; W. L. Champion, "The Importance of Careful Chemical and Microscopical Examination of Urine in Applicants for Life Insurance," *MR* (1896) 49:642.

46. L. I. Dublin, *A Family of Thirty Million*, p. 407.

47. Alonzo Nodine, "The Importance of Dental Examination for Life Insurance," *Dental Cosmos* (1913) 55:820.

48. Ibid., p. 821.

49. Ibid.

50. Ibid., p. 822.

51. William Hunter, "Oral Sepsis as a Cause of Disease," *BMJ* (1900) I:215; Audrey B. Davis, "The Emergence of American Dental Medicine: The Relation of the Maxillary

Antrum to Focal Infection," *Texas Reports on Biology and Medicine* (1974) 32:141-56. It should be noted that the dentist had the reputation of employing superior tools and implements well into the twentieth century. An historian of the S. S. White Dental Manufacturing Company claimed in 1926: "It's no wonder American dentistry has made the progress it has. No surgical instruments are to be had which in adaptation to the use intended, in temper, or in finish, are at all comparable to the dentists.''

52. At the time when life insurance companies were beginning to rely more on the advice of medical practitioners, accident insurance was introduced, which lessened the financial burden to be borne by the life insurance company. Faced with the realities of an industrializing society, insurance companies first wrote accident insurance policies in the mid-nineteenth century. In 1845, eleven British insurance companies combined to provide insurance for those injured while riding or working on the railroad. Five years later, The Accidental Death Company provided benefits to the families of those whose death was caused by an accident. The distinction between life insurance and accident insurance was not clarified in this period. Death by accident was not the only criterion that life insurance companies used to determine when to pay off a policy. German life insurance companies, for instance, paid out on policies issued to individuals after they had lost both hands in an accident. H. W. Dingman, *Insurability Prognosis and Selection*, p. 13 and "Life Insurance in Germany," *MR* (1894) 46:416.

53. G. M. Cox, "Let the Good Work Go On," p. 277. Tuberculosis was the leading fatal respiratory disease during the period of rapid growth of the insurance companies. While tuberculosis began to decline in England beginning in 1838, in New York, Philadelphia, Boston, and Paris it did not show any dropping off before 1880. Review of Thomas McKeown's *The Modern Rise of Population* (New York: Academic Press, 1976) in *Science* (1977) 197:650 by Etienne Van de Walle. By 1880, the U.S. census showed that consumption produced 12 percent mortality, while in England and Wales it comprised 9 percent of all reported deaths. Figures on death due to tuberculosis vary, but a variety of reporters seemed to agree that it was a leading cause of death. In his report to the Metropolitan Life Insurance Field Force in 1916, Louis I. Dublin, company statistician, claimed that of the company's 10 million policyholders, the principal cause of death, or 17.7 percent of all policyholders' deaths (18,913 individuals), was tuberculosis. The increased rate among industrial policyholders was ascribed to the laborers' exposure to conditions that predisposed them to this disease.

Life insurance companies continued to stress physical examinations to detect the presence of lung diseases. One study of a thousand deaths reported in the records of a New York Life Insurance Company between 1850 and 1873 showed that 27 percent (268 individuals) died of consumption, while in the country at large 15 percent of the deaths were from this disease. Medical insurance directors collected and studied numerous statistics on consumption, and Edgar Holden of the Mutual Benefit Life Insurance Company of New Jersey reported in 1884 that death from the

disease increases with age, a fact not previously established. He also showed that some American life insurance companies were able to select individuals who lived longer. E. J. Marsh reported that, to arrive at his conclusions, Holden had used Marsh's data which had been published in 1877 in "Experience of the Mutual Life Insurance Company of New York." Henry B. Baker of Lansing, Michigan found that his statistics collected in "The Vital Statistics of Michigan in 1870" and published in 1872 agreed with those of Holden. Holden replied that he claimed no originality in his report but wanted to assert the significance of the data and help establish the fact that consumption was a constant threat at all ages. See also Audrey B. Davis, "Life Insurance and the Physical Examination: A Chapter in the Rise of American Medical Technology," *BHM*, fall 1981.

54. Medical Director, "The Physical Examination," *MR* (1873) 9:414.

55. W. Detmold, "Examination for Life Insurance," p. 82.

56. Editorial on paper read by Charles Dennison, "The Mutual Interest of the Medical Profession and Insurance Companies in the Prolongation of Life," *BMSJ* (1893) 129:226.

57. W. Detmold, "Examination for Life Insurance," p. 97.

58. "Value of Cardiosphygmography for the Determination of Cardiac Valvular Conditions and of Aneurism, particularly for Examiners of Life Insurance," *AJMS* 84:119, 128. See also chapter on the pulse.

59. H. Sieveking, *The Medical Advisor*, p. 38.

60. Ibid.

61. John Hutchinson, "On the Capacity of the Lungs and on the Respiratory Functions," *Medico-Chirurgical Times* (1846) 24:37; J. C. G. Balfour, "Contributions to the Study of Spirometry," *M-CT* (1860) 38; H. M. Lee "Comparative Chest Measurements," *MR* (1899) 56:159, 160. He found the chest circumference of 800 men between the ages of 18 and 50 to be two and a half inches greater than generally taken as the average. Albert H. Buck, "An Inquiry into the Causes of Deaths," *MR* (1874) 9:49. See also Bryan Gandeira, "John Hutchinson in Australia and Fiji," *Med Hist* (1977) 21:365-83.

62. W. Gleitsman, "The Spirometer—Its Value and Utility to Life Companies," *MR* (1874) 9:555.

63. Ibid., pp. 555, 556.

64. H. Sieveking, *The Medical Advisor*, p. 615.

65. A. S. Aloe, *Catalogue*, pp. 640, 641.

66. Editorial, "The Mutual Interest of the Medical Profession and Insurance Companies in the Prolongation of Life," *BMSJ* (1893) 129:225.

67. Grahme M. Hammond, "On the Proper Method of Ascertaining the Chest Expansion by Measurement," *MR* (1894) 47:380, 381.

68. Theo. A. Weed, "A New Cyrtometer," *MR* (1881) 20:164.

69. "On Stethometry: Being an Account of a new and more exact Method of Measuring and Examining the Chest, with some of its Results in Physiology and Practical Medicine," *AJMS* (1876) 72:250.

70. Ibid., pp. 90, 100, 103. See also Richard Quain, "The Stethometer: an instrument for ascertaining the difference in the mobility of opposite sides of the chest, and thus facilitating diagnosis," *London JM* (1850) II:292-94.

71. Richard Hogner, "Contemporary Uni-Bilateral Stethokyrtographical Examinations," *MR* (1894) 45:260. The stethokyrtograph consisted "of a double slot of metal in which two self-registering cylinders of equal weight run side by side by means of cords and metal discs, which can be adjusted on suitable places around the thorax; also of a neck-band in which the apparatus hangs over the sternum. The double slot is 145 mm long, 38 mm broad (each slot 18 mm, besides the thickness of the partition) and the upper end provided with a hook to attach it to the cords from the perpendicular to a more or less horizontal position. At the foot of the apparatus is a small catch to hold the registering paper underneath the slots in a free position."

72. E. Holden, "A Discovery in Physical Diagnosis," pp. 23, 24.

73. Edgar Holden, "A Practical Pneumatometer," *MR* (1878) 13:438.

74. Note "A Pocket Clinical Pneograph by Dr. Mortimer Granville," *JAMA* (1888) 11:672.

75. J. M. Howe, *A Treatise on Mediate Auscultation . . .* (London, 1846).

76. Howard von Rensselaer, "The Pathology of the Caisson Disease," *MR* (1891) 40:180. See this article for a capsule history and excellent bibliography.

77. C. Theodore Williams, "Lectures on the Compressed Air Bath and Its Uses in the Treatment of Disease," *BMJ* (1881) I:824, 825.

78. E. Darwin Hudson, "Present Status of the Pneumatic Treatment of Respiratory Diseases," *MR* (1886) 29:29.

79. J. R. Buchanan, "Mechanical Control of the Circulation," *MR* (1892) 41:82, 83. For illustration of Junod's Boot, see Audrey B. Davis, *Triumph Over Disability* (Washington, D.C.: Smithsonian Institution Press, 1974), p. 18.

80. Including: Andral, Bouillard, Velpeau, Nélaton, Rostan, Ricord, Malgaigne, Louis Dubois, Baudelocque, Cruveilhier, Trousseau, Piorry, Casenave, Boyer, Voisin, Rayes, and Fouquier.

81. J. R. Buchanan, "Mechanical Control of the Circulation," p. 83.

82. E. Darwin Hudson, "Present status of the Pneumatic Treatment of Respiratory Diseases," *MR* (1886) 29:29.

83. "Effects of High Atmospheric Pressure," *MR* (1886) 29:30.

84. C. T. Williams, "Lectures on the Compressed Air Bath," p. 825.

85. Abstract by Try Margate, "Aérothérapie by Bath of Compressed Air," *MTG* (1872) I:404.

86. E. D. Hudson, "Present Status of the Pneumatic Treatment," p. 29.

87. Ibid. "The inhalation of condensed air was indicated in all cases of stenosis of the upper air passages, in contraction of air passages, obstruction, occlusion, or collapse of terminal tubes and air-sacs; the expiration into rarefied air was demonstrated to be the correct method indicated for the treatment and radical cure of emphysema."

88. A. Rose, "Treatment of Diseases of Respiration and Circulation by the Pneumatic Method," *MR* (1875) 10:578.

89. *Catalogue of the Special Loan Collection of Scientific Apparatus at the South Kensington Museum*, 3d ed. (London, 1877), p. 946. Numerous modifications of Waldenburg's instrument were made by Berkart in London, Von Cube and B. Frankel in Berlin (1874), and Philip Biedert of Worms. Frankel and Biedert used the principle of the bellows as applied to the accordion. Frankel's modified accordion was composed in the following manner: "On one side a metal tube is inserted, 2 cms in diameter, which carries the mouth-piece; the latter may consist of an inflating rubber cusion, [sic] similar to a pessary. If the bellows is expanded by drawing the accordeon [sic] apart, the air contained in it will be rarefied; if it is compressed, the air is condensed. If the patient during the expansion or compression applied his mouth to the cusion, the effect of the rarefaction or condensation of the air will communicate itself to the intrathoracic air. The apparatus is without valves; as it is very easy to apply or withdraw the mouth from the cusion at the right moment, any such arrangement as valves is therefore not necessary. If expiration is to be made into rarefied air, the mouth should be applied to the cusion and the belows expanded. After the expiration the mouth is withdrawn from the cushion, and while inhaling the free air the patient closes the bellows for expiring, the apparatus is found empty and ready." A. Rose, "Treatment of Diseases," *MR* (1875) 10:583.

90. Barbara Duncum, *The Development of Inhalation Anesthesia* (London and Oxford: The Wellcome Historical Museum and Oxford University Press, 1947), pp. 60-69.

91. Herbert F. Williams, "Antiseptic Treatment of Disease by means of Pneumatic Differentiation," *MR* (1885) 27:57.

92. Ibid.

93. Ibid., p. 58.

94. For technical details see Joseph Ketchum, "The Physics of Pneumatic Differentiation," *MR* (1883) 29:31-34. See also Herbert F. Williams, "The Progress of Pneumatic Differentiation," *JAMA* (1886) 7:169-72. Advertisements were placed in *JAMA* during 1867. Reprints and information were offered to those requesting them.

95. C. T. Williams, "Lectures on the Compressed Air Bath," p. 30.

96. I. H. Platt, "The Physics and Physiological Action of Pneumatic Differentiation," *MR* (1886) 29:606.

97. "The Annual Museum," *BMJ* (1887) II:468.

98. *JAMA* (1887) 9:21 for advertisement. The Douglas Cabinet was sold by the Cincinnati Medical and Surgical Supply Co.

99. H. F. Williams, "Antiseptic Treatment of Disease," p. 169.

100. "A New Method of Intra-Pulmonary Medication, with Remarks upon its use with Pneumatic Treatment," *JAMA* (1887) 9:109.

101. Ibid., p. 110.

102. H. F. Williams, "Antiseptic Treatment of Disease," p. 171.

103. Editorial, "The Pneumatic Cabinet," *JAMA* (1886) 7:211.

104. Editorial, "The Pneumatic Cabinet Again," *JAMA* (1886) 7:435, 436.

105. H. F. Williams, "Antiseptic Treatment of Disease," p. 172.

106. B. Duncan, *The Development of Inhalation Anesthesia*, London: The Wellcome Historical Museum and Oxford Univ. Press, 1947) p. 361.

107. Ibid., p. 362.

108. J. Leonard Corning, "The Use of Compressed Air in Conjunction with Medical Solutions in the Treatment of Nervous and Mental Affection," *MR* (1891) 40:225.

109. Ibid., pp. 228, 229.

110. Editorial, "The Pneumatic Cabinet," *MR* (1894) 46:377.

111. Charles Dennison, "The Toothpick in Respiratory Gymnastics," *MR* (1893) 44:768.

112. Charles Purdy, "The Comparative Values of the Newer Tests for Albumin in Urine," *JAMA* (1884) 2:57; C. Dennison, "The Mutual Interest of the Medical Profession," p. 227.

113. C. Purdy, "The Comparative Value," p. 57.

114. Ibid.

115. "Urinary Examination and Life Insurance," *MR* (1896) 49:642.

116. "The Bearing of the Presence of Albumin or Sugar in Urine on Life Insurance," *JAMA* (1886) 4:129.

117. Douglas Powell, "The Insurance of Impaired Lives," *BMJ* (1896) I:14.

118. S. Oakley Vander Poel, "The Medical Examiner for Life Insurance and His Responsibilities," *MR* (1900) 57:211.

119. W. A. Hutchinson, "The Evolution of Life Insurance." *Trans. of Actuarial Society of Am.* 21 (part ii): 43, 44; *Readings in Life Insurance: A Compendium* (New York: Life Office Management Association,1934).

120. E. M. Brockbank, *The Conduct of Life Insurance Examinations* (London: H. K. Lewis and Co. Ltd., 1931), p. 105.

121. *Readings in Life Insurance*, p. 120.

122. Oscar H. Rogers and Arthur Hunter, "The Numerical Method of Determining the Values of Risks for Insurance," *Readings in Life Insurance*, pp. 69, 70.

123. Ibid., pp. 70, 71.

124. William C. Wey, "Additional Thoughts Concerning Inebriety and Life Insurance," *MR* (1875) 10:53.

125. H. W. Dingman, *Insurability Prognosis and Selection*, p. 21.

126. Ibid., p. 359.

127. James Cuming, "The Control of Pathological Research by Clinical Observation," *BMJ* (1884) II:202; "Therapeutics as Based on the Study of Tendencies," *MR* (1880) 18:315-17.

128. Roger I. Lee, "The Physical Examination of Apparently Healthy Individuals: Its Importance, Limitations and Opportunities," *BMSJ* (1923) 188:931.

129. "The Physical Requirements of Factory Children," *JR Stat Soc* (1876) 39:682; "Medical and Physical Examination of School Children," *Am Stat Assoc* (1911) 12:558-65; see also Audrey B. Davis, "Human Technology: Emerging Medical Practices in the Nineteenth Century," (in press).

130. J. Paterson MacLaren, *Medical Insurance Examinations: Modern Methods and Rating of Lives* (London: Baillière, 1927), p. 83.

131. Lewis F. Mackenzie, "Blood Pressure with a Special Reference to the Diastolic," *Proc. Assoc. of Life Insurance Directors* (1915), p. 227.

132. A. Schott, "An Early Account of Blood Pressure Measurements by Joseph Struthius (1510-1568)," *MH* (1977) 21:305-309.

133. Andre Cournaud, introduction, *Statical Essays: Containing Haemastaticks* by Stephen Hales (New York: Hafner Publishing Co., 1964), p. vii.

134. For a capsule history of blood pressure instruments see Arthur Master, Charles I. Garfield, and Max B. Walters, *Normal Blood Pressure and Hypertension* (Philadelphia: Lea and Febiger, 1952), chap one. For details on those invented up to 1902 see N. Vaschide and J. M. Lahy, "La Technique de la Mésure de la Pression Sanguine," *Gén de Méd* (Sep., Oct., Nov., Dec.). ii 1902, pp. 349-83, 480-501, 602-39.

135. J. P. MacLaren, *Medical Insurance Examinations*, p. 85.

136. E. M. Brockbank, *The Conduct of Life Assurance Examinations*, p. 66.

137. R. M. Goepp, "Blood Pressure as a Prognostic Factor," *PMJ* (1919) 22:304. "Blood pressure findings alone are often of little value; especially is this true if we are trying to determine a man's physical fitness," Bernard Smith, "Blood Pressure Studies of Five Hundred Men," *JAMA* (1918) 71:174. Smith used the Tycos mercurial sphygmomanometer.

138. Albert Reibmeyer, "A New Era in the Treatment of Internal Diseases," *MR* (1886) 29: 70, 71.

139. Richard Shryock, "Quantification in Medical Sciences," *Isis* (1961) 52:228.

140. Knud Faber, *Nosography*, 2d ed. (New York: Paul B. Hoeber, AMS Press, Inc., 1978), p. 113.

141. Theodore Caldwell Janeway, *The Clinical Study of Blood-Pressure* (New York and London: D. Appleton and Co., 1904); Henry Jackson, *The Value of the Pulse in Diagnosis and Prognosis* (Boston, 1899).

142. A. Master et al., *Normal Blood Pressure and Hypertension*, p. 46.

143. Mackenzie, "Blood Pressure with a Special Reference to the Diastolic," p. 223.

144. Ibid., p. 221.

145. Ibid., p. 222.

146. Ibid., p. 8.

147. Richard Cabot, *Physical Diagnosis of Diseases of the Chest* (New York: William Wood and Co., 1903), p. 63.

148. Harvey Cushing, "On Routine Determination of Arterial Tension in Operating Room and Clinic," *BMSJ* (1903) 158:252.

149. Christopher Lawrence, "Physiological Apparatus in the Wellcome Museum 3. Early Sphygmomanometers," *MH* (1979) 23:477.

150. A. Master et al., *Normal Blood Pressure and Hypertension*, p. 27.

151. Ibid., p. 28.

152. R. M. Geopp, "Blood Pressure as a Prognostic Factor," p. 296.

153. Ibid.

154. A. Master et al., *Normal Blood Pressure and Hypertension*, p. 30.

155. H. W. Cook, "Report of the Committee on Blood Pressure Tests," *Trans. of the Assoc. of Life Insurance Medical Directors* (1921) 8:39.

156. Ibid., p. 42.

157. *JAMA* (1939) 113:294.

158. H. W. Cook, "Report," p. 39.

159. J. W. Fisher, "The Diagnostic Value of the Sphygmomanometer in Examinations for Life Insurance," *JAMA* (1914) 63:1752.

160. Ibid.

161. G. A. Van Wagenen, "Report of the Committee on the Blood Pressure Test," *Trans. Assoc. of Life Insurance Med. Directors of Am.* (1913-15), p. 241.

162. Ibid., p. 260.

163. Ibid.

164. Ibid., p. 243.

CHAPTER 9

1. S. Weir Mitchell, *The Early History of Instrumental Precision in Medicine* (New Haven: Tuttles, Morehouse and Taylor, 1892), p. 7.

2. Anon., "Industry and Medical Service," Review of *Diseases of Occupation and Vocational Hygiene* by George M. Kober and William C. Hanson (London: William Heineman, 1918), *Lancet* (1918) II:244.

3. To the Editor, "School Hygiene," *MR* (1878) 14:32.

4. E. G. Loring, "An Improved Means of Oblique Illumination—a Corneal Condenser," *MR* (1882) 22:614. Dr. Noyes invented the condenser, which was made by W. F. Ford and C. H. Ford of New York.

5. Editorial, "The Influence of the Medical Profession," *MR* (1876) 11:655.

6. Anon., "National Association for the Promotion of Social Science," *BMJ* (1884) II:582.

7. To the Editor, "Brain Pressure in Public Schools," Report of Crichton Brown, *MR* (1884) 26:492.

8. Editorial, "The Sanitary Bearing of Tall Buildings," *MR* (1896) 49:126, 127.

9. Editorial, "A New Danger in Tall Buildings," *MR* (1896) 49:595.

10. J. R. Black, "The Profit to Life Insurance Companies in Promoting Public Health Measures," *MR* (1875) 10:140.

11. Abstract from *Versicherungs Zeitung* of Berlin, *MR* (1874) 9:560. Refers to "Life Insurance and Sanitary Regulations," in *Insurance Times* (1874).

12. Alonzo Nodine, "The Importance of Dental Examination for Life Insurance," *Dental Cosmos* (1913) 55:821.

13. Frank Van Fleet, "We are Drifting Whither?" *MR* (1896) 49:478.

14. Ibid., p. 479.

15. Ibid.

16. William Thomson, "On Colour Blindness," *Med News and Abstr* (1880) 38:706.

17. W. M. Beaumont, "A Discussion of the Vision of Railway Servants," *BMJ* (1891) II:460. See also J. Ellis Jennings, *Color-Vision and Color-Blindness: A Practical Manual for Railroad Surgeons*, 2d ed. (Philadelphia, 1902). Jennings gives an account of Wilson in England, Helmholtz and Seeback in Germany, Foure in France, Holmgren in Sweden, and Jeffries and Thomson in the United States. All of these individuals urged the testing of railway employees for color blindness.

18. Letter of Joseph Priestley, *Smithsonian Reports* (1877) p. 132; M. L. Duncan, trans. from French of Holmgren "Color Blindness in its Relation to Accidents by Rail and Sea."

19. Letter of Joseph Priestley, *Smithsonian Reports*, pp. 131, 135.

20. Ibid., p. 179.

21. W. Thomson, "On Colour Blindness," p. 707.

22. *Smith Reports*, p. 133.

23. Ibid., p. 181.

24. Ibid., p. 180.

25. Ibid., p. 132.

26. Ibid., p. 132.

27. W. Thomson, "On Colour Blindness," p. 708.

28. George L. Collins, "Bulletin on Color Blindness," *Public Health Reports* (1918) 33:911.

29. Daniel Lewis, "The Achievement of the Pennsylvania Railroad Company," *MR* (1885) 27:129.

30. Ibid.

31. W. Thomson, "On Colour Blindness," pp. 710-711.

32. W. M. Beaumont, "A Discussion of the Vision," p. 467.

33. W. A. Brailey, "Vision of Railway Servants," *BMJ* (1891) II:470.

34. Malcolm M. McHardy, "A Review of the Tests for Color Blindness," *BMJ* (1891) II:468.

35. Ibid.

36. F. W. Edridge-Green, "The Relation of Light Perception to Colour Perception," *Proc Roy Soc. of London*, Section B (1910) 82:458.

37. Ibid., p. 471.

38. A. E. Wright, "Color Blindness and a Practical Remedy for It," *MR* (1892) 41:577.

39. F. W. Edridge-Green, "The Essentials of a Test for Color Blindness," *BMJ* (1901) II:1262.

40. Thomas Bickerton, "The Holmgren Wool Test," *BMJ* (1900) I:621.

41. Ibid., p. 622.

42. F. W. Edridge-Green, "The Hunterian Lectures on Colour Vision and Colour Blindness," *Lancet* (1911) I:285-90, 358-63.

43. Ibid., p. 358.

44. Ibid.

45. Ibid.

46. Ibid.

47. Ibid., p. 360.

48. Ibid., p. 363.

49. G. L. Collins, "Bulletin on Color Blindness," p. 911.

50. F. W. Edridge-Green, "Colour Vision and Colour Blindness," p. 363.

51. E. Jackson, "Tests for Visual Acuteness; Their Illumination; and the Standards of Normal Vision," *JAMA* (1891) 16:157-58.

52. Edward W. Heckel, "A Combination Test Card," *MR* (1894) 45:308.

53. D. W. Hunter, "A Combination Test Card," *MR* (1892) 42:579.

54. William Dennett, Editorial, "Accurate Test Types," *MR* (1885) 28:183. Meyrowitz Bros. of New York produced the charts to Dennett's specifications for mounting in the classroom.

55. "A Combined Visual and Astigmatic Eye—Remarks on Astigmatism, Characteristic Mannerism," *JAMA* (1884) 2:209-11.

56. J. L. Thompson, "Suggestions on the Examination of the Eyes of Applicants for Pension," *JAMA* (1884) 2:62.

57. Ibid., p. 63.

58. E. M. Brockbank, *The Conduct of Life Assurance Examinations* (London: H. K. Lewis and Co. Ltd., 1931), p. 8. Brockbank acted as an insurance examiner for more than sixty years and examined over 10,000 individuals.

59. B. Joy Jeffries, *Color-Blindness; its Dangers and its Detection* (Boston, 1879), p. 178.

60. Editorial, "International Medical Congress," *MR* (1876) 13:599.

61. Editorial, "The International Congress of Medical Science," *MR* (1879) 16:397.

62. E. Seguin, "Uniformity in the Practice of Physic," *MR* (1876) 13:554.

63. William Hiallard and Herbert T. Wade, *Outlines of the Use of Weights and Measures and the Metric System* (London and Toronto: The Macmillan Co., 1906), pp. 191-98.

64. Anon., "An International Pharmacopoeia," *BMJ* (1878) II:487.

65. Abstr. from *BMJ*, *MR* (1880) 17:252.

66. W. Hiallard and H. Wade, *Outlines of the Use of Weights and Measures*, p. 41.

67. George N. Kreider, "The 'Americanized' Metric system," *MR* (1880) 18:474.

68. M. S. Buttles, To the Editor, "The Metric System and Its Practical Application," *MR* (1879) 16:21, 22.

69. "Dose Dispensing Simplified," *MR* (1878) 13:184. See also R. M. F. "A Convenient Method of Dosage and Administration," *MR* (1882) 21:311-13.

70. Letter to Editor of S. M. T. "The Sin of Substitution," *MR* (1895) 47:125.

71. E. Seguin, "Uniformity in the Practice of Physic," *MR* (1876) 13:556.

72. Ibid.

73. Book review "The Physician's Visiting List," *JAMA* (1887) 8:27.

74. W. Harvey Smith, "The Application of the Graphic Method to Hearing," *MR* (1894) 46:510.

75. Annual Museum, *BMJ* (1887) II:469.

77. "Ready-Made Illustrations," *MR* (1885) 28; *BMJ* (1886) II:453.

78. Charles McManus, "On the Present Needs of the Profession—A History," *Dental Cosmos* (1898) 40:20.

79. A Medical Director, "Imperfect Reports of Medical Examiners," *MR* (1873) 8:248.

80. "New Medical Examiner's Blanks," *MR* (1873) 8:583, 584.

81. "The Card Index or Card Catalogue as adapted to History-Taking in Private Practice," *MR* (1894) 46:808, 809.

82. R. C. M. Page, "An Easy Method for Teaching Physical Diagnosis," *MR* (1885) 27:66.

83. "Nursing Charts," *BMJ* (1891) I:764. Students and young surgeons were also given charts depicting the instruments and appliances routinely used in a number of operations. L. Hepenstal Omsby, "The Annual Museum," *BMJ* (1887) II:468.

84. A. S. Aloe, *Catalogue*, pp. 394, 395.

85. Henry Bernal, "Ledger Book," *JAMA* (1888) 5:16.

86. E. Seguin, "Uniformity in the Practice of Physic," p. 556.

87. E. Seguin, *Suggestions on Thermometry*, part two of the translation of *Medical Thermometry and Human Temperature* by C. A. Wunderlich (New York: William Wood and Co., 1871), p. 234.

88. Note, "The Westminster School of Medicine New Building," *BMJ* (1885) II:666; see also Malcolm T. MacEashern, *Medical Records in the Hospital* (Chicago: Physicians' Record Co., 1937).

89. Extract from *Pop. Sci. Mo.* "Exact Dosage in Exercise," *MR* (1896) 49:628.

90. Audrey B. Davis, *Triumph Over Disability* (Washington, D.C.: Smithsonian Institution Press, 1974), p. 27.

91. "Notes on Books," A review of *The Technique of Ling's System of Manual Treatment as Applicable to Surgery and Medicine* (Edinburgh and London: J. Pentland, 1890), *BMJ* (1891) I:809.

92. A. D. Rockwell, "On the Dosage of the Galvanic Current," *MR* (1887) 31:630.

93. Ibid., p. 631.

94. Frederick B. Noyes, "Personal Recollections of a Leader, Greene Vardiman Black: His Development and Influence" Presidential Address Delivered before Institute of Medicine of Chicago, 7 December 1943, reprint.

95. See for example: Editorial, Karl Braun "On One Hundred Laparatomies and Techniques," *JAMA* (1884) 2:355-57.

96. Barbara Duncum, *The Development of Inhalation Anesthesia* (London and Oxford: The Wellcome Historical

Museum and Oxford University Press, 1947), pp. 14, 15, 24.

97. W. Stanley Sykes, *Essays on the First One Hundred Years of Anaesthesia*, vol. 1 (Edinburgh and London: E. and S. Livingstone Ltd., 1960), p. 25.

98. B. Duncum, *The Development of Inhalation Anesthesia*, p. 125, 181 for contrast between instruments in England and the United States.

99. E. Julius Gurlt, "Collective Investigation on Anesthetics," *MR* (1892) 42:79.

100. B. Duncum, *The Development of Inhalation Anesthesia*, p. 16.

101. Ernest Muirhead Little, compiler, *History of the British Medical Association, 1832-1932* (London: British Medical Association, 1932), pp. 301-305.

102. Ibid., pp. 304, 305.

103. Isambard Owen, "Meeting of Staffordshire Branch, *BMJ* (1885) I:742.

104. Tyson, "Meeting of Collective Investigation Committee of the BMA, *BMJ* (1885) I:806.

105. "Meeting of the Collective Investigation Committee," *BMJ* (1886) I:269.

106. Stephen MacKenzie, "Memorandum on Chorea," *BMJ* (1887) I:432.

107. Isambard Owen, "Supplement to the Memorandum on Collective Investigation," *BMJ* (1888) II:266.

108. W. P. Herringham, "Letter," *BMJ* (1884) II:1166.

109. John S. Billings, "Address in Medicine," *BMJ* (1886) II:316; *MR* (1886) 30:174.

110. John S. Billings, *The National Medical Dictionary*, vol. I (Philadelphia: Lea Bros. and Co., 1890), pp. xxii, xxxiii.

CHAPTER 10

1. Nöel and José Parry, *The Rise of the Medical Profession* (London: Croom Helm Ltd., 1976). See also M. Jeanne Peterson, *The Medical Profession in Mid-Victorian London* (Berkeley: University of California Press, 1978).

2. John Duffy, *The Healers: The Rise of the Medical Establishment* (New York: McGraw-Hill Book Co., 1976), p. 275.

3. Ibid., p. 274.

4. Richard W. Wertz and Dorothy C. Wertz, *Lying-In A History of Childbirth in America* (New York: Schocken Books, 1979), pp. 64, 65.

5. Norman Bridge "The New Science of Medicine," *JAMA* (1884) 2:312.

6. Editorial "Precision in Diagnosis," *JAMA* (1890) 14:276.

7. T. Gaillard Thomas, "Laparotomy as a Diagnostic Resource," *JAMA* (1886) 7:603-05.

8. Lawson Tait, "A Series of One thousand Cases of Abdominal Surgical Diagnoses," *MR* (1885) 27:1-3; also Lawson Tait, "Methods of Diagnosis," *MR* (1886) 29:141.

9. S. Weir Mitchell, "The Early History of Instrumental Precision in Medicine," *Trans. Am. Physicians and Surgeons Congress* (1892), p. 164.

10. Note, "A Suffering Patient with a Statistical Bent," *MR* (1893) 44:704.

11. Editor, "The Spitting Habit," *MR* (1892) 42:135.

12. Royston Lambert, *Sir John Simon (1816-1904) and English Social Administration* (London: Macmillan and Kee, 1963).

13. Sir Rickman Godlee, *Lord Lister*, 3d rev. ed. (Oxford: At the Clarendon Press, 1924), pp. 15, 16.

14. John Shaw Billings, "American Inventions and Discoveries in Medicine, Surgery and Practical Sanitation," *Smithsonian Reports* (1892), pp. 618, 619.

15. A. K. Stone, "The Hygienic Argument for Cremation Considered from a Bacteriological Standpoint," *BMSJ* (1893) 129:434.

16. Ibid., p. 463.

17. T. Spencer Wells, "Remarks on Cremation or Burial," *BMJ* (1880) II:461-63.

18. T. Spencer Wells, "A Discussion on the Disposal of the Dead," *BMJ* (1891) II:627, 628.

19. Acts of Parliament Sponsored by Lord Monkswell (Lords) and Sir Walter Foster (Commons), BMJ (1902) II: 908, "The Cremation Act, 1902."

20. Note, "Cremation in England," *MR* (1894) 46:651.

21. Editorial, "The Millenial of Cremation," *MR* (1893) 44:241.

22. Edward John Bermingham, *Disposal of the Dead* (New York: Bermingham and Co., 1881), p. 61; (1885), p. 48.

23. Andrew H. Smith, "The Family Physician of the Future," *MR* (1887) 32:699.

24. Ibid.

25. James Hobson Aveling, *The Chamberlens and the Midwifery Forceps* (1882), reprint (New York: AMS Press, 1977).

26. Editorial, "Medical Patents," *MR* (1876) 11:816.

27. Ibid.

28. J. Ben Robinson, "Eighteenth Century Dentistry in America, data secured from Eighteenth Century Newspapers in the Rare Book Room of the Library of Congress," typescript, Division of Medical Sciences, National Museum of American History, Smithsonian Institution.

INDEX

Abortion, 33
Abrams, Albert, 93, 109
Accession records, 27
Accidents, 35. *See also* Medical errors
Accommodation, 213
Acetometer, 69
Acoustics, 93, 99, 102, 107
Acquisition, 29
Acupuncture implements, 11
Adams, Francis, 117
Addison, William, 43, 87
Advertise(ments), 22, 23, 26, 46
Aeginata, Paulus, 17
Aesthesiometer, 82, 93, 176, 177, 178
Aid(s), 37, 141, 213; mechanical, 236
Air bath, 198, 199
Aitkin, William, 69; thermometer, 70, 77
Albucasis, 17
Albumin in urine, 201, 204
Alcock, 91
Alcohol: thermometer, 65; solution, 79
Alison, Scott, 107
Alkindi, 65
Allbutt, Thomas Clifford, 63, 70, 73, 75, 77, 130, 161; thermometer, 72
Allen, Dr. Frederick, 29
Allen, Dudley P., 55
Allen and Hanbury's, 44, 107
Allen and Howard, 75
Aloe, A. S., 34, 78, 94, 126, 127, 150, 151, 173, 174, 196, 202, 218, 219, 222, 223
Aluminum, 7, 10, 99, 101, 195
Alverez, Walter, 207
Amalgams, 228
Amaurosis, 150
Amber, R. B., 118
Amber, 101
Ambulances, 43
American Actuarial Society, 185
American Association of the History of Dentistry, 48
American College of Radiology, 22
American Congress of Rehabilitation Medicine, 33
American Dental Association, 55

American Medical Association, 44, 131, 148, 221, 224, 238
American Museums' Association Guide to Museums, 27, 40
American Ophthalmological Society, 55
American Public Health Association, 238
American scale, 226
American Society of Anesthesiologists, 30, 56
American Sterilizer Company, 10
American system of manufacturing, 12
American Urological Society, 55
Amputating saws, 9
Amputation(s), 17, 47, 182; sets, 56
Analgesis, 30
Anal speculum, 102
Anatomical Institute of Bologna, 32
Anatomic specimens, 31, 39
Anatomic waxes, 32
Anatomy, 26; wax model, 56
Ancient drugs, 16
Andral, Gabriel, 81
Andrews, E., 40
Anemia, 142
Aneroid sphygmomanometer, 208
Anesthesia(tic), 6, 18, 180, 200, 229; devices, 22, 30, 56; local, 10, 30
Aneurism, 91, 144
Angle, Edward, 48, 243
Annual Museum, 42, 43, 44, 77, 176, 200, 225
Anthropologist, 28
Anthropometric equipment, 7, 174, 178; measuring aids, 53; laboratory, 165
Anthropometry, 169, 172
Antibacterial solutions, 242
Antipyretic drugs, 158
Antique dealer, 39
Antisepsis, 9, 11, 180, 241
Antiseptic medicinals, 199
Apex rectal thermometer, 77
Apothecary shop, 39
Apparatus, 16, 18, 20, 37, 40, 44, 45, 46, 47, 183, 200, 224, 238; chemical, 42; mechanical, 43; scientific, 44

Appliances, 6, 20, 30, 42, 43, 44, 47, 182, 183, 213, 225; hygiene, 43; sanitary, 43
Appolonius, 17
Aquapendente, Fabrizio d', 18
Archeologist(s), 28, 37
Archigenes, 119
Archives, Smithsonian Institution, 48
Aretaeus of Cappadonia, 87
Aristoxenus, 119
Armed Forces Institute of Pathology Museum, 22, 29, 30, 51, 53, 55, 242; formerly U.S. Army Medical Museum, 31, 42
Armor, Samuel G., 200
Army medical chests, 42
Arnaldus de Villanova (Arnold of Villanova) 65
Arnold and Sons, 20, 44, 76, 77, 79; conversation tube, 101
Arnott, Neil, 20
Artifact(s), 16, 27, 37, 39, 46; dental, 46
Artificial body parts, 37
Artificial curiosities, 39
Artificial eyes, 47
Artificial kidney(s), 33
Artificial limbs, 37, 42, 213; arm, 56; hand and arm, 47
Artificial teeth, 10, 48
Artisan(s), 37
Asclepius, 37
Aseptic, 10
Ashmolean Museum, 29
Ashmolean School of Natural History, 16
Aspirin, 158
Association of Life Insurance Medical Directors, 190, 208
Astigmatism, 215, 219
Astigmatism dial, Green's, 219
Auenbrugger, Leopold, 88, 89, 90, 93, 145
Aurelianus, Caelius, 87
Auscultation, 82, 88, 91, 92, 102, 110, 131, 153, 155, 160, 186, 192-194, 195, 196, 208; intrathoracic, 94; mediate, 89, 91; sign, 109
Autenreith, Johann H. F., 143

Auzoux, Louis Thomas Jerome, 32; papier maché, 53
Axillary temperature, 62; axial thermometer, 67

Babbage, Charles, 162, 184
Babey-Brooke, A. M., 118
Bacteria(l), 8, 9, 64, 77, 184, 186, 192, 201, 237, 238, 241
Bacteria-free, 10
Bactericides, 199
Bacteriology, 180, 181, 211; apparatus, 131
Baillie, Matthew, 146, 182
Baker and Browning, 147
Baker and Holborn, 73
Bakken, Earl, 56
Bandages, 17, 18, 21
Barclay, 100
Baretta, Louis, 32
Barium compounds, 37
Barker, Lewellys F., 176
Barnard, Harold, 208
Barnes, Surgeon General Joseph K., 31
Barnes spirometer, 194
Barometer, 66
Barry, John, clinical thermometer, 85
Basch, Samuel R. von, 206; sphygmoma-nometer, 208
Bath: cold, 64; mud, 6; sun, 6
Baton, 87, 97
Battery(ies), 19; electric, 20; Jerome Kidder's, 49
Bausch and Lomb, 22
Baxter, J. H., 165, 178
Bayle, Gaspard Laurent, 91, 186
Beaumont, W. M., 213
Beaumont, William H., 215
Beck, R. and J., 146-147
Beck-Lee electrocardiograph, 136
Beddoes, Thomas, 199
Bedini, Silvio, 39
Bed pan(s), 23, 56
Bell, Luther Vose, 90
Bellevue Hospital, 91
Bellini, Angelo, 69
Bellows, 144
Bell stethoscope, 95
Bennion, Elisabeth, 31
Berlin wool, 214
Bernal, Henry and Company (St. Louis), 226
Bernard, Claude, 63, 144, 153, 162, 163, 164, 179
Bert, Paul, 200, 201
Bertillon, Alphonse, 165, 166, 167, 168, 170, 171, 174
Bertin, E., 198
Berzelius, 224
Bianci, Guiseppe, 65
Bichat, François Xavier, 146, 159, 163
Bickerton, Thomas, 216
Bicycle, 7
Billings, Frank, 10

Billings, John Shaw, 29, 53, 55, 231, 238
Bills of Mortality, 148
Binaural, biaural stethoscope, 95, 102, 107
Biological Museum, 42
Biometer, 188
Biometry, 188, 204
Biopsy, 147
Bird, Golding, 104
Birkitt, 80
Black, Greene Vardiman, 26, 45, 48, 228, 229, 243
Blackwell, T. C., 107
Blake, John, 48
Block's thermometer, 79
Blood, 6, 23
Blood cell counts, 12
Bloodletters, 39
Bloodletting, 17
Bloodletting instruments, 21, 31, 47, 48, 56, 206; charts, 18
Blood pressure, 11, 16, 124, 125, 131, 142, 157, 184, 185, 186, 205, 206, 208, 209, 225, 236, 237, 239; abnormal, 5, 204; instruments, 129, 131; standards, 207, 210
Blood Pressure Committee, 208; tests, 209
Blood testing equipment, 5, 179
Blood vessels, 32, 35
Bock, Heinrich, 108
Boden, H. C. and Co., 217
Bodily (or body) fluids, 7, 206
Bodily functions, 240
Bodily tissues, 228, 236, 237
Body build, 184, 203
Body measuring instruments, 178
Body weight, 184
Boerhaave, Hermann, 63, 67, 68, 161
Bone, 55, 67
Bone setters, 39
Bonet, Theophile, 145
Borelli, Alphonse, 205
Boston Medical and Surgical Journal, 79
Botanical drugs. See Drug(s)
Botanical Institute of the University of Florence, 32
Bouillard, J. B., 68
Bouillaud, Jean-Baptiste, 152
Boulitte, G., 176
Bourdon tube, 64
Bowditch, Henry I., 90, 125, 200
Bowditch, Henry P., 145
Bowles, Robert C. M., 95; patent chest piece, 95
Box, 9
Boxwood, 97; calipers, 169
Bracegirdle, Brian, 29
Bradbury, John B., 62, 161
Brainard, 40
Brambilla, Giovanni Alessandro, 6
Brand Bath, 187
Brass, 231
Brass scale, 169
Brass tubes, 194
Breaking, 35

Brecker, Ruth and Edward, 16
Bridge, Norman, 235
Bright, Richard, 150, 182
Bright's disease, 145, 150, 151, 161, 201
British Board of Trade, 215
British Dental Association, 46
British Medical Association, 42, 62, 77, 153, 159, 161, 162, 176, 200, 225, 229, 235, 239, 242
British Medical Journal, 43
British Oxygen Company, 30
British Society of Arts, 42
Broca, Paul, 80
Bronchoscope, 52
Bronze surgical instruments, 39, 46
Broussais, F.-J.-V., 152, 162
Brown-Sequard, 176
Bruce, J. Mitchell, 181
Bruit de soufflet, 92
Brunton, Thomas L., 64, 207
Bulkeley, Gershom, 57
Burch, George, 16, 133
Burr, 11
Buss, Carl Emil, 64
Buttle, M. S., 224
Byrd, Henry L., 155

Cabanis, Pierre-Jean-Georges, 87
Cabinet(s), 10, 199; pneumatic, 200
Cabot, Richard C., 93, 110, 156, 207
Caesarian section, 18
Calamai, Luigi, 31
Calcari, Francis, Museum of, 39
Caldani, Leopold M. A., 143
Calibration, 22; instruments, 239; service, 75; thermometer, 73
California Pacific International Exposition (San Diego), 44
Calipers, 169, 174; compass, 165; rule, 170; thoracic, 195
Calorimeter, 131, 144
Cambridge Instrument Company, 133, 169, 178
Cammann, D. M., 104, 107, 108; stetho-scope, 105
Campani, Giuseppi, 55
Campbell, J. Menzies, 33
Cancer, 29
Canguilhem, Georges, 179
Cannon, Walter, 179
Cannulas, 144
Carbolic acid, 238
Carbon arc lamp, 136
Card catalog syndrome, 28
Cardiac instruments, 5
Cardiac sounds, 92, 93
Cardiometer, 93, 94, 115
Cardiosonics Medical Instrument Co., 96
Cardiosphygmomagraphy, 193
Cardiovascular instruments, 137
Carious teeth, 16
Carrick, George, 107
Carroll, 176

Carter, William, 62
Carvings, 16
Casella, Louis P., 69, 75, 76
Case(s), 9; of disease, 149; thermometer, 70
Casts, 32, 42, 43, 53
Catalogue cards, 27, 31
Catalogue(s), 42, 43, 48, 53, 56, *See also* Manufacturer(s); Trade fair(s); name of museum or exhibition
Cataracts, 6
Catheter, 7
Caustic stick, 236
Cauteries, 16
Cauterization, 17
Cauterizing irons, 17
Cedar, 99
Celluloid, 101
Celsius, Anders, 17, 66
Celsius scale, 68
Celsus, Aurelius Cornelius, 164
Centennial (1876), 42, 48, 53
Centigrade scale, 66, 143
Ceramic pharmacy objects, 31
Cerebral temperature, 80
Chamberlen(s) (Peter), 241; obstetric instruments, 56
Chamber of Life Insurance, 190
Chamois, 32
Champion, W. L., 210
Chandler, Alfred, 48
Charlatan(s) (quack), 23
Charrière, M. F., 20, 21, 175
Charts, 32, 42, 193, 207, 225, 226, 227, 228, 240; acupuncture, 11; diet, 225; mapping teeth, 229; temperature, 225
Chemical analysis, 7, 160; of urine, 237
Chemical apparatus, 42
Chemical drugs, 141. *See also* Drugs
Chemical tests, 7, 155, 156, 160, 183, 186, 192, 201
Chest girth, 204
Chest measuring device, 195
Chest piece, 95
Chest rule (stethometer), 195
Chests, 46; army medical, 42
Chinese, 27, 118, 123; pulse doctrines, 129; surgery, 11
Chinese physicians, 11
Chitwood, W. R., 98
Chloroform, 30, 229
Chloroform Committee Report (1864), 229
Chrome-plated, 99
Circulation, 63, 164
Circumcision knives, 47
Clarity of vision, 217
Clark, Andrew, 91, 107
Clark, James, 90
Clarke, Edwin, 29
Classification of disease, 148, 160
Clay, 16, 32
Clepsydra, 119, 120
Clinical Pathological Conference (CPC), 156

Clinical polygraph, 130
Clinical thermometer, 71
Closets, 40
Cloth, 194; wet, 6
Cobwebs, Professor D. R. V., 40
Cockburn Barrow and Machine Company, 201
Codman and Shurtleff, 77
Cohn, Alfred E., 135
Coins, 16
Cold baths, 64
Coles, George Charles, 228
Collection(s), 5, 13, 27, 28, 29, 30, 37, 39, 40, 46, 47, 57, 76, 207; wax, 32
Collective Investigation Committee of Disease, 157, 163, 229, 230, 231, 235
Collector(s), 5, 13, 21, 31, 39, 44, 55
College of Physicians (Philadelphia), 40, 53
Collin of Paris, 98
Collin, Adolph, 21
Collin, Robert, 21, 175
Collin, Victor, 110
Collins of London, 147
Color-blindness, 7, 213, 214, 215, 216, 237; tests, 7, 216
Color-blind person, 216
Color vision, 213, 214, 231; testing, 215; tests, 214, 216
Columbian Exposition (Chicago), 42
Colver, Charles M., 217
Comins, Nicholas P., stethoscope, 102, 103
Committee on Standardization of Blood Pressure Readings of the American Heart Association, 209
Compacted wood, 99
Comparative instrumentology, 40
Compass, 176
Computer, 27, 28, 29, 156
Computer cataloguing, 28, 29
Concept of local disease, 61, 62; changing concept of disease, 5
Conservation-analytical laboratory, 28
Conservative surgery, 130
Conservatory of Arts and Measures (Paris), 42
Continued fever, 148
Contour mapping, 187
Contraceptive, 33
Conversation tube, 101, 102
Convex lens, 221
Cook, H. W., 207
Cooley, Denton, 48
Cooper, Astley, 182
Coral, 101
Corning, J. Leonard, 201
Corning Normal, 75
Corvisart, Jean-Nicolas, 88, 89, 145, 146
Cost, 29
Cotes, Roger, 66
Cotton, 70, 104
Cotyla (pulsilogia), 122
Counting red blood cells, 142
Coxeter, 169

Crawford, Adair, 63
Crellin, John, 46
Craftsmen, 37
Cremation, 42, 238
Cremation Society, 239
Crematories, 42, 239
Creosotate compounds, 64, 158
Crichton (thermometer maker), 73
Crisp, Sir Frank, 29
Croce, Andrea della, 18
Crooks, 17
Crouch, 147
Crown and bridge bench, 45
Crude drugs, 41, 48
Cruveilhier, Jean, 159
Cryer, Matthew H., 53
Cryoscopy, 152
Crytometer, 197
Cullen, William, 148
Culpepper microscope, 27
Cuming, James, 149, 161
Curator, 27, 29, 47, 48, 56
Curette, 32
Curie, Madame, piezoelectrometer, 53
Currie, James, 148; thermometer, 83
Curtis, 73
Cusanus, Nicolaus Krebs, 120
Cushing, Harvey, 177, 207
Cutting instruments, 144
Cuvier, Georges, 40
Cylinder, 97
Cylinder thermometer, 79
Cyrtometer, 195
Cystoscope, electric, 154; Nitze, 155
Czermak laryngoscopes, 56

DaCosta, Jacob, 149, 226
DaCosta, James M., 94
Dalton, John, 213, 214
Dam(s), 10
Danielsson and Co., 225
Darton, F., 77
Darwin, Charles, 178
Darwin, Erasmus, 178
Das, Sir Kedarnath, 16
Daukes, S. H., 47
Da Vinci, Leonardo, 97
Dawson, J. B., 95
Deaf, 214
Dealer, 29
Decoration, 29
Decorative handle(s), 10
Delafield, Francis, 150
Denison, Adam Benjamin, 55
Dennett, William S., 217, 219
Dennison, Charles, 95, 105, 109, 193, 194, 201
Dental advertisements, 241
Dental cabinet, 24, 25
Dental chair, 45, 48
Dental engine, 10, 45
Dental instruments, 10, 48, 55, 56
Dental museum catalogue, 33

Dentistry, 10; mechanical, 191
Dentists, 22, 26, 39, 191, 225, 241, 242; office, 56
D'Epine, 153
Dermatographic pencil, 174
Dervieu, Jules de, 102
Design(er), 83, 97, 102, 104, 107, 241
Desnoues, Guillaume, 31
Desormeaux's endoscope, 154
Detmold, William, 190, 192
Deutsches Museum of Science and Industry, 47
Device(s), 7, 20, 21, 22, 23, 26, 33, 34, 37, 40, 42, 82, 101, 110, 118, 130, 141, 146, 148, 154, 156, 158, 162, 164, 174, 176, 180, 181, 183, 185, 186, 187, 198, 199, 200, 201, 208, 211, 213, 224, 233, 238, 240, 241, 243; electrical, 146; therapeutic, 6. See also Bicycle
De Waterville, 200
Dhonden, Yeshi, 11
Diabetes, 29, 204
Diagnosis, 141
Diagnostician, 6, 26
Dickinson, Robert, 226
Dicrotic pulse, 120
Diet(s), 142, 154, 181, 188, 206, 226; special, 6
Differential diagnosis, 154
Differential stethoscope, 107, 108; thermometer, 73
Diphtheria vaccine, 35
Disability pensions, 219
Dissecting instruments, 54
Dittrick, Howard, Museum of Historical Medicine, 30-31, 55
Diving bell, 196
Doctors' office(s), 40, 55, 56
Donné test, 151
Donor, 29
Doran, Alban, 30
Drainage tubes, 20
Dresden shop, 39
Dressing(s), 10, 18
Drill(s), 10, 11, 48
Drug(s), 6, 7, 23, 34, 35, 37, 43, 46, 63, 65, 102, 187, 206, 224; ancient, 16; botanical, 6; chemical, 6; crude, 41; manufacturers, 44; treatment, 142
Dry cells, 40
Du Bois-Reymond, Emil, 125
Duddell, 135
Dudgeon, Robert E., 126
Dudgeon sphygmograph, 127, 129, 130
Dudley, 40
Duncum, Barbara M., 30
Dunglison, Robley, 148
du Val of Paris, 66, 75
Dynamographs, 19, 172
Dynamometers, 19, 82, 162, 165, 169, 172, 173, 174, 175, 176, 178

Earpiece, 102

Ebers Papyrus, 87, 119
Ebony, 99, 103; carved, 9, 95; ebonite, 101
Ebstein, Erich, 66, 79
Economics, 34
Eddons, Alfred, 77
Edgar, J. Clifton, 32
Edinburgh Royal Infirmary, 90
Editorials, 23
Edridge-Green, F. W., 215, 216; lantern, 217
Edwards, Joseph, 80
Ehrle, Carl, 81
Electrical machines or devices, 7, 22, 44, 93; apparatus, 178; stimulators, 144
Electricity, 22
Electric recorder, 110
Electric shocking, 7
Electric stethoscope, 109; multiple, 111
Electrocardiograph, 131, 164; Victor, 137
Electron microscope, 55
Electropathological Museum, 56
Electrophoresis apparatus, 154
Electrosurgery, 228
Elliotson, John, 100
Emetics, 206
Endoscope(s), 131, 186
Endoscopist, 240
Engineering skill, 35
English scale, 226
Equipment, 22, 182, 187
Equitable of England, 188
Erasistratus, 145
Erbe, C., 81
Eskridge, J. T., 80
Ether, 30, 229
Etten, H. Van, 65
Ewart, William, 107, 153
Exercise, 6, 172, 179, 181, 187; apparatus, 7; machines, 228; periods, 212; strenuous, 163. See also Device(s)
Exhibit catalogue, 27
Exhibits (Exhibition), 33, 37, 40, 44, 56, 77; medical, 42; public health, 44; trade, 22, 29
Experimental psychology laboratories, 217
Extractors, dental, 48
Eye chart, 217
Eye examinations, 213
Eye glasses, 213, 215
Eye testing equipment, 221

Facial prostheses, 51
Factory(ies), 174, 211, 212, 213, 214, 236, 237, 238
Faculty Research Department of Anesthesiology of the Royal College of Surgeons (England), 30
Fahrenheit, Daniel Gabriel, 66, 68
Fahrenheit scale, 66, 67, 193
Fahrney, C., 75
Faichney of Watertown, N.Y., 77
Fannin and Co., 69, 74, 226
Farr, William, 188
Farsightedness, 212, 221

Faught pocket sphygmomanometer, 194
Febrifuge(s), 63
Fehling's urine test set, 151
Feick Bros., 217
Felt, 229
Female catheter, 80, 102
Fenwick, E. Hurry, 154
Ferdinand II, Grand Duke, 67
Ferguson, Eugene M., 16, 17
Ferguson, William, 100
Ferris and Co., 105
Ferris and Evans, 77
Fever(s) (pyrexia), 62, 63, 69, 82, 122, 157, 158, 159; hospitals, 158
Fick, A., 125
Filling and capping teeth, 191; fillings, 10
Finlayson, James, 70, 73
Finsen, Niels, 180
Finsen light, 180
Fir, 97
Fishbein, Morris, 44, 207
Fisher, J. W., 207, 209
Fisher, William, 161
Fisheries Exhibition, 41
Fleet, Frank Van, 212, 213
Flint, Austin, 90, 92, 103, 125, 150, 153, 154, 226
Flint, James, 48
Flitner, Bogdan, 80
Florentine Museum, 32
Flouroscope, 112. See also Stethoscope
Floyer, Sir John, 118, 122, 123, 124, 164
Fludd, Robert, 68, 120, 121
Fontana, Felice, 31; models, 32
Forbes, John, 87, 90, 236
Forceps, 21; history of, 15; midwifery, 47; obstetrical, 16
Fordyce, 182
Foreign bodies 6, 35, 37, 53, 211
Fossils, 39
Fossil trusses, 40
Foster, Michael, 144, 145, 146, 160
Fothergill, John, 148
Foucault, Michel, 152
Fox, Cornelius, 73
Fracture(s), 40
Frank, François, 80, 81
Frank of Halle, 81
French, Herbert, 156
French scale, 226
Frerichs, 207
Frey, Von, 176, 177
Friedenwald, Harry, 55
Froeschels stethoscope, 108
Froriep, L. F. V., 18
Fuller, Robert M., 224

Gadget(s), 6, 182
Gaetano, Abate, 31
Gairdner, W. T., 182, 183
Galen, 62, 65, 68, 87, 117, 119, 120, 145; Corpus, 118; preparations, 224
Galileo, Galilei, 120

Galileo's thermometer, 67
Gall, J., 79
Galton, Francis, 163, 165, 169, 239
Galton whistle, 169, 172, 176
Galvanic batteries, 40
Galvanometers, 19, 135
Gamble, C. S., 110, 111
Gant, F. J., 163
Ganther, Dr., 42
GaNun and Parsons, 217
Garengeot, Réné Jacques Croissant de, 18
Garfield, Charles I., 16, 207
Garlick, Theodatus, 56
Garrison, Fielding H., 16, 90
Gasometer, 144
Gauges, 226
Gaujot, Gustav, 16
Gaussian Law of Errors, 165
Gebhard, Bruno, 42, 44
Geddes, L. A., 125
Geison, Gerald, 144
Geissler, Charles F. and Sons, 77, 81
General Electric, 137
Genetic defects, 33
Geoffrey Kaye Museum of Anesthestic
   Apparatus, 30
Gerard of Cremona, 17
Gernier, Paul, 125
German silver, 21
Germ theory, 8, 9, 10, 30, 180
Gersdorff, Hans von, 17
Gibson, F. W., 61
Gilbertson, H. and Sons, 226
Giron, Sales, 200
Glasgow Pathological and Clinical Society,
   182
Glass, 74, 97
Glazing, 21
Gmelin's test, 151
Godlee, Rickman J., 30
Goepp, R. Max, 208
Goiter, 154, 155
Goldbeater's skin, 97
Golden Gate International Exposition
   (San Francisco), 44
Goniometer, 195
Goodhart, J. F., 61
Goodman, John D., 91
Goodridge, Henry F. A., 64
Gordon, Alfred, 177, 178
Gottschalk, 109
Gould, George Milbry, 165, 178
Gourdon, L., 69
Gowers, W. R., 143
Graduated instruments, 82
Graduations, 76
Grafenberg, 145
Graphic pulse, 120
Grand Duke, Ferdinand II, 67
Grand Rounds, 11, 156
Granville, Mortimer, 196
Gray, L. C., 80
Great Lakes Exposition (Cleveland), 44

Green, John, 219
Greene, 100
Greenfield, W. S., 146, 160
Green's astigmatism dial, 219
Griffin, 77
Griffith, R. Eglesfeld, 162
Griffith Prize Essay, 15
Gross, Samuel, 90
Grumbridge of London, 101
Guerlt, Ernst Julius, 15, 18, 229
Guiacum test, 151
Guide(s), 42; Copenhagen, 33; Rome, 33
Guild, 39
Guilleneau, Jacques, 17
Gull, Sir William, 153, 162
Gum-elastic, 104; tube, 104
Gunz-Zwelthof, Edlen von, 102
Gutta percha, 70, 103
Guy, W. A., 164
Guy's Hospital, 32, 103, 150
Gynecologic (gynecology), 23, 235, 236

Hack, William, 77
Haden, Charles, 97
Haen, Antonius de, 68
Haldane, J., 143
Hales, Stephen, 125, 146, 205
Hammond, Grahme, M., 194
Hammond, Surgeon-General William A.,
   53, 195
Hamonic, Nöel, 47
Hamonic, Pierre, 47, 242
Hancock, John, 226
Hand tools, 45
Hanney, Alexander, 89
Hardware, 6, 37, 162. See also Instruments(s)
Harlaam, Royal Society of, 198
Harmon, John B., 56
Hartnack microscope, 147
Harvey, William, 87, 119, 122, 123, 164
Harvey and Reynolds, 44, 69, 70, 77
Hasler, Johannis, 65
Hauke, I., 199
Haviland, Thomas G., 32
Hawksley, 73, 77
Hawley, D. C., 93
Hawthorne stethoscope, 108
Hays, Isaac, 162
Health exhibition(s), 40, 238
Health museum, 42, 212
Health record, 239
Health standards, 237
Hearing aids, 21, 31
Heart action, irregular, 5
Heart pacemaker(s), 48, 56; valves, 48
Heart transplantation, 33
Heat, 22
Heat-pulse index, 68, 69
Heberden, William, 164
Heckel, Edward W., 217
Heister, Laurence, 18
Helmholtz, Hermann von, 55, 144, 222
Helmholtz ophthalmoscope, 53

Hemodynameter, Poiseuille's, 128
Hemoglobin content of red blood cells, 143
Hemoglobinometry, 143
Herbert, Theophilus, 89
Hering's theory of color, 216
Herisson, Jules, 125
Herisson, Paul, 125
Hermann, Ludimar, 143
Herophilus, 119, 120, 145
Herringham, W. P., 230
Hess, Julian H., 50
Hewson, William, 30
Hicks, James, 73, 77, 79
Highley, Salmon, 147
Hildanus, Fabritius, 18
Hill, Leonard, 208
Hilliard, Harvey, 105, 107
Hindus, 15
Hippel, Arndt Von, 20
Hippocrates, 17, 62, 81, 87, 88, 117, 119,
   164
Historical Museum of Medicine and Den-
   tistry of the Hartford Medical Society
   and Hartford Dental Society, 57
History museum(s), 27
Hitler, Adolf, microscope, 53
Hoff, Hebbel E., 125
Hogner, Richard, 196
Holden, Carter, 72
Holden, Edgar, 196
Hollister, 40
Holmgren, Frithiof, 214
Holmgren test, 215, 217
Holmgren wools, 216
Homeostasis, 162
Hook(s), 17
Hooke, Robert, 88
Hoover, C. F., 182, 183
Hope, James, 89
Horseback riding, 7
Hospital(s), 8, 23, 31, 40, 43, 44, 48, 70,
   82, 90, 131, 142, 147, 180, 181, 182, 183,
   187, 201, 204, 240, 242; clinics, 147;
   museum, 242, railroad cars, 42; records,
   235; statistics, 151. See also name of
   institution
Hospital garments, 10, 61
Hospital Saint Louis, 201
Houston, W. R., 156
Howard Dittrick Museum of Historical
   Medicine, 55
Howe, J. M., 196
Hudson, E. D., 91, 186
Hull, Thomas G., 44
Humphry, George Murray, 162, 230
Hunter, Arthur, 204
Hunter, D. W., 217
Hunter, John, 63, 146, 181, 182
Hunter, William, 10, 182, 191
Hunterian Museum, Royal College of
   Surgeons, 30
Huntington, D. L., 55
Huntington, H. A., 11

Hutchinson, Jonathan, 43, 44, 194
Huter, V., 102
Huxley, Thomas, 145, 157, 161
Hydrophone, 102
Hygiene appliances, 43
Hygiene museums, 42, 55, 212
Hygiene technology, 242
Hypodermic syringe, 53, 200
Hyrtl, Joseph, 30, 53

Iatrochemistry, 123
Iatromechanism, 122
Iatrophysics, 123
Immisch, Moritz, 77, 78
Implement(s), 17, 21, 22, 23, 26, 35, 37, 39, 183, 242; dental, 10
Incandescent lamps, 6
Incising, 17
Incubator, 50
Index thermometer, 67, 73, 74, 75, 83, 85; Phillip's, 73; water, 73
India cane, 97
Indian, 27, 118
Indiana State Medical Society, 44
India rubber, 102
Industrial exhibition, 42
Infection, 191
Ingraham, Charles Wilson, 83
Institutions, 16
Instructional stethoscopes, 109
Instrument(s), 6, 9, 10, 12, 13, 20, 27, 32; alteration of, 21; ancient bronze, 46; applications of, 17, 20; cases, 9, 169; components of, 3, 8, 17, 18, 21; construction of, 3, 16, 21, 29, 32, 35; design of, 18, 21, 22, 26, 35; devices, 6, 19, 23, 26; diagnostic, 4, 6; dull, 10; form, 3; function of, 17, 22, 26, 29, 35, 152; gadget(s), 6; hand tools, 45; hardware, 6; laborsaving, 10; line drawings of, 15; maker, 17; mucus-laden, see Thermometer; operative, 17; parts, 17, 21, 22; quality of; scale, 17, 143; shape, 3, 7, 8, 9, 10, 12, 17, 29, 32; sharp, 10, 11; size, 12, 21, 29; structure of, 22; style, 7, 9; surgical, 6; tools, 6, 10, 13, 15, 16, 17, 18, 20, 37, 39, 40; toy(s), 6; types, 21; uses of, 18; veterinary, 31. See also name of instrument
Instrumental fossils, 40
Instrument cases, 9
Instrument designer, 35
Instrument manufacturer's catalogs, 29
Instrument testing centers, 187
Insurance company(ies), 178
Insurance examination, 209, 210
Insurance examiners, 193, 208
Insurance medicine course, 192
Internal environment, 153; milieu intérieur, 179
International Committee of Weights and Measures, 75
International Congress of Medicine, 47

International Exhibition (1851), 41, 69, 102, 104
International Health Exhibition (1884), 165
International Health Exposition (New York City), 46
International Medical Congress, 79
Internist, 240
Inventor(s), 23, 26, 28, 40, 55, 90, 93, 105, 109, 139
Iron, 231
Iron chambers, 201
Isham, A. B., 193
Italian majolica jar, 46
Ivory, 9, 21, 56, 67, 97, 102, 104, 196; earpiece(s), 99, 100

Jackson, Chevalier, 48, 53
Jackson, Edward, 217
Jackson, James, Jr., 90
Janeway, T. C., 207
Japanese, 27
Javal-Schiötz ophthalmometer, 222
Jefferson Medical College, 18, 90
Jeffries, B. Joy, 221, 229
Jellinek, Stephen, 56
Jellinek Museum, 56
"Jena Normal" glass, 73, 75
Jenner, Sir William, 158
Job standards, health, 211
Johns Hopkins Medical School, 131
Johnstone, Paul, 71
Jones, Nelson, 158
Josephinium of Vienna, 32
Joseph II, Emperor, 32
Journal of the American Medical Association (JAMA), 44, 77, 79, 80, 90, 153, 200, 226, 235
Jung, R., 178
Junod, Victor-Theodore, 198

Kantrowitz, Adrian, 48
Kaye, Simon, Ltd., 31
Keeler polygraph, 132
Keener, W. T., 225
Kells, Charles, office, 242
Kelly, Howard A., 93
Kensington, South, Exhibition, 42, 67
Kerotoscope, 219
Kerr, William J., 108
Kesteven, W. B., 75
Ketcham, Elizabeth, 234
Ketchum, Joseph, 199, 200
Kew Observatory (London), 73, 75, 79
Key, Dr., 191
Kidder, Jerome, tip battery, 49
Kidney, artificial, 38
King, A. Charles, 22, 30, 154
King's College Hospital, 63
Kirchner, Athanasius, 120
Kits, 46
Klemperer, Paul, 146
Knife (knives), 17, 18, 23, 37
Knoxville Academy of Medicine, 56

Kny-Scheerer, 100, 174
Koch, Robert, 10
Koehler, F. W., 108
Koenig, Rudolph, 178
Koerner, 206
Kohl, Max, 178
Kolff-Brigham kidney machine, 38
Korányi, Alexander Von, 152
Korotkoff, N. L., 124, 208
Krebs, Nicolaus (Cusanus), 120
Kreider, George N., 224
Krohne and Seseman, 44, 130
Krumbhaar, Edward B., 147
Kuestner, Otto, 80
Kymograph, 53, 125, 132, 142, 163, 164

Laboratory: apparatus, 141, 142, 143; tests, 119, 148, 149, 150, 154, 156, 182, 183, 184, 191, 192, 210, 211, 224, 225, 233, 236
Labor-saving, 10
Lactometer, 69
Ladd and Pilsher microscope, 147
Ladies Health Protective Association of Allegheny County, New York, 238
Laennec, René-Theophile-Hyacinthe, 146, 153, 154, 182, 186; stethoscope, 53, 61, 87, 90, 91, 97, 99, 102, 108, 110, 124
Lama, Dalai, 11
Lambert, T. S., 188
Lancet, 164
Lancet, The, 158
Landois, Leonard, 143
Landouzy, Marc Hector, 97, 104, 110; patent, 109
Langenbeck, Bernhard R. C. Von, 181
Lantern, 217
Laparoscope, 35
Laparotomy, 236
Larned, Charles W., 110
Laryngoscope, 154
Latham, Peter Mere, 89
Lavoisier, Antoine, 63
Lay-biographies, 15
Laycock, Thomas, 188
Lead, 21
Lealand microscope, 147
Leared, Arthur, 92, 104
Leather, 9, 229; soft, 32
Le Fevre, Egbert, 92
Leiter, Joseph, 154
Lens(es), 159, 213
Leopold, Prince de Medici, 122
Leslie, 73
Lewis, Geoffrey, 28
Lewis, Sir Thomas, 107, 129, 179, 183
Lewis of Allen and Hanbury's, 107
Leyden, 207
Liebermeister chamber, 64
Liebig, Justus, 144
Life history album, 163
Life insurance company, 5, 155, 184, 185, 186, 187, 188, 211, 212, 221, 236

Life insurance data, 231
Life insurance examinations, 195, 209, 221
Life insurance examiners, 201, 204
Life insurance records, 82
Life table(s), 188
Ligate (ligation), 11
Ligature, 144
Lindbergh-Carrel perfusion pump, 48
Lindeboom, G. A., 67, 68
Lindsay and Blakiston, 225
Linen, 10, 23
Ling, Peter, 228
Linneaus, Carl von (Linné), 66, 148
Linnell, J. W., 129
Linseed oil thermometer, 66
Lisfranc, J., 91
Lister, Lord Joseph, 10, 30, 238; carbolic
    acid spray device, 53
Lithotomy, 47
Lithotrite, 35
Litters, 42
Little, William, 219
Littman, David, 96
Littré, Émile, 81
Loading tests, 152, 203
Local disease concept, 61
Lodge, Oliver, 216
Lombard, J. S., 80
London Clinical Society, 162
London Exhibition, Great Exhibition
    (1851), 41, 224, 242
London Hospital, 154
London Medical Gazette, 227
London Science Museum, 29, 47-48
Longsightedness, 215
Loomis, Alfred L., 79, 91, 151, 200, 226
Lord's Prayer slide, 30
Loring ophthalmoscope, 53, 161
Louis, Pierre A., 81, 90, 91, 163, 164, 186
Luciani, Luigi, 143
Ludwig, Carl, 125, 143, 145, 163
Lung capacity, 186
Lusk, William T., 154

Macalister, Donald, 157
Macmillan and Co., 163
Mackenzie, James, 128, 129, 131, 149
MacKenzie, Lewis F., 207
Mackenzie, Morell, 154, 155
Mackenzie polygraphy, 53
McCaskey, D. W., 200
McDaniel, W. B., 40
McHardy, Malcolm M., 215
McKnight, Charles, 38, 50
Magendie, François, 143, 144
Magnifying glass, 77; sound, 124
Mahogany, 9, 10, 102
Mahomed, Frederic A., 126, 153, 230
Majno, Guido, 16
Malaria, 64
Mallet(s), 48, 160
Manometer, 199
Manual skills, 233

Manufacturer(s), 19, 20, 21, 23, 26, 27, 28,
    32, 34, 56, 73, 75, 76, 79, 83, 102, 109,
    174, 178, 187, 213, 241, 243
Maragliano, Edoardo, 80
Marble, 16
Marey, Étienne Jules, 63, 125, 126, 157
Marey's tambour, 130
Markellinos, 119
Marketing techniques, 21
Marsh, 103
Marshall, John, 55
Marsh spirometer, 194
Martin, Henry Newell, 145
Martin-type microscope, 56
Mascagni, Paolo, 32
Masking laboratory, 125
Massachusetts General Hospital, 90, 110
Mass production, 12
Master, Arthur, 16, 207
Master's two-step device, 179
Material(s), 7, 21. See also Aluminum;
    Amber; Cedar; Clay; Compacted wood;
    Coral; Ebony; Ivory; Leather; Linen;
    Mahogany; Marble; Metallic alloys; Oak;
    Papier-maché; Pearl; Pine; Plaster of
    Paris; Plastic(s); Rubber; Steel; Stone
    replicas; Tin; Velvet; Veneer(s); Wood
Material-cultural specialists, 28
Mathieu, Emil L., 176; catalogue, 197
Matthews, 107
Maximal thermometer, 81
Maxwell, James Clerk, 12
Measuring tape, 169
Measuring tubes, 22
Mechanical aids, 6
Mechanical models, 157
Medical bibliography, 16
Medical director(s), 186, 201, 206, 208
Medical equipment, 10, 44
Medical errors, 34
Medical exam, 190, 226, 236, 237
Medical examiner, 188, 189, 192
Medical library(libraries), 40
Medical museum, 13, 44, 55
Medical Record, 18, 23, 46, 80, 190, 212
Medical records, 184, 204, 225
Medical report, 209
Medical society(societies), 40, 44
Medical supplies, 30; exhibition of, 40;
    physician's use of instruments, 3;
    profession, 3
Medical technicians, 146
Medical thermometer. See Thermometer(s)
Medici collection, 39
Medicinal spoons, 47
Medicine as applied technology, 3
Medtronic, 56
Memorabilia, 40
Mensuration, 88
Mercier, 69
Mercury: alloys, 228; thermometer, 66, 69
Mercy Hospital, 40
Mergier, G. E., 42

Mersenne, Marin, 122
Messe, 46. See also Trade fair(s)
Messenger, Hyram J., 212
Metal(s), 9, 35, 102, 107, 108, 194, 229
Metallic: chamber, 199; plates, 241;
    stethoscope, 9
Metallic alloys, 7, 10
Metropolitan Life Insurance Company,
    188, 192
Meyrowitz, E. B., 20, 21, 22, 216, 222, 225
Micanzio, Fulgenzio, 120
Micrometer, 178, 228
Microscope(s), 7, 20, 23, 27, 29, 47, 55, 56,
    61, 62, 75, 79, 82, 110, 144, 145, 146,
    150, 154, 156, 159, 160, 161, 181, 186,
    201, 203, 211, 230; exam, 151, 191;
    Nuremberg type, 27
Microscopial analysis, 237; specimen
    preparation, 43, 45
Microtome(s), 29, 144
Middleton, W. E. Knowles, 65, 68
Midwifery forceps, 47
Midwives, 39, 65, 235; set, 56
Milieu intérieur, 179
Military medical items, 46
Miller, 154
Miller, Willoughby Dayton, 10
Milne, John Stewart, 15
Minerals, 39
Mitchell, S. Weir, 10, 15, 110, 211, 235,
    236
Models: anatomic, 31, 32, 42, 43; building,
    92; obstetrical, 32; organs, 42, 43; sani-
    tary dwellings, 42; wax, 53; wood eye,
    161
Moeller-Christensen, V., 15
Monaural, stethoscope, 102
Monglond, 179
Moore, Sir Norman, 47
Morgagni, Giovanni, 145, 182
Morton, William G., 16
Mount Vernon Hospital, 129
Mouth gags, 9
Mud baths, 6
Mueller, Johannes, 143, 144, 146
Muetter, Thomas Dent, 53
Muetter Museum, 51, 55
Mukhopadhyoya, Girindrenath, 15
Muralt stethoscope, 108
Murphy, Leonard, 16
Museum(s), 4, 27, 37, 39, 41, 46, 240;
    biological, 42; hygiene, 42, 212, 238;
    medical, 40, 57; medical school, 31;
    neurological, 45; public health, 55
Museum, instrument collection(s), 4, 28;
    Athens, 15; Europe, 15; Naples, 15, 46
Museum at Alexandria, 39
Museum catalogue, 27, 29
Museum directory, 40
Museum of American History, National,
    21, 242, 243
Museum of Electricity and Life (Min-
    neapolis), 56

Museum of the History of Science of Oxford, 27
Mutual Benefit Life Insurance Company, 209
Myers, J. A., 178
Myths in medical technology, 5

Naples, National Museum in, 46
Nasal speculum, 102
National Dental Association, 44
National Insurance Convention, 189
National Museum of Athens, 39
Nearsightedness, 221, 237
Neckar Hospital, 110
Needle, 7
Negebauer, 35
Negretti and Zambra, 77
Nei Ching, 118
Nelson, Robert, 48
Nephritis, 151
Neurological instruments, 5, 19; museum, 45
New Jersey Medical Society, 44
Newman, Charles, 147
Newton, Isaac, 66
New York Academy of Medicine, 21
New York City Dispensary, 90
New York Life Insurance Company, 188, 208
New York World's Fair, 44
Nickel-plated, 194
Nicolai, 108
Niemeyer, Felix von, 102
Nitrous oxide, 30, 200, 201
Nitze, Max, 154; cystoscope, 155
Nobel Prize, 180
Nodine, Alonzo, 191
Nöel-Hume, Ivor, 37
Nogent, France, 21
Northrup, W. P., 19
Northwestern Mutual Life Insurance Company, 209
Nosology, 91, 148, 156, 159
Noyes, Bradford, 69
Numerical method(s), 163, 164, 203, 224, 225; terms, 230
Numerical scale, 204, 206
Numerical terms, 11, 125, 146
Nuremberg microscope, 27
Nurse(s), 18, 22, 32, 46, 62, 65, 82, 225
Nursing aids, 226
Nursing appliances, 56
Nursing bottles, 21, 56
Nursing homes, 23

Oak, 10
Obstetrical, 16
Obstetric forceps, 16, 17, 200, 235; kit, 234, 241, 242; models, 32
Obstetrics, 235
O'Dwyer, Joseph, 19
Oertel, Max Joseph, 107, 108, 206, 228
Oertman, 80, 81

Ogle, John W., 176
Ointments, 16
Oliver, Dr.: air manometer, 195; hemogynamometer, 207
Omsby, L. Hepenstal, 225
One-minute thermometer, 74
Operating: equipment, 143, room, 46, utensils, 48
Operations, trivial, 18
Ophthalmologic, 23
Ophthalmological Society of London, 219
Ophthalmologist(s), 213, 215, 229, 237, 240
Ophthalmology, 23, 213, 224, 235
Ophthalmometer, 102
Ophthalmoscope(s), 55, 150, 154, 159, 160, 161, 219, 221
Optometrist, 213, 215
Oral sepsis, 191
Oriental, 11
Orthopedic: apparatus, 16, 21; devices, 47
Osler, Sir William, 47, 90
Otis, Lt. Col. George A., 29
Otolaryngologist, 240
Otology, 224
Ott, Isaac, 63
Otto, F. G. and Son, 69, 128
Otto and Reynders, 199
Outline stamp(s), 226
Owen, Isambard, 230
Oxford University Museum, 43

Pacemakers, 48, 56
Page, R. C. M., 226
Paget, James, 187
Pain, 6, 10, 11, 152, 177, 179
Paintings, 16
Pales, L., and Monglond, 179
Pancoast, Joseph, 18
Panniers, medical, 42
Paper cylinder, 88
Papier-mâché, 31, 32, 92; models, 53
Paré, Ambroise, 18, 88
Parke, Davis & Co., 48
Parkes, Edward A., 160
Parkes, John, 63
Parrish, Laurence, 32
Parry, Nöel and José, 233
Pasquale, N. P., 16, 133
Pasteur, Louis, 10
Pastorelli, Francis, 69
Patent(s), 28, 103, 200, 204, 229, 240; specification, 4; wooden leg, 40
Pathological Society of London, 42, 182
Patient(s), 6, 7, 8, 11, 22, 28, 34, 35, 37, 39, 40, 79, 81, 82, 85, 110, 122, 125, 129, 131, 147-150, 153-159, 161, 163, 164, 174, 176, 180, 182-187, 192, 206, 208, 213, 225, 228, 231, 233, 235, 237, 239, 240, 241
Patient testimonial, 237
Paul, Constantin, 107
Payne, J. F., 47

Pearl, 9; handle, 48
Pearson, Karl, 185
Pediatrics, 235
Pendulum, 120, 123
Pennsylvania Railroad Company, 214
People's Theater (Omaha, Nebraska), 23
Percival, Thomas, 148
Percussion, 62, 82, 88, 89, 90, 91, 92, 110, 115, 131, 145, 153, 186, 192, 193, 194; hammer, 102, 146
Percussor (or pleximeter), 102
Perforating, 17, 35
Perimeter, 176; self-recording, 222
Pessaries, 21, 81, 236
Peter, M., 80
Pewter, 56; syringe(s), 47
Pharmacists, 22, 221; German, 224
Pharmacopoeias, 224
Pharmacy, 31, 56
Pharmacy jar(s), 46; objects, 56
Philadelphia Neurological Society, 177
Phillips, John, 69
Phonocardiography, 110
Phonograph records, 110
Photograph(s), 22, 27, 28, 33, 45, 46
Photomicrography apparatus, 31
Phthisis, 155, 186, 189, 199, 200
Physical agents, 6
Physical exam, 148; case, 169; check-up, 184
Physical medicine, 22
Physical signs, 41, 150, 230
Physician(s), 22, 23, 26, 28, 35, 47, 51, 64, 73, 75, 83
Physician's hat, 10
Physician's office, 8
Physikalisch-Technische Reichanstalt, 187
Pick(s), 9
Piezoelectrometer, Madame Curie's, 53
Piffard, Henry G., 151
Pill- and tablet-making machine, 224
Pilling, George, P., 19, 28, 194
Pillsbury, Oliver, 189
Piltdown man, 53
Pine, 99
Pinel, Philippe, 146
Pinnard stethoscope, 100
Piorry, Pierre Adolph, 62, 102, 108, 186
Plants, 39
Plaster of Paris, 31
Plastic(s), 7, 10; heart valves, 48; tubing, 96
Platt, Samuel Joseph, 56
Plethysmograph, 52
Pleurisy, 94, 206
Pleximeter (or plessimeter), 62, 102, 145, 192, 237
Plugger(s), 48
Pneograph, 196
Pneumatic Cabinet Company of New York, 200, 201
Pneumatic: chambers, 196; device, 199
Pneumatometer, 196, 199
Pneumonia, 230

Pocket case, 200
Poel, S. Oakley Vander, 203
Point(s), 17; pointed rod, 174
Poiseuille, Jean, 205
Poiseuille's tube, 125, 144; hemodynameter, 128
Politzer, Adam, series of tympanic membranes, 53
Polygraph, 129, 132, 142, 239
Polystethopolyscope (polyscope), 110
Pompei, 39, 46; surgical instruments, 56
Pond sphygmograph, 128
Porte-caustique, 102
Porter, W. T., 130
Positive diagnosis, 82, 224
Postmortem, 88, 181
Potain, Carl E., 207, 208
Pottery, 56
Poulain, V., 102
Poultice, 18
Powell, Douglas, 147, 153, 203
Powers, L. M., 82
Practical history, 29
Practitioner, 26
Pravaz, C. G., 198
Praxagoras, 119
Pray, Dr., 219; vision test, 220
Precision, 12, 13, 85, 115, 118, 125, 161, 163, 176, 177, 186, 187, 193, 195, 214, 224, 231, 235, 236, 239, 240; instruments of, 11, 183
Presbyterian Hospital (New York), 61
Prescriptions, 226
Preservative surgery, 130
Pressure chambers, 7, 237
Pressure gauge, 20
Preventive medicine, 239
Primavesi brothers, 77
Private collection, 39, 40
Probe(s), 16, 17
Promotional literature. *See* Trade catalogue(s)
Prosthetic equipment, 16
Prudential Life Insurance Company, 203
Psychiatric museum (St. Petersburg), 45
Ptolemy, 39
Public health, 181; museum, 55
Pulse, 92, 117, 164, 205, 208, 225, 226, 236; rate, 186
Pulse clock, 125
Pulse graphs, 239
Pulse instruments, 5, 11, 15
Pulse scale, 121
Pulse timers, 120, 123
Pulse-watch, 122, 123, 124, 164
Pulse writer, 7
Pulsilogium, 122
Pump(s), 11, 21
Purdy, Charles, 201
Purges, 206
Purtle, Helen M., 29

Quack, 23

Quain, Richard, 64, 89, 100, 158
Queen, J. W. and Co., 219
Queen Victoria, 180
Quekett, John, 30
Quetelet, Adolphe, 162, 163, 165, 184
Quimby, C., 201
Quincke, Heinrich, 100
Quinine, 64

Railroad employees, 7, 181
Railroads, 11, 174, 181, 211, 213, 214, 215, 236; cars, 42; surgeon, 181, 182; *The Railway Surgeon*, 182
Ramadge, F. H., 196
Ranney, A. L., 19
Ransome, Arthur, 195
Ransome and Randolph Co., 24, 25
Rapp, Dietmar, 143
Rational surgery, 130
Réaumur, Réné Antoine F., 66
Recording apparatus, 198
Records, medical, 141, 146, 233, 237
Red Cross Drug Company, 74
Reed, Surgeon General Walter, 79
Reese, Michael, Hospital, 50
Reflector, 102
Reformatory instrument, 146
Refraction, 212, 221
Refractive error, 237
Registrar, 29
Registration of museum objects, 27
Regnier, 162
Reichert, Philip, collection, 194, 195, 205, 207, 208
Reichert, von, 125
Reiner and Keeler, 216
Reiser, Stanley J., 4, 5, 33
Repair, 35
Replicas, 37
Resection knife, 181
Respiration, 15
Retinoscope, 219
Retractor, 17
Richardson, Benjamin Ward, 128
Riolan, Jean, 122
Ritchie, John, 147
Riva-Rocci, S., 207, 208
Roberts, Charles, 165, 169, 204
Robin, Charles, 142
Robinson, J. Ben, 48
Robson, A. W., 147
Rockefeller Institute Hospital, 135
Rockwell, A. D., 228
Roentgen ray apparatus, 131
Rogers, Oscar H., 188, 204, 208; Tycos sphygmomanometer, 205
Roman Carthaginian nursing bottles, 56
Root, Edward K., 209
Rosen, George, 89
Rosenbach, Ottomar, 152
Ross, A., 147, 199
Ross, George, 89
Royal Albert Hall, 41

Royal Berkshire Hospital, 30
Royal College of Physicians (London), 157, 158
Royal College of Physicians of Edinburgh, laboratory, 147
Royal College of Surgeons (England) 22, 144, 216
Royal Southern Hospital, Liverpool, 62
Royal Victoria Hospital (Netley), 69
Rubber, 35, 104, 105; bags, 194; case, 79; hard, 7, 10; soft, 109; soft tube, 195, 208
Rufus of Ephesus, 119
Rule, 165, 174
Rumford, Count of (Benjamin Thompson), and Leslie, 73
Rush, Benjamin, 148; medical chest, 53
Rush Rhees Library (Rochester, New York), 22
Russell, Raymond, 31
Ryff, Walther Hermann, 18

Saccharometer, 69
Saddle bags, 56, 200
St. Bartholomew's Hospital, 89
St. George's Hospital, 89, 239
St. Louis, Hospital of, 32
St. Peter's Hospital for Stone and Other Urinary Diseases, 154
Salicylate of soda, 64
Salicylic acid (aspirin), 64, 230
Salt and Son, 44, 108, 228
Salter dynamometer, 173
San Francisco Exhibition, 44
Sanitary reform, 212
Santorio, Santorio, 65, 66, 122, 123, 144
Sardy, Coles and Co., 79
Saw, 23, 37
Scale (thermometer), 65, 66, 73, 76, 77, 79, 165; Galvanic degrees of heat, 65
Scaler(s), 48
Scales, 202, 226
Scalpel(s), 9, 18, 37, 48, 181, 205, 242
Scarificators, 242
Scarlet fever, 212
Schall, 44
Schank, 145
Schieffelin & Co. (New York), 48
Schiller, Joseph, 142
Schindler, Rudolf, 48
Schmalz, Karl Gustavus, 91
School(s), 81, 181, 211, 212
Schoot, Frederick Otto, 73
Science museum(s), 39; *See* individual names
Scissors, 20
Scudamore, Charles, 92
Scultetus, Johannes, 17, 18
Seebeck, 214
Seguin, Edouard, 68, 69, 73, 75, 80, 81, 82, 117, 125, 176, 221, 224, 225, 226, 228
Seidel, Victor, 33
Self-registering thermometer, 64, 69, 70, 74, 77

Self-sterilizing thermometer case, 79
Seller, William, 159, 160
Selzer, Richard, 11
Semiology, 149
Semmelweis, Ignaz, 56
Semmelweis Medical Historical Museum,
    Library, and Archives of Budapest, 33,
    56
Sensory instruments, 5
Seppili, Guiseppe, 80
Sewell heart pump, 48
Shaft, 17
Sharp and Smith Surgical Instruments, 71,
    85, 106, 133
Shaw, Sebastian, 130
Shepard and Dudley, 73, 196
Sherman, Orran T., 75
Shoemaker's rule, 176
Shortsightedness, 215
Shrady, George, 23, 80
Shrewsbury, Edwyn Andrew, 70
Shryock, Richard, 206
Sieveking, Edward Henry, 176, 193
Sigerist, Henry, 15, 16
Sign(s), 149, 231, 236, 237
Silk, 104, 107
Silver, 80, 228; German, 21
Silver plating, 21
Sim, Patrick, 56
Simon, John, 151, 238
Simpson, Alexander R., 154
Skeel, F. D., 222
Skoda, Joseph, 93
Slides(sliders), 30
Smallpox, 212; hospital, 158
Smellie forceps, 56
Smith, Andrew H., 198, 239
Smith, Thomas W., 238
Smith and Beck, 77
Smith Papyrus, 119
Smithsonian Institution, 22, 40, 55, 242;
    archives, 48; Division of Medical
    Sciences, 31, 48, 53; National Museum
    of American History, 21, 29, 32, 33, 46,
    48, 53
Smith-Turner dental museum, 46
Snellen, Herman, 217; eye test type, 218
Snelling, Dr., 105
Snow, John, 30
Societal forces, and medical technology, 34,
    81, 82, 191, 243
Société Genèvoise d'Instruments de
    Physique, 12
Society of Life Assurance Medical Officers,
    203
Solger stethoscope, 102
Somatoscope, 102
Soranus, 17, 87
Sorré, M., 179
Sound(s), 21, 236
South Kensington Exhibition, 67
South Kensington Museum, 199
Spallanzani tubes, 144

Spatula(s), 8
Spearman aesthesiometer, 177
Special diets, 6
Specialized instruments, 229
Specola Museum, 31, 32
Spectacles, 217
Spectroscope, 154, 216
Speculum, 200, 236
Spencer, Dr., 105
Spencer Lens Company, 29, 107
Sphygmograph, 82, 125, 126, 129, 131, 132,
    142, 164, 193, 224, 230, 236, 237, 239;
    Pond, 53, 128
Sphygmography, 126, 132
Sphygmology, 117
Sphygmomanometer, 7, 125, 184, 193, 204,
    206, 208, 209, 236, 239; clinical, 207
Spirit thermometer, 66
Spirometer(s), 178, 185, 186, 193, 194, 224,
    237; Barnes, dry, 196; wet, 196
Spirometry, 199
Spittal, Robert, 90
Splint(s), 34, 56
Sponges for ether, 229
Spoon, medicinal, 47
Sprague, Howard B., 95
Spring manometer, 209
Squibb, Edward R., 74
Standard(s), 85, 120, 182, 184, 186, 187,
    206, 213, 216, 219, 231, 236, 239;
    dentistry; 191; hygiene, 238; tables, 240
Standardization of blood presure, 209;
    data, 224; instruments, 5; of body
    temperature, 62
Standardization resulting from instruments,
    5, 12
Standard nomenclature, 221
Starling, 125
Statistics, 235; statistical, 81, 188
Statue(s), 39
Stebbins, Roswell O., 10, 11
Steel, 10, 21
Stereostethoscope, 108
Sterilization, 9, 181
Sterilized, 8, 9, 10, 77
Sterilizers, 10
Sternberg dynamometer, 169
Sterne, Albert, 183
Stethograph, 195
Stethokyrtograph, 195
Stethometer (chest rule), 195
Stethophone, 110
Stethophonometer, 109
Stethophonometry, 93
Stethoscope(s), 5, 6, 7, 8, 9, 27, 56, 61, 62,
    79, 87, 124, 130, 131, 137, 146, 153, 155,
    160, 182, 192, 193, 208, 230, 236, 239,
    240; multiple, 110; paper, 90; teaching,
    103
Stickler, J. W., 61
Stillings, Dennis, 56
Stillman, Ralph, 184
Stitches, 16

Stokes, William, 87, 89, 181
Stone replicas, 16
Stratton, Samuel W., 187
Strength tests, 184
Stretchers, 42
Struthius, Joseph, 118, 120, 122, 205
Stuffed animals, 39
Succussion, 88
Sun baths, 6
Surface thermometer, 80
Surgeons, 15, 22, 26, 28
Surgery, 15
Surgical dressings, 23
Surgical instruments, 10, 15, 16, 17, 18, 23,
    27; Greek, 47; Japanese, 47; Roman, 47;
    sets, 47
Surgical procedures, 17, 23; sets, 242
Surgical staplers, 48
Swift, James and Son, 23, 147
Sydenham, Thomas, 81, 236
Sylvester's method for artificial respiration,
    225
Symballophone, 108
Symes, Sir James, 30
Symptom(s), 149
Syringe(s), 21, 35, 102, 144; pewter, 47

Taberié, R., 198
Tact, 92
Tait, Lawson, 236
Tape, 169
Tay, Warren, 43
Taylor Instrument Company, 75, 76
Taylor Monroe thermometer, 84
Technical aids, 233
Technological appliances, 6
Technological devices, 6
Technological museum, 242
Technological refinements, 4
Telioux, Bartholomew, 65
Temperature records, 68
Tendon tucker, 21
Terra cotta, 56
Test(s), 35, 185; cards, 219; chart, 217;
    lantern, 216; meal analysis, 147; vision, 217-
    21. See also Chemical analysis
Testo-Reaction Matares, 178
Tetanus, 64
Texas Centennial Exposition (Dallas), 44
Teyler Museum, 29
Thayer, William Sydney, 129, 131
Theoretical, 26
Theories, 30, 62
Therapy, 12
Thermoelectric apparatus, 19
Thermograph 64, 157
Thermometer(s), 5, 7, 8, 9, 23, 61, 91, 102,
    130, 132, 144, 157, 158, 159, 186, 187,
    224, 230, 239; mucus laden, 82; scale, 74;
    shape, 67; tube, 177
Thermometric Bureau, Yale College, 73
Thermopile, 63
Thermoscope, 65, 73

Thomas, K. Bryan, 30
Thomas, T. Gaillard, 235, 236
Thompson, C. J. S., 15, 30
Thompson, Sir Henry, 154, 239
Thomson, W. H., 158, 214, 215; disc, 223
Tiemann, George, 20, 68, 77, 105, 109, 113, 114, 127, 151
Timers, 178
Tin, 21, 56
Tongue depressors, 9, 47
Tonometer, 109
Tonsillotomes, 9
Tools, 6, 16, 94, 141, 162, 182, 208, 240, 241
Toothbrush, 48
Toothpick, 48
Touch-pieces, 27
Tourniquets, 56
Towne, Joseph, 32
Townsend, Gary, 123
Toxins, 186
Toy(s). See Instrument(s)
Trade cards, 28
Trade catalogue(s), 15, 20, 21, 22, 23, 33, 46, 55
Trade fair(s), 42
Traube, Louis, 63
Trephine (trephining or trepanning), 17, 37, 47; set, 50
Trephined skulls, 16
Trocars, 47
Trotter, Wilfred, 179
Trousseau, Prof., 112
Truax, Charles, 20, 74
Trusses, 213
Tube, 35; rubber, 11
Tuberculosis, 83, 91, 155, 161, 186, 187, 189, 193, 201, 236, 237
Tubing, rubber, 108
Tuke, John, 89
Tumor, 6
Tuning fork, 176; Hartmann's, 225
Turner, Gerard, L., E., 27
Twisting, 35
Tycos thermometer, 84
Tyndall, John, 107
Typhoid fever, 158
Typhus fever, 70, 158
Typical man, 174
Tyson, Dr., 230

Uffenbach, Peter, 18
Ulcer, 6
Union College, 29
U.S. National Bureau of Standards, 75, 187
U.S. Pharmacopoeia, 225
University College Hospital, 150, 154, 179
University Museum, Oxford, 43
University of Florence, 32
University of Kansas Medical Center Museum, 27
Unorthodox practitioner, 240
Ureometer, 151

Uretal catheter, 131
Urethral instruments, 202, 226
Urethroscope, 154
Urinalysis equipment, 150, 210
Urine test(s), 191, 236; equipment, 179
Urologic, 23
Uroscopy, 183
Utensils, 9, 37
Utrecht University Museum, 29

Vaccination, 180
Vaccine therapy, 180
Valentin, Gustav Gabriel, 143
Van Buren and Keys, 226
Van Wagenen, G. A., 209
Varrier-Jones, P. C., 66
Veith, Ilza, 118
Velvet, 9
Veneer(s), 7
Verick, 147
Vernier scale, 176
Vesalius, Andreas, 17
Vibrations, 22
Victor electrocardiograph, 137
Victoria and Albert Museum, 41
Victorian medicine, 3, 5
Vidius, Vidus, 17
Vienna Institute of Medicine, 32
Vierordt, Carl, 125
Vigneron, G., Jr., 18
Virchow, Rudolf, 63, 146, 149, 157, 159, 184
Vision, 212; defective, 213; test(s), 7, 213, 215, 219
Visiting list, 225
Visual acuity, 12, 213, 215; standards, 215
Vital capacity, 12, 142, 178, 185, 194, 199, 237
Viviana, Vincentio, 122
Vivisection, 143, 144
Volta batteries, 144
Votives, 37, 39, 56

Wade, Philip S., 18
Wagenen, G. A. Van, 209
Waidner, C. W., 75
Waldenburg, L., 125, 199
Waldo, Leonard, 74
Walfardin, François Hippolyte, 69
Walfardin thermometer, 69
Walking staff (or stick), 107
Wallace, James, 217
Wallace Brothers (North Carolina), 48
Wall and Ochs, 217
Walsh, A. S., 100
Walshe, Walter Hayle, 150
Walter Reed Army Hospital, 55
Walters, Max B., 16, 207
Wappler, Reinhold, 22
Warren, John Mason, 229
Wasserman test, 182, 183
Water clock. See Clepysdra
Watt, James, 199

Weapon(s), 18
Weber, E. H., 176
Weight, 204
Weil, Adolf, 93
Weinhagen, 77
Weiss, John, 196
Welch, John, 69
Wellcome, Sir Henry, 46, 242
Wellcome Historical Library and Museum, 22, 29, 30, 32, 33, 46, 47, 242
Weller, 133
Wells, George W., 190
Wells, Horace, 57
Wells, Spencer, 239
Wet cloths, 6
Whewell, William, 12
White, Octavius A., 128
White, Paul Dudley, 95, 96, 130, 207
White, S. S., 48
Whitebread, Charles, 48
Wilks, Samuel, 107, 158
Williams, C. J. B., 89, 99, 100, 102
Williams, C. Theodore, 153
Williams, Herbert F., 199, 200
Williams, Horatio B., 135
Willis, Thomas, 63, 123
Wilson, Frank, 134, 135
Wilson, George, 214
Wilson, John Steinbeck, 235
Winchester Observatory, 73
Wingate, Charles, 212
Wodderspoon and Co., 225
Wolff, Christian, 68
Wolfley, Dr. Lewis, 233
Women physicians, 235
Women's Medical College (Philadelphia), 91
Wood, Horatio C., 63
Wood, 9, 31, 32, 35, 102
Wood, William and Co., 228
Wood Memorial Museum, 56
Woodhead, G. Sims, 66
Woodward, J. J., Assistant Surgeon General, 42
Wormull, 77
Wounds, history of 16, 18
Wright, A. E., 216
Wunderlich, Carl, 61, 62, 63, 76, 81, 187
Wykoff collection, 56

X-radiation, 16, 22, 156
X-ray equipment, 22; film, 28; machine, 48; sections, 187
X-ray tube(s), 27, 37, 186, 187

Young-Helmholtz theory of color, 214, 216
Young's optometer, 144

Zander, Gustav, 228
Zeiss, 147
Zimmermann, E., 169, 177, 178
Zinc, 194
Zumbo, Guilio, 31
Zurich Medical Society, 69
Zwaardemaker's olfactometer, 176

About the Author

AUDREY B. DAVIS is Curator of Medical Sciences at
the Smithsonian Institution in Washington, D.C. She is
the author of *The Circulation of the Blood and Medical
Chemistry in England, 1650-1680, Triumph Over Disability*, and many other publications.